PREGNANCY LOSS:
Medical Therapeutics
and
Practical Considerations

PREGNANCY LOSS:
Medical Therapeutics
and
Practical Considerations

Edited by **JAMES R. WOODS, Jr., M.D.**

Associate Professor of Obstetrics and Gynecology
Director of Obstetrics and Maternal-Fetal Medicine
Department of Obstetrics and Gynecology
University of Rochester School of Medicine and Dentistry
Rochester, New York
Formerly:
Associate Professor of Obstetrics and Gynecology
Director of Obstetrics
Department of Obstetrics and Gynecology
University of Cincinnati College of Medicine
Cincinnati, Ohio

JENIFER L. ESPOSITO

Cincinnati, Ohio

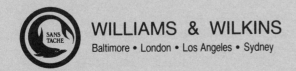

WILLIAMS & WILKINS
Baltimore • London • Los Angeles • Sydney

Editor: Carol-Lynn Brown
Associate Editor: Linda Napora
Copy Editor: Wendy Polhemus
Design: Alice Sellers
Production: Raymond E. Reter

Accurate indications, adverse reactions, and dosage schedules for drugs are provided in this book, but it is possible that they may change. The reader is urged to review the package information data of the manufacturers of the medications mentioned.

Printed in the United States of America

Library of Congress Cataloging-in-Publication Data

Main entry under title:

Pregnancy loss.
    Includes bibliographies and index.
    1. Miscarriage—Psychologic aspects. 2. Stillbirth—Psychologic aspects.
3. Fetal death—Psychologic aspects. 4. Bereavement—Psychologic aspects.
5. Pregnant women—Psychology. 6. Medical personnel and patient.
7. Medical social work. I. Woods, James R., Jr., 1943–   . I. Esposito,
Jenifer L., 1954–   . [DNLM: 1. Abortion—psychology. 2. Counseling.
3. Fetal death. 4. Grief. 5. Infant, Newborn. 6. Parents—psychology.
7. Professional—Family relations. 8. Professional—Patient relations. WQ
225 P923]
RG648,P89 1987   155.9′37   86-15769
ISBN 0-683-09256-1

                                        87 88 89 90 91
                            10 9 8 7 6 5 4 3 2 1

Preface

There is growing awareness in the obstetric community of the devastating impact that the death of a fetus or newborn has on parents. Appropriately termed a "pregnancy loss," this crisis not only involves the catastrophe of the baby's death but also shatters parents' dreams, plans, and hopes for their future child. Anyone professionally involved in obstetric care can sense the magnitude of this loss just by listening to parents say, "I never got to say goodbye," or "I never told my son I love him."

Although the general topic of death and dying is receiving increasing attention by the medical community, little is known about the impact that pregnancy loss has on the lives of those experiencing it. What happens to these people after the woman is discharged from the hospital? How do parents as individuals react to their loss? What happens to a couple's relationship with each other as a result of their baby's death? For some couples, the death of their baby may lead, for either medical or emotional reasons, to a life that will always be childless. There is a wide range of reactions that people have in response to pregnancy loss; its potential effects can alter the lives of those who experience it. What can be done to help this very high-risk group return to a normal life?

Unfortunately, the obstetric community for too long has fostered the belief that if parents do not talk about their loss they will forget about it. But, people do not ever forget a pregnancy loss. A grandmother in the presence of her daughter who has just delivered a stillbirth will say, "I had a stillborn daughter many years ago. I don't think about it much now." Pause. "You know, she would have been 19 last month."

For years, members of the clergy, nurses, and social workers have quietly shouldered the responsibility of caring for families after a pregnancy loss. Although beneficial to the individuals who come under these professionals' care, this approach is random and easily undermined. Many patients will never be offered an explanation of the type of medical care they received or hear details concerning their baby's death. The obstetric community must recognize that responsibilities to families experiencing a pregnancy loss do not end at the 6-week postpartum visit. What is needed is a systematic, comprehensive, and physician-directed support service.

PHYSICIANS' ATTITUDES

Little attention is devoted to teaching physicians how to deal with the death of a patient's baby or with a family's emotional response to the event, let alone how to help these people in the process of grieving for their loss. Physicians are taught in medical school and during residency to measure patient care on the basis of survival statistics. The probability of delivering a baby with Down's syndrome is correlated with maternal age. Successful management of premature labor is described in terms of neonatal survival. In this statistical environment, fears and concerns tentatively hinted at by patients are considered only tangentially or, worse, are ignored completely.

The medical community is not consistent in attitude or skill when caring for patients with a pregnancy loss. Patients expect that their physicians will be understanding and compassionate, especially when the worst fear has become a reality and the baby has died. Sadly, these expectations too often are unfulfilled, leaving the patient angry and confused. Medical training aggravates the problem by regarding fetal or newborn death as a deviation from standard outcome, thereby denying its significance and impact. It is not surprising that the young obstetrician entering private practice feels unprepared to deal with these challenging and personally threatening aspects of patient care. Teaching hospitals therefore must assume a particular responsibility for educating residents and medical students in this crucial area. The obstetric community needs to enhance the level of care that patients can expect when they have lost a baby.

PURPOSE

The purpose of this book is to provide a straightforward, step-by-step approach for professionals in the medical community who encounter patients with a pregnancy loss. All of the contributors to this project have had experience within this field. Each chapter therefore reflects the personal commitment of the individual contributor to this important area of obstetric healthcare.

The text is divided into 3 sections. Section 1 describes issues and events surrounding the topic of pregnancy loss. The process of bereavement is discussed, with special emphasis on unique aspects of grief in response to pregnancy loss. The impact that early pregnancy detection has on pregnancy awareness and parental bonding, which is shattered when pregnancy loss occurs, is then presented. Section 1 also examines care given to typical patients experiencing miscarriage, ectopic pregnancy, stillbirth, or neonatal death. This portion of the text emphasizes how professionals from several disciplines (physician, nurse, social worker, chaplain) interact to provide medical and psychologic care. This section does not spell out the full responsibilities of each professional group, but instead describes their roles as part of an interdisciplinary team as the patient might perceive them during her hospitalization. This portion of the text offers a clear idea of how a patient is taken through the entire support system, in which care is provided by several types of professional disciplines.

The purpose of Section 2 is to define more specifically individual professional roles. Within Section 2, Parts 1 and 2 correspond to patient management during hospitalization and follow-up outpatient care after discharge from the hospital. In-hospital care encompasses the responsibilities of physician; labor nurse, newborn intensive care unit nurse (NICU), and floor nurse; chaplain; social worker; and funeral director. Outpatient follow-up after the patient's discharge includes contact with the physician as outpatient counselor, the office nurse, the geneticist for between-pregnancy counseling, and the peer support group. The value of the autopsy and the reaction of pregnancy-loss patients to their next pregnancy are also addressed.

Section 2 also describes support service formats in 2 major hospital settings. This information may provide guidelines for those individuals who wish to set up similar systems in their own hospitals. First, a straightforward description of the Perinatal Support Service (PSS) at the University of Cincinnati is given. This description focuses on methods of long-term outpatient follow-up and provides data from demographic analysis of the patient population and patient compliance with this type of program. The Two-Roof Support Service at Children's Hospital Medical Center and Akron City Hospital, in Akron, Ohio, is then described. The goal of both programs is to anticipate long-term needs of the bereaved patient and her family after the loss of a baby and to facilitate their grieving and recovery process.

Section 3—"The Patient Speaks Out"—gives professionals an opportunity to view themselves as they might be perceived by a patient and her partner who experience a pregnancy loss. The importance of this portion of the text cannot be emphasized enough. We of the medical community have learned most about the subject of pregnancy loss by listening to those for whom we have cared; they have been able and tolerant teachers.

PREGNANCY LOSS: AN OBSTETRIC RESPONSIBILITY

There is encouraging, growing interest in the topic of the impact of pregnancy loss on patients and their families. Peer support group networks in recent years have risen up as a strong advocate for the patient and her family who suffer the loss of their baby. For too long, professionals who interact peripherally with these patients in the hospital—primarily social workers and members of the clergy—have had to assume the burden of providing emotional support. There has been no long-term support for these people undergoing such a life crisis as the death of their baby.

It is time that we who care directly for these patients begin to work with social workers, clergy, and others to provide support when our patients are suddenly confronted with an unexpected, devastating, and complex loss. We believe that the support service concept described in this book has important, critical features that make this patient care unique. It is the authors' hope that similar programs offering good, comprehensive perinatal support will be developed and that the need for obstetrically oriented and physician-directed programs will be recognized both by practicing physicians and by medical training institutions. This book is intended to serve as a resource for obstetricians, pediatricians, nurses, chaplains, social workers, and other care providers who come into contact with the patients for whom this book is written—and to whom this book is dedicated. Additionally, nursing students and medical students, as well as people specializing in counseling and bereavement, will benefit from the subject format.

Grateful acknowledgment is extended to Pamela Kuhlman for her patience, initiative, and dedication as word processor for this book.

James R. Woods, Jr., M.D.
Associate Professor of Obstetrics and Gynecology
University of Rochester School of Medicine and Dentistry
Director of Obstetrics and Maternal-Fetal Medicine
Strong Memorial Hospital
Rochester, New York

Jenifer L. Esposito
Cincinnati, Ohio

Contributors

Robert Bendon, M.D. (Chapter 13)
Assistant Professor of Pathology
University of Cincinnati College of
  Medicine
Cincinnati, Ohio

D. Gary Benfield, M.D. (Chapter 17)
Neonatologist
Children's Hospital
Akron, Ohio

Sara Berlepsch, R.N. (Chapter 11)
Perinatal Center
University Hospital
Cincinnati, Ohio

Carole Bonno (Chapter 14)
Co-Founder and Coordinator
Reach Out (Formerly Mothers
  Supporting Mothers)
Cincinnati, Ohio

Peter St. J. Dignan, M.D. (Chapter 12)
Professor of Pediatrics
University of Cincinnati College of
  Medicine
Director of Regional Genetics Center
Cincinnati, Ohio

Jenifer L. Esposito, B.A. (Chapter 18)
Cincinnati, Ohio

F. Paul Esposito, Ph.D. (Chapter 19)
Professor of Physics
University of Cincinnati
Cincinnati, Ohio

Ann Hager, C.N.M. (Chapter 2)
Certified Nurse-Midwife
University Hospital
Cincinnati, Ohio

Jerald Kay, M.D. (Chapter 1)
Associate Professor of Child Psychiatry
University of Cincinnati College of
  Medicine
Cincinnati, Ohio

Janet Kirksey, R.N. (Chapter 15)
Co-Founder and Coordinator
Support After Neonatal Death (SAND)
Alta Bates Hospital
Berkeley, California

Reverend Bert A. Klein (Chapters 7 and
  16)
Protestant Minister
Chaplain, University Hospital
Cincinnati, Ohio

Justin P. Lavin, M.D. (Chapter 17)
Director of Maternal-Fetal Medicine
Akron City Hospital
Akron, Ohio

Kate McElwain, R.N. (Chapter 6)
Labor and Delivery Nurse
University Hospital
Cincinnati, Ohio

Beverly Malone, Ph.D. (Chapter 6)
Assistant Administrator of Nursing
  Services
Director, Obstetrics and Gynecology
  and Neonatology Nursing
University Hospital
Cincinnati, Ohio

Andrea Matthews, M.S.W. (Chapter 8)
Clinical Social Work Supervisor
Chief, Perinatology Social Worker
University Hospital
Cincinnati, Ohio

O'dell M. Owens, M.D. (Chapter 2)
Formerly: Assistant Professor of
  Obstetrics and Gynecology
University of Cincinnati College of
  Medicine
Chief, Division of Endocrinology
University Hospital
Cincinnati, Ohio
[Now in private practice]

Ronald Troyer (Chapter 9)
Funeral Director
Hudson, Wisconsin

James R. Woods, Jr., M.D. (Chapters 3,4,5,10,13,16)
Formerly: Associate Professor of Obstetrics and Gynecology
University of Cincinnati College of Medicine

Director of Obstetrics
University Hospital
Cincinnati, Ohio
Currently: Associate Professor of Obstetrics and Gynecology
University of Rochester School of Medicine and Dentistry
Director of Obstetrics and Maternal-Fetal Medicine
Strong Memorial Hospital
Rochester, New York

Consultant

Reverend Kenneth J. Czillinger, Pastor
Immaculate Heart of Mary Church
Cincinnati, Ohio

Contents

SECTION

Pregnancy Loss

PART

The Issues

Chapter 1
Pregnancy Loss and the Grief Process

Pregnancy Loss and the Grief Process

JERALD KAY, M.D.

Despite the universality of grief, it is striking that scientific study of this process is only 40 years old. While it is true that Freud (1) first drew attention to the ubiquity and types of loss and to the distinction between mourning and depression, it was not until Lindemann's (2) classic study of survivors of the Cocoanut Grove fire that a detailed symptomatology of grief was presented to the health professions. Psychologic and physical effects of loss of a loved one, be it spouse, parent, or child, are now widely accepted. Yet, only very recently have the full impact and consequences of pregnancy loss become appreciated. In this chapter, the author reviews normal mourning and bereavement and then examines unique aspects of those processes that relate to pregnancy loss. Also included is a discussion of potential psychopathology that may complicate bereavement after a pregnancy loss.

The response to loss has been termed "bereavement," "grief," or "mourning," largely because many disciplines have studied this same process and its consequences. In this chapter, bereavement is defined as the entire process precipitated by loss through death; grief, the specific subjective feelings that accompany this loss; and mourning, the process through which resolution of grief is accomplished.

UNIQUE ASPECTS IN RESPONSE TO PREGNANCY LOSS

Any examination of the response to loss must acknowledge the numerous forms it may take. This is especially true for pregnancy loss. Given individual circumstances surrounding miscarriage and ectopic pregnancy, stillbirth, or neonatal death, any or all of the following may come into play: real (actual) loss of a person, threatened or impending loss of a person, loss of status (motherhood), and symbolic loss. Symbolic loss associated with pregnancy loss frequently has been overlooked, but it can be summed up by the following: "When your parent dies, you have lost your past. When your child dies, you have lost your future" (3).

Frequency of Pregnancy Loss

Although there are a number of characteristics distinctive to pregnancy loss, infrequency is not among them. Indeed, pregnancy loss is by no means uncommon. Most people outside obstetric and neonatal disciplines would be surprised to hear that approximately 40,000 neonatal deaths occur yearly in the United States and that, out of every 100 pregnancies, 2 end in stillbirth and 10 to 20 in miscarriage (4). Within the field, the sheer magnitude of pregnancy loss may help to account for the prevailing attitude that such events represent only the loss of nonviable life. Ordinarily, obstetric and neonatal interventions are directed exclusively to the emergency or crisis component of the event and not its psychologic significance as well. Rapid and highly visible technologic advances in the general obstetric, perinatal surgical, neonatal, and fertility areas also obscure the frequency of pregnancy loss.

Death is rarely predictable or expected at any but the final stage of the life cycle. For postneonatal loss, fortunately, numerous social institutions support the bereavement process. During gestation, death seems most remote of all. Thus, fetal or neonatal death may be the last type of loss to be accorded its due. Uniformly recognized or available social rituals have yet to be associated with pregnancy loss—"It is celebrated only in the tears of women" (5). Such losses frequently are referred to as "nondeaths" (6) or "nonevents" (7) of rarely named "nonpersons" (8), which negates the reality of the loss. This attitude persists despite documentation of the developmental processes of expectant parenthood (9). Full discussion of these issues is contained in Chapter 2, "Early Pregnancy Loss." The subject is also included below, however, to illustrate reasons for the intense grief response to pregnancy loss.

MOTHERHOOD AS A BIOPSYCHOSOCIAL EVENT

For the woman, expectant motherhood is a discrete biopsychosocial process that transforms and broadens her role to that of mother. This process is accomplished largely before delivery, through a host of important responses and reactions to pregnancy. These include the following:

Psychologic Process of Becoming a Parent

Feelings of procreativity or generativity;

A sense of continuity through the generations;

Responses to quickening and bodily changes;

Fears and expectations about the coming baby;

The impact of this exciting process on expectant parents' relationship at home;

Changes that the baby will bring to their careers and to their lives in general.

The pregnant woman experiences a unique psychologic state, a turning inward, wherein she focuses significant emotional energy on herself, her baby and the baby's father, the future, and her relationship with her own mother, both past and present. Through pregnancy, a woman comes to "know" her baby intimately as a consequence of rich fantasies, fears, and dreams.

It should also be noted that sonograms and amniocentesis increase prenatal bonding significantly (10). In an ongoing study of the psychologic impact of knowledge of fetal sex on expectant parents, the author has learned that information gained antenatally from such procedures gives rise to richer fantasies and expectations, early naming, and well-developed responses from children in the family.

EXPECTANT FATHERHOOD

The mother is not alone in her response to prospective parenthood. Recently, Herzog (11) has delineated eloquently three psychologic approaches to fatherhood. His study of 103 fathers-to-be reveals that there are most, less well, and least attuned groups of expectant fathers, with attunement essentially corresponding to a man's empathic intimacy with the pregnant woman. Intimately involved fathers-to-be, the "most attuned" group, passed through characteristic stages of expectant fatherhood. These involve a getting-ready period, a time of fullness and ecstasy after conception, a refocusing on the relationship with his own father, and a reworking of his own caregiving ideas and expectations as intimacy with his partner intensifies.

PHASES OF MOURNING

Numerous clinicians and researchers have documented characteristics of normal grief (2, 7, 12–16). A degree of uniformity has been found sufficient to merit the designation of mourning as a syndrome with an expected course and a resolution. Three approximate phases have been described: protest, disorganization, and reorganization. The description of these stages must be preceded by the caveats that variation among grieving individuals is considerable and that the process is more fluid than an ordering of discrete phases would seem to imply. As has happened with the misapplication of Kübler-Ross' (17) stages of death and dying, the clinician must guard against inappropriate expectations of the patient.

Protest

Protest, the initial phase of mourning, lasts from a few hours to several days. It is marked by a desperate and frantic attempt to reinstitute the relationship with the lost person. This is likely to consist of an immediate, pervasive sense of shock, numbness (lack of emotional reaction), disbelief, and denial. In most instances, the apparent inability to grasp what has transpired is short-lived. It is soon followed by distress, which is manifested by weeping and sighing.

These immediate responses, as well as those that follow, probably emanate from childhood attachment behavior. Premature separation of a child from his mother is accompanied by crying, which is both an attempt to recover her and a protest against her loss. The child's response is striking in its similarity to adult grief. Our capacity to bond or affiliate with others is precisely what leaves us vulnerable to grief when a relationship is abruptly ended. Anger and hostility are frequently present during the initial phase of mourning. Both may be directed at physicians and nurses in the hospital setting. Or they may be toward oneself, specifically for having failed to do something to avert the loss.

Disorganization

The second phase, disorganization, introduces developing awareness of finality. Emotions become explicitly painful and are accompanied by profound sadness and deep yearning in search of the lost person. Feelings of intense loneliness, isolation, and meaninglessness are the rule. Freud (1) made an enduring distinction between these normative, although very disruptive, feelings on the one hand and pathologic grief or melancholia on the other. Only the latter involves a prominent lowering of self-esteem, which often is expressed through self-reproach. Because of certain features unique to pregnancy loss, however, Freud's distinction may not be as valid in this case as it is for more typical reactions to loss of an adult or an older child.

Somatic expressions of grief, frequently evoked by memories or comments about the lost person, may include any or all of the following: decreased appetite, difficulty in sleeping, weakness, tightening of the throat, empty feeling in the stomach, choking sensations, sighing, lethargy, and anergy. Also prominent during the stage of disorganization is a significant withdrawal from the outside world. This withdrawal is evidenced by introversion, lack of spontaneity and warmth, and disinterest in eating and grooming.

The most characteristic feature of this phase is preoccupation with thoughts of the deceased while the mourner relives his or her relationship with the lost one. These memories are intrusive, unbidden, unwanted, and painful; they constitute, however, the necessary grief work that eventually helps the mourner relinquish the important attachment. Denial frequently reappears in an attempt to hold on to things as they were previously. The person's attitudes and behaviors reflect this effort, and there are wish-fulfilling dreams and daydreams wherein the deceased returns. Characteristically, there is a restlessness and aimlessness during this phase. The mourner often finds it difficult to sit still or concentrate. He or she must make an effort to function, performing chores routinely and automatically, many times without paying conscious attention.

Reorganization   In the third phase of mourning, reorganization, the bereaved person slowly reinvests interest in the world. This process varies greatly in duration from individual to individual. Painful memories become less frequent and are replaced by more positive ones. New activities are begun. New relationships are entered into, and old ones are reestablished. There may, however, be transitory feelings of guilt about having survived the loss and enjoying life in spite of it.

As is true in all phases of human development, a life crisis can bring on despair and regression or it can promote growth through acquisition of new insights, attitudes, strengths, and values. This is true of successful bereavement. Traditionally, the process just described extends for at least one to two years. Bereavement nears completion as the survivor becomes operational, enjoys life again, and looks to the future.

MATERNAL GRIEVING AND PREGNANCY LOSS

An understanding of the experience of expectant parenthood provides the groundwork for appreciating the intensity of the response to pregnancy loss. The richness of the psychologic journey eventuating in strong attachment to the unborn baby speaks loudly against a superficial and one-dimensional biomedical view of pregnancy loss as nothing more than the loss of nonviable "products of conception." Moreover, intense grief following pregnancy loss should not be viewed suspiciously as a histrionic overreaction. Rather, it should be seen as an indication of the mature capacity for relatedness and affiliation, which ultimately are a function of a cohesive sense of self and an effective self-esteem regulation.

Regardless of the nature of a pregnancy loss, the bereavement process is both universal in many respects and uniquely varied for the individual. In particular, a woman's capacity to adapt to pregnancy loss is a function of those same factors determining her capacity to deal with uncomplicated pregnancy—her personality structure or character, coping skills, life setting, and family constellation (18).

Component Losses of Pregnancy Loss

Pregnancy loss has a number of important component losses. Not only is there a real and fantasized loss of a baby, but there are significant self-esteem losses as well. These include loss of being pregnant and of the sense of oneness with the fetus, loss of anticipated motherhood, loss of the special attention and care frequently accorded a pregnant woman, and loss of prenatal medical care. In addition, there is a crucial loss of self-esteem resulting from the woman's inability to rely on her body and successfully give birth. How one experiences one's body is a fundamental constituent of a person's total identity and sense of self. A closely related phenomenon occurring in expectant parents whose pregnancy loss is associated with fetal anomalies is the lowering of self-esteem from carrying defective genes.

Early versus Late Gestational Losses

Maternal grieving after pregnancy loss follows the typical process described earlier. There is, however, one important distinction between early pregnancy loss (miscarriage, ectopic pregnancy, or elective abortion) and stillbirth or neonatal death. In the latter instances, the mourning process can be facilitated by the presence of a body and/or pictures of the stillborn fetus or dead neonate. To mourn for a baby lost early in the pregnancy, whose existence goes unrecognized by so many, often is more complicated because there is no recognizable body to visualize. A stillbirth or a neonate who was alive only for a short time nevertheless can be viewed, held, and photographed by his or her parents, thus permitting a much more concrete attachment by parents with resultant prominent memories. In this respect, in the author's clinical experience and that of others (19), although close-to-term pregnancy loss may usher in a more intense first phase of grieving, it can also result in an earlier and more definitive reorganization phase than that for an early pregnancy loss.

PROCESS OF MOURNING A PREGNANCY LOSS

The initial phase of maternal grief is marked by emotional numbness and denial. There is shock even when the loss is anticipated, as is the case in some stillbirths or neonatal deaths.

This shock may be more pronounced when an unexpected death occurs at or shortly after the time of delivery. However, even when fetal death is diagnosed prior to delivery, and therefore anticipatory grieving is possible, there generally is still very strong shock and disbelief at the time of delivery (20). "Instead of the expected cry of the healthy baby within the delivery room, there is only silence" (19).

Blame and Anger

An increasing acceptance of the death characterizes the second or disorganization phase of mourning. The woman more freely experiences her feelings of loss, sadness, emptiness, anger, inadequacy, blame, and jealousy. There are almost always significant feelings of guilt centered around fantasies of having either caused or contributed to the pregnancy loss in some fashion. Concerns over excessive exercise or heavy lifting, improper diet or consumption of alcohol, insufficient rest, and too-frequent sexual relations are commonplace. In cases where a woman has undergone a previous elective abortion, the author has never failed to uncover some well-circumscribed belief linking it somehow to the pregnancy loss. In such instances, there is the belief that the current loss is a punishment for the abortion or in some other, "medical" way consequent to it. Blame and anger frequently accompany pregnancy loss, as a response to intense feelings of helplessness. This can be directed toward the woman's partner, doctor or midwife, religion, and, of course, herself. With regard to anger at the physician, Wolff et al. (21) have reported that, of those women in their sample conceiving after a stillbirth, 50% changed obstetricians. It would be highly speculative to assume that such a change of physician indicates only unresolved anger from the pregnancy loss. However, this finding may speak to numerous insensitivities experienced by pregnancy loss patients, and it may be reasonable for women to opt for such a change.

Envy and Jealousy

Envy and jealousy toward other pregnant women are ubiquitous following a pregnancy loss. Although these feelings are generally more intense toward relatives and friends, it is not at all uncommon for women who have experienced pregnancy loss to report envious and jealous feelings toward pregnant strangers or toward mothers they meet on the street or in social encounters. In the early months following pregnancy loss, many women avoid social situations in which they would have to interact with others who are pregnant or who have recently become mothers.

Return of Menstruation

One event generally perceived as helpful in the process of resolution or reorganization is the return of menstruation. The first period after pregnancy loss ushers in hope that pregnancy can again be attempted. Also, menstruation offers women reassurance, to varying degrees, that reproductive processes are functioning correctly. It should be noted, however, that subsequent periods are received more ambivalently, because these mark the failure to conceive and may aggravate feelings about the pregnancy loss.

The final stage of the mourning process is characterized by the diminution of feelings of self-reproach, loneliness, and emptiness. The woman, and those in her life as well, note a return to "normality." She can enter the room and handle the clothes once designated for the baby without becoming overwhelmed. Renewed interest in activities and in others is evident. She can once again be around babies and engage them without undue painful emotional consequences. For many women, however, a complete sense of acceptance or integration of the loss comes only with the subsequent delivery of a healthy baby. (See Chapter 15, "Impact of Pregnancy Loss on Subsequent Pregnancy.")

VARIATIONS AMONG INDIVIDUALS IN THE DEGREE OF RESOLUTION

A critical clinical point about bereavement following pregnancy loss is that the degree to which resolution is achieved varies from individual to individual. Psychoanalytic literature in particular has addressed a mother's unique loss of a child in terms of discontinuity or broken connection of the generations. Such losses are understood to be more difficult to work through when compared with other more typical losses (22, 23).

"Shadow Grief"

Peppers and Knapp (4) allude to this characteristic of the postmourning process through use of their term "shadow grief." Although physical sensations such as dull ache or unresponsivity can be associated with any loss of a loved one, this manifestation of grief is an especially apt way to note the tendency for painful memories and sensations to arise on anniversary dates such as the stillborn baby's due date and delivery date or the neonate's death date and/or birthday. These events are marked by tears, mild sadness, emptiness, and occasional low levels of anxiety which leave the person with a sense that something is "not quite right." Although no formal studies exist on this particular facet of bereavement with regard to pregnancy loss, it is the author's contention that shadow grief is very much related to the profound sense of isolation (from physicians, nurses, partners, relatives, friends, and others) experienced by women suffering pregnancy loss. Many have addressed this "conspiracy of silence" that surrounds perinatal death, wherein a mother is not encouraged to explore her feelings about her loss and is even discouraged from doing so (24). She is discouraged from appropriate mourning by unempathic comments from doctors, nurses, family, friends, and even her partner; by remarks about her alleged ability to have another child; by use of sedatives and minor tranquilizers; and by the failure of others to allow her to have contact with her baby and to be involved in funeral or burial activities (5, 21, 25).

Unique Aspects of Pregnancy Loss

Circumstances surrounding two particular types of pregnancy loss are worthy of mention at this point, because they often constitute more intense forms of shadow grief but frequently go unrecognized because of the conspiracy of silence. In the first, with the loss of one of a set of twins, even less support appears available for the mother than usual (26). The most frequent response by everyone, except the grieving mother, is that she should be thankful for the survival of one of the babies. The second case involves the instance in which complicated decisions about prolonging neonatal life are necessary and/or there is some debate about whether or not to intervene medically or surgically with a baby in whom there is likelihood of severe handicap. Recent media attention on legal aspects of such decisions perhaps has created even more confusion that distracts healthcare professionals and the immediate family from their primary obligation to the mother.

IMPACT OF PREGNANCY LOSS ON THE FAMILY

The bereavement process following pregnancy loss is not limited to the mother. Although not nearly as intimate or direct, the expectant father's emotional experience is analogous to his partner's during her pregnancy. Even though the expectant father is likely to have the least attachment to the baby following a miscarriage, his attachment may be great in the case of neonatal death. This is especially so if he can catch up with his partner's bonding process when time permits him to interact with the newborn prior to death.

Incongruent Grieving

Peppers and Knapp (4) have described potential difficulties between a man and woman resulting from incongruent grieving, a natural outcome of incongruent bonding. The woman often perceives her partner as having escaped the full emotional burden of the loss. Possibly, she may even see him as uncaring. This may be because of role expectations in our society whereby the man is supposed to remain composed, rational, and, thus, available to his partner as protector and consoler.

IMPACT OF PREGNANCY LOSS ON MARITAL STABILITY

A father's calm exterior is commonly misinterpreted by his partner as an absence of feeling or response to pregnancy loss.

As he begins to be in touch with his feelings of loss, the man may himself experience a strong sense of isolation, and he may feel that there is no one with whom to share his grief. He may be in conflict about sharing his loss with his partner for fear of upsetting or depressing her. Frequently, a man may feel angry toward his partner when she, because of her own grief, fails to respond to his efforts at intervention and support. Absence of mutual support and sharing during grieving is the most significant contribution to complicated bereavement following pregnancy loss.

A Woman's Sense of Failure

The more general feelings of disappointment felt by bereaved expectant parents often obscure a nearly universal sense of failure experienced acutely by the woman. This sense of failure takes the form of having disappointed her partner because she has been unable to give birth to a healthy baby. She has failed in her attempt at loving procreation. Although many women may not be able to articulate this fear to their partners, they nevertheless are intensely worried that their partners do indeed hold such a view. These feelings are not limited to fantasy, for frequently a woman has accurately interpreted her partner's attempt to rationalize the tragic loss through blaming another—her. The degree to which committed partners can address these troublesome thoughts and fantasies will enhance their ability to assist each other in their acute grief.

It is important to recognize that not all couples experiencing pregnancy loss automatically go on to an intense state of dysfunction in their relationship. In fact, the opposite may be more common. Harmon et al. (27), in a recent study of 38 women grieving from neonatal loss, found that at both 3 and 9 months postloss these women reported more closeness with their partners than previously. Only 10% stated that the pregnancy loss had created difficulties for them with their partners. Nevertheless, most clinicians agree that the potential for conflict for a couple is very great after pregnancy loss.

RESPONSE OF CHILDREN TO PREGNANCY LOSS

Children in the family also react to pregnancy loss (28). What determines the child's response to the loss depends for the most part on two factors: his or her cognitive development and therefore the capacity to understand death; and the response of his or her parents, especially the mother, to the loss. Wass and Corr (29) point out that concepts of death develop in four stages. No specific ages can be attached to these stages, since many factors determine when a particular child will advance to the next stage.

A Child's Developing Concepts of Death

In the first stage, during infancy, a baby has no concept of death. Although babies can form internal images, these images are of things found in their immediate world such as people, food, or toys. The second developmental stage in the concept of death occurs in early childhood. The child's own experiences govern his or her understanding of events. Children at this stage believe that everything in the world, including tricycles and stones, is alive and that everything is manufactured for people's convenience. They believe that whatever is desired or wished for will happen, that anything is possible. They also believe that events happen for personal reasons. A bad dream may happen because a child has been bad. Three-, four-, and five-year olds have difficulty comprehending that death is final and that they have no control over the event.

In the third stage, during late childhood and preadolescence, death is understood to be an irreversible event. However, children at this stage hope to escape the process entirely themselves or at least to delay any experience with death for a very long time. They begin to find the physiology of death, dying, and decomposition a source of interest. The fourth, mature, stage in understanding death is achieved in adolescence. Death finally is understood to be irreversible and inevitable. Adolescents are able to develop personal, abstract, and theological views toward death and are aware of the meaning of the experience for others.

As does the expectant father, children have varying degrees of involvement and attachment to the fetus or neonate. When pregnancy loss occurs, children may develop symptoms (anger, depression, aggression, phobic behavior, anxiety, sleep disturbances) because the loss actualizes for them the ambivalence with which they have regarded the expected sibling. It is one thing to feel that the forthcoming baby is a rival and intruder and appropriately wish it dead; it is quite another and scary event to have that wish come true. Yet, in the very concrete and egocentric world of the young child, this is precisely the scenario. Some children may blame the mother for the loss of their new sister or brother, and they become quite resentful, especially toward the mother. This is exquisitely painful to a grieving woman.

Impact of Mother's Preoccupation with Mourning

Ultimately, what makes children vulnerable is that they are very dependent on the adults in their environment. A mother's quite normal depression after her pregnancy loss temporarily renders her emotionally less accessible and responsive to her children. It is this perceived withdrawal that is most threatening to a child. Thus, it is advisable to call upon other familiar adults in the extended family or neighborhood to be available to children during the period of mourning.

PREGNANCY LOSS AND PSYCHOPATHOLOGY

Bereavement as a Factor in Illness Onset

The remarkably limited literature on pregnancy loss contains primarily two subjects: (1) complicated maternal bereavement following neonatal death and (2) the impact of the hospital milieu and doctor-patient relationship on parental grieving. There remains significant controversy in adult psychiatric literature as to whether or not increased physical morbidity and mortality are associated with bereavement. Clayton (30) concluded from her prospective studies of widows and widowers that there is no appreciable increase in mortality or morbidity in the bereaved. However, Rees and Lutkins (31) and Parkes (14) have been able to demonstrate significantly higher morbidity and mortality rates in the bereaved, and Engel (32) and Holmes (33) have singled out bereavement as a major factor in illness onset.

Risks of Experiencing Prolonged Grief

Similarly, with regard to psychopathology following pregnancy loss (excluding the questionable literature on emotional responses to spontaneous abortion), Wolff et al. (21) found that, of 40 women who lost a baby at or shortly after birth, there were no psychiatric sequelae at 3-year follow-ups. Jensen and Zahourek (34) studied 25 women who experienced neonatal death and found that, after 1 year, a significant number of them were still depressed. One-third of Cullberg's (35) neonatal loss subjects demonstrated serious mental symptoms including psychosis, phobias, anxiety attacks, and severe depression at 1- to 2-year follow-ups. In a retrospective study by telephone interview 10 to 20 months after pregnancy loss, 23% of mothers were diagnosed as having prolonged grief reactions. Those with a surviving twin or subsequent pregnancy less than 5 months following the death were at higher risk of prolonged grief reactions than were those without subsequent pregnancy or pregnancy more than 6 months later (36). Harmon's (27) neonatal loss study found at 3- and 9-month follow-ups that mothers described their baby's death as having a major impact on their wellbeing and functioning. At 3 months approximately four-fifths, and at 9 months approximately three-quarters, of their sample indicated that their lives had been substantially changed directly by the loss. Nearly 75% admitted to being depressed at 9 months and attributed it again to the neonatal death. At the 9-month follow-up, approximately one-half reported irritability and crying episodes. More than a third were still angry at healthcare professionals for their alleged role in that loss.

ABNORMAL GRIEF REACTIONS

Most bereaved persons are sufficiently supported by their social milieu so that bereavement is successfully concluding within a year or so. The results of a number of studies, however, suggest that abuse of alcohol is frequently correlated with negative bereavement outcomes (30, 14). One of the strongest predictors of complicated bereavement is a history of poor psychologic functioning prior to pregnancy loss. A comprehensive personal and marital history could alert healthcare professionals as to when enhanced likelihood of future difficulties in mourning exists. In general, the woman who is psychologically vulnerable prior to pregnancy loss and who is without adequate emotional support from those around her especially deserves close follow-up after pregnancy loss.

Prolonged Grief

Complicated bereavement or abnormal grief reactions after pregnancy loss generally take one of these two forms: (1) chronic, prolonged grief or (2) absent grief. It is important to note that there has been little systematic study of abnormal grief reactions after pregnancy loss. Nevertheless, it has been the author's experience that the most frequent form of abnormal grief is that of prolonged grief or persistent and intense grieving despite passage of time. People experiencing this reaction appear to be trapped in their mourning, which at times may serve as a defense against even more painful feelings of hopelessness. Excessive guilt, anger, self-reproach, and continued preoccupation with the loss are typical of such presentations, as are unmistakable symptoms of a major depressive episode. Major depression is defined as presence of a persistent dysphoric (sad) mood or loss of interest in activities and pasttimes, as well as presence of at least four of the characteristics listed in Figure 1.1.

Absent Grief

Lack of any apparent grief response, particularly to stillbirth and neonatal death, should raise suspicions about another form of pathologic mourning, absent grief. Although this form of abnormal grief is relatively infrequent, it is sometimes difficult to diagnose because the person reports no feelings of distress

Significant change in appetite with either weight loss or weight gain

Sleep disturbance (insomnia or hypersomnia)

Psychomotor agitation or retardation

Decrease or loss of interest and pleasure in activities and sex

Anergy and fatigue

Feelings of worthlessness and lowered self-esteem

Decreased ability to think and concentrate

Recurrent thoughts of suicide and death

Figure 1.1.   Characteristics of major depression.

and takes great pride in carrying on with his or her life in spite of the apparent importance of the deceased. However, astute observation will reveal that there is almost always heightened irritability and tension in these people. It is common for those with absent grief reactions to present with a multiplicity of somatic complaints to their physicians or emergency rooms.

Posttraumatic Stress Disorder

There is one other potential category of psychologic complications with which healthcare professionals should be familiar, the posttraumatic stress disorder (PTSD). Diagnosis of this anxiety disorder depends on the "existence of a recognizable stressor that would evoke significant symptoms of distress in almost anyone" (37). Persons suffering from PTSD re-experience psychologic trauma as manifested by repetitive and unwanted memories and/or dreams of the event. There may be the sudden acting or feeling as if the trauma were reoccurring. After the trauma, persons with PTSD typically have a numbing of responsiveness to or reduced involvement with the world, as indicated by decreased interest in one or more significant activities, feelings of detachment or estrangement from others, and/or constricted affect (the capacity to experience only a limited number of feelings). There may be a hypervigilance or startle response, sleep disturbance, survivor's guilt, difficulty in concentrating or remembering, avoidance of activities reminiscent of the traumatic event, and intensification of symptoms by exposure to events that either symbolize or resemble the traumatic event. Many of the characteristics of PTSD can be commonly observed in complicated bereavement. This is especially true when dramatic circumstances surround the pregnancy loss, as in instances of neonatal death from prematurity in which labor was induced by a traumatic psychologic or physical event such as a car accident or an assault. In such cases, mourning can be complex and protracted with many or all of the features of PTSD. Patients with such responses can be readily treated with intensive psychotherapy and should be referred to a psychiatrist.

CONCLUSION

It is apparent from this chapter, and indeed this entire book, that the tragedy of pregnancy loss goes largely unrecognized by significant segments of healthcare professions, as well as by society at large. Many grieving mothers and fathers are very much left on their own to navigate this bereavement process. The author hopes that the account in this chapter of the normal process undergone by almost all who have experienced such loss will enable professionals to be more empathic with these patients. Often, what is most poignant about events surrounding pregnancy loss is the absence of professional empathy, which unnecessarily traumatizes patients even further. Although it is true that anger and hostility are normal reactions to such a loss, it is also true that such feelings are sometimes appropriate responses to insensitivity of hospital staff to the personal meaning of these experiences for the individuals involved. The response by others in the environment to a traumatic episode may be equal to, if not more important than, the precise nature of the overwhelming event itself. A pregnancy-loss patient in particular is at high risk for sustaining psychic trauma and for suffering the painful loss of care providers who should be but are not emotionally available. Care providers of all disciplines will become eminently more successful and will grow professionally when they can respond in depth to an individual patient's plight.

REFERENCES

1. Freud S: *Mourning and Melancholia. The Standard Edition of the Complete Psychological Works of Sigmund Freud, vol 14, London, 1917.* Hogarth Press and Institute for Psychoanalysis, 1957.
2. Lindemann E: Symptomatology and management of acute grief. *Am J Psychiatry* 101:141–149, 1944.
3. Luby E. In Schiff HS (ed): *The Bereaved Parent.* New York, Penguin Books, 1977, p 23.
4. Peppers LG and Knapp RJ: *Motherhood and Mourning: Perinatal Death.* New York, Praeger Scientific, 1980, p 14.
5. Friedman R and Cohen KA: Emotional reactions to miscarriage. In Notman MT and Nadelson CC (eds): *The Woman Patient.* New York, Plenum Press, 1982, vol 3, pp 173–187.
6. Phipps S: Mourning response and intervention in stillbirth: an alternative genetic counseling approach. *Soc Biol* 28:1–13, 1981.
7. Bowlby J: *Loss: Sadness and Depression—Attachment and Loss.* New York, Basic Books, 1940, vol 3, p 123.
8. Lewis E: The management of stillbirth: coping with an unreality. *Lancet* 2:619–620, 1976.
9. Anthony EJ and Benedek T: *Parenthood: Its Psychology and Psychopathology.* Boston, Little, Brown & Company, 1970.
10. Fletcher JC and Evans MI: Maternal bonding in early fetal ultrasound examinations. *N Engl J Med* 308:392–393, 1983.
11. Herzog JM: Patterns of expectant fatherhood: a study of the fathers of a group of premature infants. In Cath SH, Gurwitz AR, Ross JM (eds): *Father and Child: Development and Clinical Perspectives.* Boston, Little, Brown & Company, 1982, pp 301–314.
12. Pollock GH: Mourning and adaption. *Int J Psychoanal* 42:341–361, 1961.
13. Clayton P, Desmarais L, Winokur G: A study of normal bereavement. *Am J Psychiatry* 125(1):64–74, 1968.
14. Parkes CM: Broken heart: a statistical study of increased mortality among widowers. *Br Med J* 1:740–748, 1969.
15. Parkes CM and Weiss RS: *Recovery from Bereavement.* New York, Basic Books, 1983.

16. Raphael B: *The Anatomy of Bereavement.* New York, Basic Books, 1983.
17. Kübler-Ross E: *On Death and Dying.* New York, Macmillan, 1969.
18. Bibring GL, Dwyer TF, Huntington DS, Valenstein AF: A study of the psychological processes in pregnancy and of the earliest mother-child relationship I and II. In *Psychoanalytic Study of the Child, vol 16,* New York, Inter University Press, 1961, pp 9–24.
19. Harmon RJ and Graham-Cicchinelli D: Fetal and Neonatal Loss. In Simons RC (ed). *Understanding Human Behavior in Health and Illness,* ed 3. Baltimore, Williams & Wilkins, 1985, pp 151–157.
20. Kirkley-Best E and Kellner K: The forgotten grief: a review of the psychology of stillbirth. *Am J Orthopsychiatry* 52:420–429, 1982.
21. Wolff JR, Nielson PE, Schiller P: The emotional reaction to a stillbirth. *Am J Obstet Gynecol* 108:73–77, 1970.
22. Gorer G: *Death, Grief and Mourning.* New York, Doubleday, 1965.
23. Videka-Sherman L: Coping with the death of a child: a study over time. *Am J Orthopsychiatry* 52:688–698, 1982.
24. Lewis E: Mourning by the family after a stillbirth or neonatal death. *Arch Dis Child* 54:303–306, 1979.
25. Stringham J, Riley JH, Ross A: Silent birth: mourning a stillborn baby. *Social Work* 27:322–327, 1982.
26. Wilson AL, Fenton LJ, Stevens DC, Soule DJ: The death of a twin: an analysis of parental bereavement. *Pediatrics* 70:587–591, 1982.
27. Harmon RJ, Glicken AD, Seigel RE: Neonatal loss in the intensive care nursery: effects on maternal grieving and a program for intervention. *J Am Acad Child Psychiatry* 23:68–71, 1984.
28. Cain AC, Erickson ME, Fast I, Vaughan RA: Children's disturbed reactions to their mother's miscarriage. *Psychosomat Med* 26(1):58–66, 1964.
29. Wass H and Corr C: *Helping Children Cope with Death—Guidelines and Resources.* Washington, DC, Hemisphere, 1984.
30. Clayton PJ: The sequalae and nonsequalae of conjugal bereavement. *Am J Psychiatry* 136:1530–1534, 1979.
31. Rees WD and Lutkins SG: Mortality of bereavement. *Br Med J* 4:13–16, 1979.
32. Engel GL, A life setting conducive to illness. *Ann Intern Med* 69:293–300, 1969.
33. Holmes TH: Life situations, emotions and disease. *Psychosomatics* 19:747–751, 1978.
34. Jensen J and Zahourek R: Depression in mothers who have lost a newborn. *Rocky Mountain Med J* 69:61–63, 1972.
35. Cullberg J: *Psychosomatic Medicine in Obstetrics and Gynecology (Third International Congress).* London, Basel and Karger, 1972, pp 326–329.
36. Rowe J, Clyman R, Green C, Mikkelson C, Haight J, Ataide L: Follow-up of families who experience perinatal death. *Pediatrics* 62(2):166–170, Aug 1978.
37. *Diagnostic and Statistical Manual of Mental Disorders,* ed 3. Washington, DC, American Psychiatric Association, 1980, pp 236–238.

The Events

Early Pregnancy Loss: Miscarriage and Ectopic Pregnancy

ANN HAGER, C.N.M.
with a contribution by
O'DELL M. OWENS, M.D.

From a medical and nursing perspective, a first-trimester pregnancy loss is a routine emergency. It may involve only an office visit or a brief hospitalization for dilation and curettage. Generally, it is not life threatening, treatment is relatively simple, and recovery is rapid. Historically, care providers have treated this event in a medically efficient manner with the basic kindness and consideration shown to any patient. There has been little recognition that an early pregnancy loss represents a major life crisis or that it often precipitates a grief reaction in the woman, her partner, or her children. Clichés that abound in the lay population—"It was too early for her to be attached" or "Well, at least she conceived; she can always have another child"—have contributed to this oversight.

In the 1970s, the medical community began to recognize that parents grieve for stillborn babies and neonatal deaths. In the 1980s, studies began to confirm what women have always tried to communicate to the medical profession: Miscarriage is as much a pregnancy loss as is the death of a fetus or newborn.

The purposes of this chapter are twofold. Psychologic tasks of pregnancy are explained. These tasks, in fact, are integral to the first trimester of pregnancy, and they account for the strong grief response to a first-trimester loss. Emotional reactions to miscarriage can be understood better when factors contributing to the impact of such an event are acknowledged. In this chapter, the authors also describe the experience and interventions that are common as a woman progresses along the continuum from threatened abortion to the actual event and subsequent recovery. Ectopic pregnancy and early elective abortion are included in the discussion because they are forms of early pregnancy loss whose impact on the patient and her family is similar to that of miscarriage. (Note that the authors use the word "miscarriage" rather than the clinically more precise "abortion," in order to distinguish between a spontaneous and an elective abortion.) Much of the difficulty that women experiencing an early pregnancy loss encounter is a result of the general assumption that it has happened "too early" to affect her or her family.

PSYCHOLOGIC TASKS OF PREGNANCY

Pregnancy as a Fantasy

For a woman, pregnancy begins psychologically long before it occurs in her body. Peppers and Knapp (1) point out that bonding with the baby may start with fantasy thoughts of what it would be like to be a mother and that attachment to the baby officially starts when birth control is stopped. Planning may not be a requirement for bonding, but this activity may speed up the process.

Ambivalence

If planning the pregnancy is the first event in formation of a mother-infant bond, confirmation of pregnancy constitutes the second step (2). With the advent of accurate home pregnancy tests, radioimmunassay blood tests, and ultrasound, confirmation of pregnancy may occur earlier now than in the past. Once pregnancy is confirmed, a woman begins to assess her situation and to accomplish the key task of the first trimester, acceptance of pregnancy. Although a positive pregnancy test removes any of the woman's doubts regarding her fertility, the wish to be pregnant is not always the wish for a child (3). Most authors agree that, even in planned pregnancies, there is ambivalence. Grimm (4) found that 50 % of women surveyed at the beginning of a pregnancy did not want the baby.

In the first trimester, both positive and negative feelings may be exaggerated by physical signs such as nausea, vomiting, fatigue, mood swings, and a decrease in sexual desire. Although they are reassuring as proof of pregnancy, these physical and emotional changes may become the focus of attention. The woman may resent the baby for imposing itself into her normal routine. She may feel that she has become a different person suddenly, and she may also feel some panic about new responsibilities that she has assumed by becoming pregnant (3, 5, 6).

Conflicts of Self-Image

Although an expanded relationship with the father of the baby may begin to be of concern, the woman's relationship with her mother undergoes serious examination. She may wish to be a better mother than her own mother was, but she also may be afraid to admit her pregnancy to herself or others, for fear of having to compete with her mother. Even in these early weeks, long before she looks pregnant, the woman begins to formulate a unique mothering identity separate from that of her own mother.

During this time of acceptance, the woman perceives her baby as an extension of herself. "The embryo at this time is there by intimation, not as a separate entity" (p. 217) (3). The first trimester becomes a time of incorporation. The woman integrates and merges with this foreign body and turns it into an integral part of herself. However, since it is not apparent that she is pregnant, she can withhold the fact selectively, not discussing it if she prefers not to mention it. Despite her increasing acceptance of the pregnancy, she may choose to keep it a secret.

Quickening Introduces the Fetus as Separate

The second trimester is a time of differentiation (5) or of perceiving "the otherness within" (3). The key event is quickening. Bibring et al. (7) point out that "quickening disrupts the narcissistic process and undeniably introduces the baby as the new object within the self." At this point, the woman usually begins to fantasize about the baby and to weave a mental image of her child. Names mentioned casually in the first trimester are considered and baby items purchased. The sensation of movement brings relief, reaffirmation of pregnancy, fulfillment, and delight. However, ambivalent feelings also linger. Although she may be delighted to wear maternity clothes, the woman may worry about her changing body image. Difficulty accepting her lack of control over the intruder inside is counterbalanced with concern that everything the woman does affects her baby (8).

Loss of Control

As the woman realizes that she cannot control many of the changes happening to her, she may search for someone to take care of her. Her mother may be the obvious figure, and the woman may be flooded at this time with memories of her mother's maternal qualities (4). At the same time, the woman also wants to turn away from her past. She may look to contemporaries as role models and to the father of the baby as someone on whom to depend (8). During the second trimester, the major psychologic task for the woman becomes that of asserting her role as wife and assuming the identity of a mother, as a confident, mature adult. Dreams during this period reflect

Sources of Anxiety

renewed investment in her partner. Although in the first trimester she might dream of harm to herself, during the second trimester she may dream that her partner has been hurt or killed. During daytime hours, she will be concerned for his safety (5).

Concerns in the Third Trimester

As the third trimester begins, the woman enjoys special interest that she receives because of her pregnancy. She may be the center of attention among her group of friends. Pride and anxious anticipation dominate the early part of this trimester. However, as weeks pass, fetal movement, once reassuring, may become irritating. Physical complaints abound, and body image is a major concern. These thoughts and physical signs help accomplish the task of the last trimester, which is separation of the fetus from the mother (that is, the loss of oneness). The third trimester is an anxious time for the woman. She worries about labor, the possibility of losing her baby, and added responsibilities she must assume. In her dreams, babies sometimes are misplaced or injured. In addition to excitement and worries, there is increasing realization that she and her baby will move apart.

The task of separation is completed as labor begins. There is now acceptance by the woman that delivery is inevitable, even though "she is being carried along against her will by a run-away organ" (p. 70) (5). Although her desire to see the baby may be overwhelming, subconsciously the woman may see labor as a test of her personal competence and a challenge to her womanhood.

Birth

The baby's birth begins the emotional work of the postpartum period. The woman must resolve the conflict between her idealized and her real infant, accept the parent role, and form an attachment to her newborn. This attachment is defined by Klaus and Kennell (2) as "the unique relationship between 2 people that is specific and endures through time" (p. 2). The atmosphere surrounding the birth and touching and caring for the baby aid in the attachment process.

FATHERS: PSYCHOLOGIC TASKS OF PREGNANCY

There are significant psychologic adjustments for men during and following pregnancy. Fortunately, the body of literature on fathers is growing, with such books available as *Parent-Infant Bonding* by Klaus and Kennell (2) and *Expectant Fathers* by Bittman and Zalk (9).

On Becoming "Number Two"

For the father, psychologic tasks to be accomplished as pregnancy progresses parallel those of his partner. In the first trimester, confirmation of a planned or unplanned pregnancy will give most men a sense of relief and pride. Virility has been proved. At the same time, a man may feel remote from the tiny conceptus whose presence is not yet apparent in his partner. In the early months of pregnancy, the man may be confused by the mood swings and emotions exhibited by his partner, whose feelings of happiness may be mixed with periods of irritability or sickness. Moreover, he may notice that she is the focus of attention and feel that he is now "number two," even to his own mother. During the early stages of pregnancy, he may look at his past, reevaluate his present, and dream of his future. Peer relationships and professional plans come in for review. Fears, anxieties, and new responsibilities may seem overwhelming, and avenues for expressing these feelings are few.

Demands of the Second Trimester

In the second trimester, more demands are placed on him. The woman looks to him for love, affection, and protection as she turns away from her mother. The payoff for these increased responsibilities is feeling the baby's movements. Peppers and Knapp (1) feel that paternal bonding does not begin until this event. However, although movement creates a link with the baby, it may also create problems in the area of sexuality. Someone has literally come between them. Moreover, while delighted about the baby's movements, the father may also be envious that he cannot carry a baby.

Bonding May Be Incomplete Until Birth

Men's and women's emotions during the third trimester are very similar. The man may be very involved in home preparations and childbirth classes and he, too, is increasingly anxious to see the baby. He may look forward to labor and delivery but has anxieties about and fears for his partner's safety. The financial and emotional responsibilities of parenthood also can no longer be denied. The parental bonding process for the man appears to be ongoing throughout pregnancy. Based on interviews with 40 couples, however, Peppers and Knapp (1) (1980) found that bonding between father and baby may remain incomplete until birth.

DEFINITIONS

A *spontaneous abortion* is the preterm delivery of a non-viable fetus before the 28th week of pregnancy (10). However, because the majority of spontaneous losses occur in the first trimester, discussion in this chapter will be limited to pregnancy losses occuring in this time period. In Chapter 3, pregnancy losses after 13 weeks are discussed.

A *threatened abortion* is presumed when any bloody vaginal discharge or vaginal bleeding appears in the first half of pregnancy. "A threatened abortion may or may not be accompanied by mild cramping pain resembling that of a menstrual period or by low backache . . ." (p. 472) (11). Most threatened abortions occur in the 12 weeks following the last menstrual period.

An *inevitable abortion* occurs in the presence of cervical dilation and is usually accompanied by gross rupture of the amniotic membranes. The products of conception are expelled by uterine contractions that begin soon after the initial event.

An *incomplete abortion* is the incomplete expulsion of fetal and/or placental tissue and may result in significant bleeding. It usually entails some hospitalization (even if only for a matter of hours) and a dilation and curettage.

A *missed abortion* has been defined as the retention of products of conception in utero for 8 weeks or more after the fetus has died (10).

Habitual abortion refers to women who have had 3 or more consecutive first-trimester losses.

A woman chooses prenatal care from among a variety of healthcare professionals. She may see an obstetrician, a certified nurse-midwife or nurse practitioner, or a family practitioner. In addition, professionals from other disciplines such as nursing or social work may contribute to her care at some stage in her pregnancy, at the time of delivery, or after delivery. It is for this reason that the term *care provider* is used in this chapter (and throughout the text) unless a more specific term is indicated.

MISCARRIAGE THREATENS: THE PROCESS

The Woman's Emotions

Reaction to Bleeding

A woman who is pregnant for the first time or who has had a previous uneventful pregnancy usually expects that conception will lead to the birth of a healthy baby. It is understandable, therefore, that when the first symptoms of miscarriage appear— usually bleeding—the woman is very fearful. Fliegelman and Rosenau (11) point out that, because of the bleeding, the woman instinctively may fear for her own health as well as that of her baby. Often, she may deny physical signs and symptoms rather than confront the threat of pregnancy loss and her sense of vulnerability.

Focusing Blame

Women also describe feelings of helplessness and anger. A woman may feel helpless because she is unable to alter events that are occurring in her body. Furthermore, she might not be able to comply indefinitely with her care provider's orders. If a miscarriage threatens over a period of days or weeks, a woman instructed to remain off her feet may need to return to her household duties or job. In an effort to reestablish some sense of control, she may look for someone to blame. Blame or anger frequently is directed at the care provider, especially if that person minimizes the woman's symptoms or her concerns about them. The woman and her partner may be doubtful about the care provider's advice and actions. Although there are no known techniques for reversing the miscarriage process, the care provider's failure to act may be misinterpreted as ineptitude and become a focus for the couple's anger.

Intervention

For psychologic as well as medical reasons, a woman with presumptive or positive signs of pregnancy must be taken seriously when she reports symptoms consistent with threatened miscarriage. The care provider must gather as much information as possible to determine the location and duration of and the prognosis for the pregnancy, as well as the emotional wellbeing of the woman.

Response of Care Providers

As many as 30–40% of all women experience some spotting during the early weeks of pregnancy. Most women, however, cannot be reassured over the telephone that bleeding, no matter how little, is of no clinical significance. If spotting is minimal and there is no uterine cramping, an emergency room visit in the middle of the night may be inappropriate. Nonetheless, a woman with such spotting should be seen as soon as possible during regular office hours to gather pertinent information about the bleeding episode and to minimize her uncertainty about what is happening to her.

If a benign cause for bleeding is not apparent, the episode should be managed as a threatened abortion and appropriate studies ordered. Clinical evaluation should be combined with other tests to evaluate the status of the pregnancy. Unfortunately, while attention has been given recently to tests that can predict early pregnancy failure (11–16), no test or combination of tests can completely predict pregnancy outcome (13).

Use of Clinical Tests

Results from real-time ultrasound and a hormone or biochemical marker provide helpful information as to pregnancy status. Although the type of hormonal marker may be dictated by laboratory facilities, radioimmunassay (RIA) for the Beta

TABLE 2.1
Laboratory Values for B-hCG Correlated with Length of Gestation

CONCEPTUAL AGE	MILLIUNITS PER ML
1st week	10–30
2nd week	30–100
3rd week	100–1,000
4th week	1,000–10,000
2nd to 3rd month	10,000–100,000
2nd trimester	10,000–30,000
3rd trimester	5,000–15,000

subunit of human chorionic gonadotropin (B-hCG) is frequently utilized. If the woman has accurate dates for her pregnancy, comparison of her B-hCG level with normal laboratory values is useful. Values for the University of Cincinnati Medical Center are shown in Table 2.1.

In addition to the B-hCG measurement, a real-time ultrasound is of great value. By 4 to 5 weeks from the last menstrual period (LMP), a gestational sac is visible. The beating fetal heart is seen by 7 weeks past the LMP. At 9 weeks, human features are discernible (17).

In a threatened abortion, ultrasound may reveal a relatively inactive fetus, a lack of expected growth of the gestational sac, poor sac outline, and/or positive cardiac activity but no spontaneous movement. Moreover, the sac may have detached in an *inevitable abortion*, and it can be seen in the lower uterine segment.

When a *blighted ovum* (a fertilized ovum whose development has ceased at an early stage) is present, the gestational sac may be seen by ultrasound but it is empty. The sac also is too small for expected gestational age. The fetal pole and the area of thickening that would become the placenta are absent. If evidence suggests a blighted ovum but the woman is unsure of her dates, a follow-up ultrasound scan is indicated in 1 to 2 weeks. A gestational sac that fails to increase by 75% in the course of 1 week probably contains a blighted ovum (18).

If a woman describes a large amount of bleeding and cramping, followed by a decrease in bleeding, ultrasound may show a normal-shaped uterus with a central line representing a decidual reaction. No products of conception or sac are seen. Sanders and James (17) feel that this represents a complete abortion and that the woman does not need dilation and curettage (D & C), that is, an evacuation of the uterine contents. Under these circumstances, however, ectopic pregnancy as an etiology for the physical and ultrasound findings should be considered and ruled out.

Management

Ultrasound should be performed by someone who is capable of interpreting findings immediately to the woman. In most cases, this is a physician. After the physical examination, ultrasound, and laboratory tests have been performed, all findings should be explained to the woman. For example, although no absolute predictions can be made, an appropriate B-hCG level with evidence of cardiac activity can be offered as reassurance, whereas a low B-hCG and the absence of a sac in the uterus, suggesting an ectopic pregnancy, should be explained in terms of their implications.

Providing Information to the Patient

Examination and test results should be discussed with the woman in the presence of a support person. This meeting should take place in a private room. If a physical examination precedes this meeting, the woman first should be allowed to dress in her own clothing again. Delay in talking with the woman should be avoided at all costs. Wall-Haas (19) relates the comments of a woman in her study:

> My male physician was not very supportive; he kept my husband and myself waiting for two hours after the ultrasound confirming the loss. He continued to see all of his other patients first. (p. 53)

Formulating a Plan

If a D & C is indicated, the reasons and procedure should be described in nonmedical terms. Care should be taken to avoid emotionally charged words. "Scraping" the uterus may sound routine to a professional's ear, but it may be regarded by the woman as a "painful intrusion of the womb where she has carried the potential child" (p. 121) (20). The D & C is discussed in more detail in the next section.

If there is no definitive diagnosis, a repeat ultrasound and B-hCG titer may be scheduled in 1 week. The woman then is sent home, if her bleeding is not significant enough to warrant hospitalization. Before she leaves, she needs to know where and whom to call if there is a change in her condition or if increased bleeding, fever, and severe cramping—all of which warrant immediate action—occur. She should be familiar with the names of those who may be on call for her care provider and prepared to explain her situation briefly. Finally, she should be advised to collect any pregnancy tissue that she may pass at home, to be examined later. For this purpose, she might be given a specimen container with a lid (available in most offices), which saves her from having to rummage through her kitchen for a suitable container. Frequently, tissue and blood clots are passed into the toilet. A small kitchen strainer can be used to transfer them from toilet bowl to container. Because distinguishing between clots and tissue would place an unnecessary burden on the woman, she should be instructed to collect everything.

Values and Limitations of Bedrest

Bedrest has been a traditional prescription for a threatened miscarriage. This recommendation adheres to the medical dictum to "do no harm." In reality, there is little evidence that bedrest makes any difference in the outcome. Psychologically, it may help a woman feel that she is doing something to help her baby—"I did all I could." However, bleeding may continue for a long enough period of time that bedrest is no longer possible. No sexual activity and refraining from lifting are commonly advised. These activities probably have no effect on the outcome, although intercourse could increase the chance for infection if the cervix were open. Unfortunately, sexual activity mistakenly may be associated with miscarriage by the couple if an increase in bleeding occurs coincidentally with or soon after intercourse. To avoid guilty feelings on the part of either partner, it may be wise if they abstain from intercourse until the immediate danger is resolved.

THE EVENT: THE ACTUAL MISCARRIAGE

Emotions

Patient's Reaction

For some women, the process and event of miscarriage occur together, so there is no time to adjust or prepare emotionally or physically for the loss. Shock and disbelief may dominate when miscarriage occurs without warning. At the time of the actual miscarriage, the emotions that women describe are very similar. In its pamphlet, *The Emotional Impact of Miscarriage*, the organization RESOLVE (21) warns that

> fear of the unknown and the helplessness of being unable to control the situation are two of the most common feelings. Some women admit later that they had fears of dying or believed they were hemorrhaging and would require a hysterectomy.

Women also worry about what it will be like to pass the fetus. "I had no idea of what to expect from the 'baby' I was going to pass through my vagina. Would I see a whole baby, parts of one, or something very malformed?" (p. 26) (22).

Intervention

Dilation and Curettage (D & C)

Hospitalization. If the decision is made that a pregnancy is not viable, elective D & C may be recommended. In this case, the woman has some time to plan and to prepare herself emotionally. Unfortunately, the decision to perform a D & C more often is forced on the care provider and his or her patient because of heavy vaginal bleeding or incomplete passage of the contents of the uterus. Confronted with these events and concerned about infection or further blood loss, the care provider and patient, after proper informed consent, view the D & C as the only reasonable plan of management. Emotionally, this surgical procedure still may appear to the woman as an invasion of her body, because she hopes without hope that her pregnancy may not have to end yet.

Location of the Procedure. In many institutions, the patient's D & C procedure and recovery occur in the labor and delivery unit rather than in a surgical suite. Consequently, many couples complain that seeing and hearing other people's happy outcomes add to their distress. If the procedure must be done in labor and delivery, then a private labor room for pre- and postoperative care is essential. Moreover, care providers must think to protect the patient from overhearing statements that are directed at other patients on the floor but that may intensify the anxiety and grief experienced by the woman. Given the option, most women would not choose to undergo a D & C in labor and delivery after a miscarriage but instead would prefer the neutral atmosphere of a surgical suite.

Type of Anesthesia. For many patients, local anesthesia for D & C is quite acceptable, because it is simple, convenient, quick, and safe (23). Because she is awake, the patient may feel more in control and in contact with her care providers. General anesthesia may increase risks of perforation, blood loss, and anesthesia-related complications. It is important, however, to consider the woman's wishes. One patient, for example, was adamantly opposed to being awake, albeit sedated, during the procedure. She did not wish to hear sounds associated with her D & C and was willing to incur risks associated with general anesthesia. Another patient reported significant pain awareness during D & C, despite 50 mg of Demerol, 5 mg of Valium, and a paracervical block.

Presence of a Support Person

Value of a Support Person

In most labor and delivery settings today, the presence of the patient's partner or another support person is welcomed. Even for a cesarean section, someone usually is encouraged to remain with the patient throughout. Yet, this is not widely accepted in the case of early pregnancy loss, because miscarriage generally is not perceived as labor and delivery of a baby. The woman and her support person often are separated as soon as she enters the surgical or obstetrical area, even if she will be awake for the procedure. Women report that the experience would be less painful if the woman could have her partner or another support person with her during the procedure and in the recovery room (24). In their study of 93 patients who presented to an obstetrical unit with an inevitable abortion followed by D & C, Seibel and Graves (25) found that 58% of the women would have preferred to have someone in the room with them. Although the presence of a support person is not a usual occurrence in the operating room, this option should be available to patients who request it and who will be awake for the procedure. The support person may be allowed in after the woman has been draped. Virtually none of the D & C can be viewed by a person sitting at the head of the table, where he or she can best be positioned to comfort the patient. Of course, this option is not appropriate if even one of the participants—the woman, her partner, or the surgeon—is uncomfortable, but it should not be dismissed "because we have never done it that way."

Location for Recovery from the D & C

Women exposed to the sounds of crying babies, while they are recovering on the ward from a pregnancy loss, later express anger at the insensitivity of care providers. Friedman and Gradstein (24) note that many women wish to be placed on a nonmaternity floor, want the option of a private room, and want their partners with them overnight. Flexible visiting hours are also important.

Preventing RHO(D) Isoimmunization

The administration of RHO(D) Immune Globulin (RHIG) following delivery of a RHO(D) positive baby from a RHO(D) negative unsensitized woman is standard practice in obstetrics. Because an estimated 4–5% of RHO(D) negative women become sensitized after induced abortion (26), this same practice must be instituted following an early pregnancy loss. According to the ACOG Technical Bulletin (27), the dosage of RHIG will vary according to the stage of gestation at which the loss has occurred. A dose of 50 μg RHIG is recommended for patients with ectopic pregnancies or those whose miscarriages occur prior to 13 weeks gestation. For pregnancy losses beyond 13 weeks gestation, the standard 300 μg dose is recommended.

Importance of Viewing the Products of Conception

Viewing the Removed Pregnancy Tissue

In *Coping with a Miscarriage* (22), the contributor Rothchild encourages parents to look at what the woman has passed. In the Seibel and Graves study (25), almost a third of the patients said that they would like to have seen the products of conception. Very often, though, the woman has difficulty articulating this need, or she may not think of it herself, but would be eager to see her "baby." The simple question, "Would you like to see the tissue?" gives the woman her choice in this matter. In the authors' experience, patients have derived comfort and resolution from doing so. After spontaneously passing an early but complete embryo, R. M. said, "At least now I feel as if I had really been pregnant." M. K. had a D & C at 10 weeks with her husband present. She expressed a desire to see the tissue, although she understood that it would not look like a baby. She and her husband reacted appropriately and felt that this experience reinforced the finality of the event.

Friedman and Gradstein (24) also note that many women wish to participate in the decision about disposal of the fetal tissue. Although histopathologic examination may intervene between the actual event and the time of disposition, it need not preclude input from parents. Most often, they primarily wish to know what will happen to their baby. Less commonly, parents may wish to have a religious service and bury their baby's tissue, after specimens for pathology have been obtained and examination has been completed.

COUNSELING

Care providers must continue to provide support and understanding for the woman after miscarriage. The concepts are described in Chapter 10, "Obstetrician as Outpatient Counselor," and Chapter 11, "Office or Clinic Nurse's Role." In their study of 22 women, Leppert and Pahlka (20) showed that following a miscarriage the grief reaction was as intense as that noted from women experiencing a stillbirth or neonatal death. These women felt intense relief upon learning that their reaction to the miscarriage was normal. After the initial shock and sorrow of the event, the woman progresses to new feelings and begins the grieving process described in Chapter 1. Each woman will experience a set of feelings unique to her personal life situation and support network. For some women, for example, a miscarriage may be a relief if the pregnancy had been unplanned. In such a case, the woman may move quickly toward resolution of any grief she experiences in response to her loss. For others, the miscarriage may represent the most significant personal crisis of her life. Studies and personal anecdotes identify anger, guilt, sadness, fear, and sense of failure as reactions usually experienced by women who miscarry.

MEN'S RESPONSE TO MISCARRIAGE

Although a man's emotional attachment to the baby may lag behind that of his partner's, it is important to recognize that he, too, is affected by a miscarriage. His initial feeling will probably be concern for her wellbeing. If the couple is separated because of hospital rules, his imagination may run rampant: "What if she bleeds to death? What if she never wakes up?" Powerlessness and helplessness are overwhelming feelings at this time.

Reaction Correlated with Length of Gestation

Once reassured about his partner's safety, the man may find that sadness or disappointment set in. This progression of emotions may be contrasted with the acute sense of loss that the woman feels. Leppert and Pahlka (20) found that, while women experienced intense grief regardless of the gestational age at the time of pregnancy loss, the magnitude of men's emotions seems to correlate directly with length of gestation at the time when the loss occurred. Because of these differences between men and women, the man may be bewildered by the intensity of his partner's reaction to a very early pregnancy loss.

Guilt may be experienced by men also. They may feel especially guilty if they worry that the miscarriage was related to sexual intercourse. As the woman reviews her habits, diet, and activities, so too does the man.

Feelings noted by several authors (1, 22, 24, 28) were:

Disbelief—How could this be happening?

Anger and frustration—Why me? Why us? We really wanted this baby. Why do I have to be strong—I'm hurting too.!

Pessimism—Will we ever be able to have a child?

Blame—What did *she* do? She was the one carrying the baby, not me.

Relief—The pregnancy came at a bad time, we hadn't planned it.

In summary, a man's reactions to pregnancy loss may be varied and individual, but sincere and intense. Men welcome an opportunity to express their feelings and to have them acknowledged. Men often cry if given "permission" or encouraged to do so. If not encouraged to express their feelings, they may find that resentment and frustration inhibit the grieving process that they too must go through.

RESPONSE OF OTHER CHILDREN

For families with a child or children at home, there are other important relationships to consider. Children are keenly

Child's personality structure and current level of development

Quality of the child's awareness of the pregnancy and the miscarriage

Child's attitudes toward and hopes for the unborn child

Child's response to pregnancy *per se*

What the child sees, hears, or is told regarding the miscarriage

Complexities of parents' response

Parents' response to the child's initial reactions

Figure 2.1. Factors influencing a child's reaction to miscarriage. (Reproduced from Greer et al.: Psychological consequences of the therapeutic abortion. *Br J Psychiatry* 128:74–79, 1976.)

aware of everything that goes on in a family and can read very subtle cues. During a miscarriage, they react to emotional upheaval in the home and to the absence of their mother, if hospitalization is required for her. More important, within their developmental limits, they also react afterward to the miscarriage itself. Cain et al. (29) note that a child's reactions to a miscarriage are determined by the factors listed in Figure 2.1. General principles that can guide parents to help their children are given in Figure 2.2. In short, children should be included in, not excluded from, the event. Because they are a part of the family, they should share in the reaction and recovery as the family unit confronts this unique life crisis. (The reader is referred to Chapter 1, "Pregnancy Loss and the Grief Process," and Chapter 8, "Social Worker: Hospital Advocate for the Immediate and Extended Family," for more discussion on this topic.)

FAMILY AND FRIENDS

The loss of a baby not only affects the woman and her family, it also affects others. Many people are supportive, especially if they have experienced pregnancy loss or a recent death themselves. They can say, "I know how you feel." Talking and crying with these people can be therapeutic for the couple.

Unfortunately, for every friend or relative who offers meaningful support, there may be as many others who lack the ability to give support. Worse, they actually may make insensitive remarks. It is helpful to warn the couple about typical remarks and the reasons for them. Common clichés or remarks about miscarriage are listed in Figure 2.3.

Listen and ask open-ended questions to determine what the child is feeling and thinking.

Give simple, direct, and honest answers

Speak in a gentle, soothing voice and show affection.

Avoid communicating anxiety, but be open to showing emotion and sadness.

Use precise words such as "death" and "died." Avoid incorrect terms such as "gone to sleep," or "lost the baby," which can mislead a child.

Reassure the child that he or she is not responsible, is in no danger of death or abandonment, and is loved.

Accept the child's feelings of sadness and disappointment in the loss of a potential sibling and playmate.

Make use of books designed for children to explain death. Wass and Corr (1984) have a large annotated bibliography. They feel that the books listed by Friedman and Gradstein (1982) are excellent.

Respect a child's defenses. He or she may not want to talk about the loss immediately.

Continue to offer time for expression, reflection, and questions.

Be on the lookout for danger signs such as anxiety attacks, nightmares, aggressiveness, stuttering, death phobias, outbursts of fear, and depression.

Enlist the help of your pediatrician, family physician, or nurse practitioner if the child seems to have regressed or to have developed behavioral problems.

Figure 2.2. Guidelines for parents helping their children following pregnancy loss. (Reproduced from Wass H, Corr C: *Helping Children Cope with Death: Guidelines and Resources.* Washington, DC, Hemisphere Publishing Corp, 1984.)

ELECTIVE ABORTION

The Woman's Feelings Concerning Elective Abortion

An Emotionally Charged Event

Regarding psychologic aspects of abortion, Fleck (30) points out that every surgical procedure has some psychologic component that may have long-lasting effects. "Abortion is but one such intrusive assault, a very special one because pregnancy involves directly the core of femininity, a woman's creativeness in the most literal sense, her sexuality, her mothering capacities, and her new family" (p. 44). It is important for care providers to recognize that elective abortion, as well as spontaneous abortion, is an emotionally charged event.

— It's for the best; the baby wouldn't have been right.
— You weren't far enough along to be attached.
— At least you didn't know the baby.
— You can always have another baby.
— Be thankful you have other children at home.
— Don't think about it and you'll get over it faster.
— It was God's will.
— Pull yourself together. You need to be strong for
_____'s sake.
— You have a little angel in heaven.

Figure 2.3.   Clichés about miscarriage.

Sense of Isolation

Freeman (31) studied 106 women who elected to terminate a pregnancy. The decision to abort was not a casual decision for these women. Thirty-seven per cent had been certain before learning of the pregnancy that they would never decide to have an abortion. The irreversibility of the decision and the limited timespan in which to make it create a great deal of stress. Women find the matter difficult to discuss with family, friends, or even their partners, which leads to a sense of emotional isolation.

While the woman considers her decision, the availability of thorough, balanced counseling is critical. Her partner should be included if at all possible. Client-centered, nonjudgmental counseling should direct the woman's attention to issues she may have overlooked. She needs to explore her attitudes toward herself, her baby, the father of her baby, and current and future social circumstances. In Freeman's (31) study, most women expressed ambivalence about the decision; but this, in itself, is not a contraindication to the procedure. However, if marked ambivalence has been expressed by the woman or perceived by the counselor, the procedure should be postponed. If after adequate counseling the woman's decision is unchanged, the procedure should take place as soon as possible.

Type of Abortion Procedure

D & E versus Prostaglandin-Induced Labor

While the type of abortion procedure chosen depends on many factors, care providers must recognize that there may be important psychologic components attached to different methods. These components may affect the nursing staff and physician as well as the woman. In a small study, Kaltreider et al.

(32) compared 30 patients who had mid-trimester abortions by dilation and evacuation (D & E) with 20 patients who had intra-amniotic prostaglandin abortions. Utilizing an attitudinal questionnaire and a Profile of Mood State Scale prior to and after the procedure, they found significant differences between the two groups. Women who had a D & E under general anesthesia viewed the experience as minor surgery. They were able to utilize denial mechanisms, saw the process as "out of their hands," and perceived general anesthesia as a dream-like experience. In short, they felt that an unpleasant experience had been made bearable. The group receiving intra-amniotic prostaglandin reported significantly more anger, lingering guilt, and depression than did the other group. They viewed the abortion as long and painful and described the product of the labor as a "baby." Pain was described as more intense than any that had been experienced in a previous labor. Additionally, many women were angry because the attending physician was not present.

Grief Is Often Similar to Other Pregnancy Losses

Not all patients find the concept of a D & E preferable to induction of labor and vaginal delivery for a second-trimester abortion. By necessity, a D & E requires that the fetus be dismembered during surgical extraction. Following the procedure, the physician must identify all fetal body parts in order to assure completeness of the procedure. For some patients, the mental picture of this approach to their abortion is unacceptable. For others, their inability to hold or even view their aborted baby following a D & E may lead them to choose labor induction and vaginal birth. Many care providers may be surprised that a patient electively undergoing a second-trimester abortion would express intense grief, a desire to hold the baby, and the need to collect mementos and other items that memorialize the baby. For some, the grieving process is identical to that which occurs after a stillbirth. The need for long-term psychologic support also may be similar in both groups of patients. (For information regarding patient management, the reader is referred to Chapter 3, "Stillbirth," for a description of methods of induction of labor.)

Mixed Reactions from Staff

Elective abortion is so complex because there are additional issues that may create difficulty on the staff's part. In the study by Kaltreider et al. (32), the nursing staff expressed distress over labor induction and vaginal birth for a second-trimester abortion. They regarded the procedure as a form of abandonment by the medical staff. Their resentment also reflected the fact that reluctant nursing staff may be required to participate in care during more lightly staffed evening and night shifts. In contrast, operating room nurses may have more of a choice to be involved in the procedure or the patient's care. Moreover, in the latter setting, the professional with primary responsibility, the physician, is always present. Another source of conflict is that, at the same time that elective abortions are being performed, prematurely delivered babies of only slightly greater gestation are being taken to and aggressively cared for in the hospital's neonatal intensive care unit. Because the weight differences between a late second-trimester aborted fetus and a potentialy viable newborn may differ by only 100–200 grams, this contradictory utilization of medical and nursing skills can create anger and bitterness among staff (32).

Because only four physicians were involved in the Kaltreider et al. study, generalizations are impossible. The study does suggest that physicians may welcome the relative noninvolvement of labor induction and vaginal delivery. The two physicians who performed D & Es admitted that they experienced occasional strong emotional reactions, but they believed the procedure to be safer, less painful, quicker, and more appropriate than intra-amniotic prostaglandin abortions for most patients.

Postabortion Feelings

Freeman (31) found that 65% of women who underwent an abortion could not say if they would choose abortion again. Most had some degree of conflicting emotions. Twenty-four per cent reported that the hardest part of the experience was dealing with the feeling that they had lost a child. In pre- and postabortion counseling, the word "fetus" was used by professionals, but women used the more emotionally charged word "child."

In a larger study, Greer et al. (33) measured psychosocial, marital, interpersonal, and sexual adjustments of 216 women 1 week prior to their first-trimester abortion and at follow-up 3 and 18 months later. Although 37% of women reported feelings of guilt and depression prior to the procedure, there was marked resolution at 3 months. These results indicate that women who had a legal abortion prior to 12 weeks gestation have immediate significant improvement in areas of distress, such as guilt or depression. The women in this study had minimal risk of psychologic or social problems at the 2-year follow-up.

Emotional Instability Prior to Abortion: A Risk Factor

In a follow-up article, Belsey et al. (34) found that postabortion women at risk for marital, sexual, or interpersonal problems had poor emotional support at home and difficulties of a similar nature *before* the abortion. Most women who have an elective abortion simply need supportive counseling; it is important, however, to identify the woman with poor family ties, few friends, and problems with her partner, because it is likely that she will need greater help.

Termination of Pregnancy for Maternal/Fetal Indications

Peck and Marcus (35) studied 50 white middle-class women who were seeking abortion for therapeutic reasons. One half had fetal or maternal indications for the termination. More than one third of this group had depressive reactions within 6 months after the procedure. These women had desired their pregnancies and had been in good mental health prior to abortion. Even though they understood the validity of the reason for terminating pregnancy, they felt sad and guilty, and they missed the baby acutely. They had dreams of losing the baby and felt rejected by their families. Their reactions were similar to those of women who have stillbirths (for this discussion, the reader is referred to Chapter 3). Fortunately, these feelings were resolved within 6 months without psychiatric treatment. However, this study and other anecdotes remind us that postprocedure support and counseling may be as important as that given prior to the procedure.

Subsequent Pregnancy after Elective Abortion

Increased Depression and Anxiety May Occur in Subsequent Pregnancy

Kumar and Robson (36), evaluating the psychologic health of women having their first babies, obtained extensive interviews throughout 117 women's pregnancies. Twenty-one of these women had had a previous elective abortion. Thirty-eight per cent of women having had an elective abortion were clinically depressed or anxious at some point during the subsequent pregnancy versus only 8% of those women never having experienced an elective abortion. Even in the absence of obvious depression or anxiety, the authors observed that these women admitted having intense anxieties about fetal abnormalities, unresolved feelings of guilt, and fears of retribution. Women with a history of miscarriage did not show such a correlation. The authors advocate watching women with a history of elective abortion closely for signs of distress during a subsequent pregnancy. Although the majority of women with good support systems appear to have no severe emotional sequelae as a result of elective abortion, healthcare providers need to view them as a group at risk. The same support, counseling, and interventions given to women who spontaneously miscarry should also be available to these patients.

ECTOPIC PREGNANCY

"Loss of a Baby" Minimized

One of the most neglected areas in gynecology is treating the woman with an ectopic pregnancy with empathy and compassion. Emotional support and good patient education should be a reflexive response by the care provider treating a woman with such a pregnancy loss. It is essential to maintain or establish a strong positive relationship between patient and care provider when this type of loss becomes apparent. Care providers should be prepared to facilitate the expression of normal grief and to identify and manage abnormal mourning if it occurs.

Historically, the situation has been responded to as a surgical emergency because the patient would present in shock or near death. The gynecologic surgeon focused his or her attention and skills on saving the woman's life. Because of the nature of the problem and the anxiety generated by the care provider's grave approach, the woman and her family also feared for the woman's life. Understandably, the loss of the baby was minimized or completely disregarded.

After surgery, with the woman on her way to normal convalescence, the pregnancy and its loss may never again have been acknowledged. Care providers often directed discussion toward the critical nature of the problem and claimed, "We have saved your life." The woman at some point came out of shock and took in what had happened—she was stable now, but her baby was gone. Her care providers' failure to sympathize and to address the issue of the baby's death may have left her confused about what she was feeling.

"We Have Saved Your Tube"

Today, ironically, this confusion may be more common than formerly. With the use of ultrasound, more women's ectopic pregnancies are detected before rupture. Therefore, fewer acute patients are diagnosed and treated. Because there seems to be less of an emergency, a woman and her family may fail to perceive the urgency of her condition. Surgical management of an unruptured ectopic is much less frantic; at times, it may involve a small incision and the use of the laparascope. The surgeon afterward is pleased because early diagnosis was made or because the incision was small or because everything "went well." This sense of accomplishment is what is communicated to the woman. Emphasis shifts away from the issue of pregnancy to "We have saved your tube."

This elation by care providers leaves the patient confused and upset. She has learned recently that she had a positive pregnancy test. She has been experiencing the earliest stages of bonding with her pregnancy and already may have begun to fantasize about details of the delivery and her baby's appearance. Suddenly, there has been this urgent diagnosis and she has undergone surgery. A woman with an unruptured ectopic pregnancy who was not sick, not in shock, and not near death feels confused. She wants to know why her physician could not transplant the pregnancy "back into the uterus." There is no talk of the baby she was expecting. Everyone tells her how lucky she is that she is alive or that she still has her fallopian tube. A support structure for her grieving process is either never developed or never facilitated for the ectopic-pregnancy patient.

The woman with an ectopic pregnancy should be told as much as possible about what has occurred with her pregnancy. Medical explanations should be tempered with sympathy and compassion. Loss of the pregnancy should be presented openly, and it should remain a point of focus for discussion. Before the woman can begin to work through her grief, she must be helped by her care providers to express any sense of guilt or anger. She may feel guilty about having used an IUD or because she had a pelvic infection. With sufficient explanation and sympathetic support from her care providers, the woman can better begin to make the transition from being ecstatic about the baby she and her family were expecting to accepting the reality of ectopic pregnancy.

FOLLOW-UP CARE

Emotional Issues

In follow-up visits with families who have suffered a miscarriage or an ectopic pregnancy, care offered must address both physical and emotional issues. A number of visits may be required to address these issues. Follow-up visits should be scheduled weekly until both parties feel that further consultation is no longer necessary. Most couples attend one or two counseling sessons only (see Chapter 16).

The reader is referred elsewhere in the text for more extensive discussion of support and counseling once the patient is discharged home:

Pregnancy Loss and the Grief Process, Chapter 1

Chaplain's Ministry When a Baby Dies, Chapter 7

Social Worker: Hospital Advocate for the Immediate and Extended Family, Chapter 8

Funeral Director, Chapter 9

Obstetrician as Outpatient Counselor, Chapter 10

Genetics and Pregnancy Loss: Value of Counseling between Pregnancies, Chapter 12

Value of the Perinatal Autopsy, Chapter 13

Peer Support Group Network, Chapter 14

Impact of Pregnancy Loss on Subsequent Pregnancy, Chapter 15

Perinatal Support Service at the University of Cincinnati, Chapter 16

Management of Grief in a Two-Roof Perinatal Center, Chapter 17

Why Did It Happen?

Technically, even for a woman with her first miscarriage, there are many possible reasons why a miscarriage could have occurred. See Figure 2.4 for possible causes of miscarriage. For the apparently healthy woman experiencing her first loss, most of the items in Figure 2.4 are unlikely reasons for a miscarriage. Substance abuse and environmental causes must be seriously considered; but statistically, the most likely reason for a miscarriage is genetic abnormality. Unfortunately, chromosomal analysis of the products of conception often is not requested by care providers, and pathology reports do not provide a great deal of information as to the cause. Therefore, most often the couple does not learn the answer to their question, "Why did it happen?"

When to Investigate Causes of Miscarriage

For the woman experiencing her first miscarriage, searching for the cause by means of extensive physical and laboratory testing is seldom warranted. Clinicians may recommend testing (such as parental karyotyping) after a second loss; most believe that extensive testing is appropriate after a third consecutive

Uterine body abnormalities (such as fibroids, adhesions, or a bicornate uterus)

Cervical incompetence (usually associated with second-trimester losses)

Hormonal/endocrine dysfunction (thyroid deficiency or luteal-phase defect)

Endometrial infections (Mycoplasma, Listeria, or viral infections such as herpes or rubella)

Presence of an IUD

Systemic disorders (e.g., lupus erythematosus)

Sperm abnormalities

Substance abuse (e.g., cigarettes, alcohol, and drugs)

Environmental causes (e.g., chemical exposures through occupation or hobby)

Genetic abnormalities

Figure 2.4.   Possible causes of miscarriage.

loss (37). In light of the cost and emotional strain that these tests impose on a family, this recommendation seems to be reasonable and most satisfactory for all parties concerned. (The reader is referred to Chapter 12, "Genetics and Pregnancy Loss," for a more complete discussion of this issue.)

"Was I to Blame?"

In most cases, a woman can recite a litany of things she did and things she should not have done during her pregnancy. Women examine everything that happened during the pregnancy after it concludes with a loss. All that her care providers can do is reassure her when there is no reason to link these "causes" to her miscarriage.

With respect to substance abuse and hazardous environmental exposures, however, there sometimes may be a "cause" to which pregnancy loss may be attributed. Spontaneous abortions have been linked with smoking and alcohol use (38, 39). Some chemicals such as xylene used in hobby spray paints are suspected teratogens (40), and job-related chemical exposures may also be suspect (41). Women whose miscarriages can be traced to such causes deserve to have the reason acknowledged. They should be aware of any problems linked to hazardous exposures so that these can be avoided during a future pregnancy.

When Can I Try to Get Pregnant Again?

The issue of when to attempt another conception is a complicated one. The reader is referred to Chapter 15, "Impact of Pregnancy Loss on Subsequent Pregnancy," for a thorough discussion of this topic.

Preconception Counseling

Planning and Preventive Medicine

In addition to discussing birth control and the timing of a subsequent pregnancy, couples can benefit from preconception advice. The time to tell a woman about the dangers of smoking, alcohol, and chemicals is before she conceives. In the time following a pregnancy loss, it is helpful to have the woman and her partner fill out a preconception health appraisal questionnaire similar to the one developed by Moos and Cefalo (42) at the University of North Carolina. Although the questionnaire covers many items included in a routine complete history, it also elicits additional subtle information, such as ownership of a cat or types of hobbies. Before another pregnancy is attempted, the woman should undergo a screening test for rubella and be immunized if she is found to be susceptible. Even with a history of the disease or of immunization, it is wise to consider this inexpensive test, since approximately 14% of women today are susceptible (43).

Models for Preconception Safety

The issue of reproductive epidemiology and hazards in the workplace is a complex one requiring sophisticated knowledge. Fortunately, for the average consumer, there are private and governmental agencies that offer advice regarding risks associated with the workplace or with hobbies.* Care providers do not have to know everything, but they are legally and ethically obligated to find out about or refer the consumer to the appropriate place to answer all questions that are raised. Preconception clinics and programs, such as those described by Moos and Cefalo (42), Chamberlain (44), and Queenan (45), provide excellent models for obstetrical care providers to emulate. The Preconception Clinic at the University of Cincinnati is directed by a perinatologist and includes a nurse-midwife and a registered nurse on the staff. Specialists in reproductive epidemiology, genetics, and pharmacology are available as needed. The client may be referred by her primary care provider, or she may elect to come on her own. A health appraisal questionnaire is used, and handouts on preconception nutrition, smoking, drugs, and alcohol are distributed when appropriate (42).

*The National Institute of Occupational Safety and Health (NIOSH) will perform a health-hazard evaluation of the workplace if requested by the employer or employee. A form to request such an evaluation may be obtained by writing or calling NIOSH, Hazard Evaluation and Technical Assistance Branch, 4676 Columbia Parkway, Cincinnati, OH 45226, (513) 684–4382. The Center for Occupational Hazards in New York City, (212) 227–6220, will provide information on hobbies that might be dangerous to the developing fetus.

REFERENCES

1. Peppers L and Knapp R: *Motherhood and Mourning*. New York, Praeger Publications, 1980.
2. Klaus M and Kennell J: *Parent-Infant Bonding*, ed 2. St. Louis, The C.V. Mosby Company, 1982.
3. Jessner L, Weigert E, Foy J: The development of parental attitudes in pregnancy. In Anthony IE and Benedek T (eds): *Parenthood*. Boston, Little, Brown & Company, 1970.
4. Grimm E: Women's attitudes and reactions to childbearing. In Goldman G and Milman D (eds): *Modern Woman*. Springfield, IL, Charles C Thomas, 1969.
5. Colman A and Colman L: *Pregnancy: The Psychological Experience*. New York, Heider and Heider, 1971.

6. Boston Women's Health Book Collective: *The New Our Bodies, Ourselves.* New York, Simon & Schuster, Inc., 1984.

7. Bibring G, Dwyer T, Huntington D, Valenstein A: A study of the psychological processes in pregnancy and of the earliest mother-child relationships. I. Some perspectives and comments. *Psychoanal Study Child* 16:9–27, 1961.

8. Lichtendorf S and Gillis P: *The New Pregnancy.* New York, Praeger Publications, 1979.

9. Bittman S and Zalk S: *Expectant Fathers.* New York, Hawthorn Books, Inc., 1978.

10. Pritchard J, MacDonald P, Gant N (eds): *Williams Obstetrics.* Norwalk, CT, Appleton-Century-Crofts, 1985.

11. Fliegelman E and Rosenau A: Psychological aspects of the lost pregnancy. *The Female Patient* 7:40–45, 1982.

12. Westergaard J, Sinosich M, Bugge M, Madsen L, Teisner B, Grudzinskas J: Pregnancy-associated plasma protein A in the prediction of early pregnancy failure. *Am J Obstet Gynecol* 145(1):67–69, 1983.

13. Hertz J: Diagnostic procedures in the threatened abortion. *Obstet Gynecol* 64(2):223–229, 1984.

14. Balzer F, Weiner S, Corson S, Schloff S, Otis C: Landmarks during the first forty-two days of gestation demonstrated by the beta-subunit of human chorionic gonadotropin and ultrasound. *Am J Obstet Gynecol* 146(8):973–979, 1983.

15. Masson G, Anthony F, Welson M, Lindsay K: Comparison of serum and urine hCG levels with SP and PAPP-A levels in patients with first-trimester vaginal bleeding. *Obstet Gynecol* 61(2):223–226, 1983.

16. Duff G, Evans J, Legge M: A study of investigations used to predict outcome of pregnancy after threatened abortion. *Br J Obstet Gynecol* 87:194–198, 1980.

17. Sanders R and James A (eds): *The Principles and Practice of Ultrasonography in Obstetrics and Gynecology,* ed 3. Norwalk, CT, Appleton-Century-Crofts, 1985, pp 423–434.

18. Robinson HP: The diagnosis of early pregnancy failure by sonar. *Br J Obstet Gynecol* 82 (11):849–857, 1975.

19. Wall-Haas C: Women's perceptions of first trimester spontaneous abortion. *J Obstet Gynecol Neonat Nurs* Jan/Feb: 50–53, 1985.

20. Leppert P and Pahlka B: Grieving characteristics after spontaneous abortion: A management approach. *Obstet Gynecol* 64(1):119–122, 1984.

21. RESOLVE: *The Emotional Impact of Miscarriage.* Belmont, MA, RESOLVE, Box 474.

22. Pizer H and Palinski C: *Coping with a Miscarriage.* New York, A Plume Book, 1980.

23. Van Lith DAF, Wittman R, Keith LG: Early and late abortion methods. *Clin Obstet Gynecol* 11(3):585–592, 1984.

24. Friedman R and Gradstein B: *Surviving Pregnancy Loss.* Boston, Little, Brown & Company, 1982.

25. Seibel M and Graves W: The psychological implications of spontaneous abortions. *Reprod Med* 25(4):161–165, 1980.

26. McMaster Conference on prevention of Rh immunization, 28–30 September 1977. *Vox Sang* 36(1):50–64, 1979.

27. ACOG Technical Bulletin #79, August 1984.

28. Johnson J and Johnson M: *Miscarriage.* Omaha, Centering Corp., Box 3367, 1983.

29. Cain A, Erickson M, Fast I, Vaughan R: Children's disturbed reactions to their mother's miscarriage. *Psychosom Med* 26:58–66, 1964.

30. Fleck S: Some psychiatric aspects of abortion. *J Nerv Ment Dis* 151(1):42–50, 1970.

31. Freeman E: Abortion: Subjective attitudes and feelings. *Fam Plan Perspect* 10(3):150–55, 1978.
32. Kaltreider N, Goldsmith S, Margolis A: The impact of mid-trimester abortion techniques on patients and staff. *Am J Obstet Gynecol* 135(2):235–238, 1979.
33. Greer H, Lal S, Lewis S, Belsey E, Beard R: Psychological consequences of the therapeutic abortion. *Br J Psychiatry* 128:74–79, 1976.
34. Belsey E, Greer H, Lal S, Lewis S, Beard R: Predictive factors in emotional response to abortion: King's termination study. *Soc Sci Med* 11:71–82, 1977.
35. Peck A and Marcus H: Psychiatric sequelae of therapeutic interruption of pregnancy. *J Nerv Ment Dis* 143(5):417–425, 1966.
36. Kumar R and Robson K: Previous induced abortion and antenatal depression in primiparae: preliminary report of a survey of mental health in pregnancy. *Psychol Med* 8, 711–715, 1978.
37. Poland BJ, Miller JR, Jones DC, Trimble BK: Reproductive counseling in patients who have had a spontaneous abortion. *Am J Obstet Gynecol* 127(7):685–691, 1977.
38. Harlap S and Shiono P: Alcohol, smoking, and incidence of spontaneous abortions in the first and second trimester. *Lancet* 7/26/80:173–176.
39. Kline J, Stein Z, Shrout P, Susser M, Warburton D: Drinking during pregnancy and spontaneous abortion. *Lancet* 7/26/80:176–180.
40. New York Times: Art supply makers to label hazardous items. Feb 3, 1985.
41. NAACOG: *Reproductive Health Hazards: Women in the Workplace.* No. 11, Feb 1985, Washington, DC, NAACOG, 600 Maryland Ave. SW, Suite 200, 20024.
42. Moos MK: *Preconception Health Program: Improving Perinatal Health Outcome.* Chapel Hill, University of North Carolina, 1984.
43. Horstmann D: Rubella: still a problem for obstetricians. *Contem Obstet Gynecol* 13:67–83, 1979.
44. Chamberlain G: The pre-pregnancy clinic. *Br Med J* 281:29–30, 1980.
45. Queenan JT: Prepping your patients for pregnancy [editorial]. *Contem Obstet Gynecol* 21:11, 1983.

SUGGESTED RESOURCE MATERIALS BOOKS ON DEATH FOR CHILDREN (AND PARENTS)†

Primary Grades and Preschool

De Bruyn, MD: *The Beaver Who Wouldn't Die.* Chicago, Follett, 1975.

Fassler J: *My Grandpa Died Today.* New York, Behavioral Publications, 1971.

Viorst J: *The Tenth Good Thing about Barney.* New York, Atheneum, 1971.

Children 10–14 Years Old

Miles B: *The Trouble with Thirteen.* New York, Knopf, 1979.

Paterson K: *The Bridge to Terabithia.* New York, Crowell, 1977.

Parents and Children

Zim HS and Bleeker S: *Life and Death.* New York, Morrow, 1970.

Parents

Grollman E: *Explaining Death to Children.* Boston, Beacon Press, 1969.

Rudolph M: *Should the Children Know? Encounters with Death in the Lives of Children.* New York, Schocken, 1978.

Wolf AWM (ed): *Helping Your Child to Understand Death.* Child Study Association of America, 1958.

†From Wass H and Corr C: *Helping Children Cope with Death: Guidelines and Resources.* Washington, DC, Hemisphere Publishing Corp., 1984.

CHAPTER

Stillbirth

JAMES R. WOODS, Jr., M.D.

Parents experiencing an intrauterine fetal death present the care provider with a complex and multifaceted challenge. Who will tell the patient that her baby is dead? What alternatives for delivery are available? Should parents see their baby after delivery? How can this unbearable situation be made more bearable? And how can care providers confront their own anxieties about death?

The purpose of Chapter 3 is to examine the complex issues of diagnosis and management when a family experiences an intrauterine fetal death. This discussion focuses on the period of time from initial diagnosis of fetal death until the patient is delivered and discharged from the hospital. For the sake of clarity, the term "intrauterine fetal death" (IUFD) in this chapter will encompass all pregnancies of more than 12 weeks gestation. (The reader is referred to Chapter 2, "Early Pregnancy Loss," for a comprehensive discussion of the patient experiencing a first-trimester—less than 12 weeks gestation—miscarriage.)

ISSUES

Multifaceted Loss

Diagnosis and care of the patient experiencing an intrauterine fetal death can be traumatic for patient and care provider alike. For the patient and her partner, the tragedy is twofold: it is not only the death of their expected baby, but also the destruction of hopes, dreams, and plans of the couple anticipating a lifetime for their child. Preparations done for the

51

baby must now be undone. The baby's room must be dismantled; the crib, taken down. Gifts must be returned or put in storage. Friends or neighbors must be informed, a draining task often made more difficult because these encounters may occur in the supermarket or other places where privacy and intimacy are lacking. And, after all the necessary chores are completed, the family must live with their loneliness and the sadness of knowing that they will never be able to tell their baby of the hopes and dreams they had for his or her future.

Infrequent Exposure to Pregnancy Loss

The medical community is no better prepared to deal with this type of pregnancy loss than the patient herself. Few nursing, medical, or seminary schools have programs that teach the principles of responding to this type of death. As a consequence, most care providers in the medical community gain their experience with these patients case by case. Fortunately, intrauterine fetal death is an infrequent event. An obstetrician in private practice may not see a case of IUFD from one year to the next. The infrequency of this type of pregnancy loss, however, hampers the opportunity for care providers to cultivate and improve their patient management skills. When a patient whose pregnancy terminates in intrauterine fetal death presents in the office, ultrasound department, or labor and delivery unit, it is not surprising that few medical personnel are prepared to provide the type of needed care. For some, denial of death may make them keep their distance from the patient. More often, however, care providers are afraid that they will not say or do the "right thing." They either avoid the patient completely or mechanically focus on technical aspects of care to sidestep the possibility of becoming emotionally involved with the patient.

HISTORICAL PERSPECTIVE

Sedate and Isolate

Care of the patient delivering a stillbirth has changed dramatically in the past few years. In the late 1960s and early 1970s, it was common for the patient who had experienced an intrauterine fetal death to be heavily sedated in labor. Delivery often was managed under additional intravenous sedation or general inhalation anesthesia. Upon delivery, the thought of showing the baby to the mother or allowing her to hold him or her seldom arose. Taking a picture of the stillborn baby for the parents seemed even more far-fetched.

Loneliness

After delivery, the patient usually was moved to a nonobstetrical ward, to isolate her from any contact with babies. As a rule, no one mentioned what had happened, and the mother was discharged as soon as her medical condition would permit. The fortunate patient might be visited by an understanding chaplain or cared for by a supportive nurse. Unfortunately, many of these patients were left alone as they struggled to sort out their feelings and to begin to comprehend a confusing, tragic event. It is ironic that many patients may have found a housekeeping employee who came in each day to clean the room to be the most understanding and accessible.

Upon discharge, women were routinely given a 6-week outpatient return appointment for postpartum examination. It was the rare obstetrician who recognized the need to bring these patients into the office early in the postpartum recovery period for counseling. In a busy obstetrical practice, time constraints may have legitimately precluded approaching the issue of pregnancy loss in this manner. For many physicians, however, assuming the role of postpartum counselor after a pregnancy loss was not well accepted. Conducting the 6-week postpartum check-up routinely and perfunctorily is less threatening. At times, this approach may have been taken because of an obstetrician's personal insecurities concerning the issue of death.

Today, most hospitals have staff, social work, or other care providers who recognize the value of encouraging parents to see and hold their stillborn baby, to select a name, and to take a picture of their baby. Through the efforts of such individuals, some uniformity of care is now developing. Despite these personal efforts, often made by members of the nursing staff or clergy, much still must be changed in order to provide optimum support for the patient with a stillbirth.

INITIAL DIAGNOSIS IN THE OFFICE

"I Cannot Hear the Baby's Heartbeat"

That moment when no fetal heartbeat is detected can be frightening for both the patient and the physician, nurse/midwife, or nurse listening for the heartbeat. In some cases, the clinic visit may have been preceded by 1 or 2 days in which fetal movement was decreased or absent. Women may volunteer the information that something has seemed wrong. Sometimes a patient has arranged for this visit because she is afraid for her baby. The fear that a problem exists solidifies when the care provider listens unsuccessfully over different areas of the uterus, then finally admits that no fetal heart sounds are present. There is very little that can alleviate the patient's growing anxiety other than verification of her baby's health. Her obstetrician should acknowledge her concerns and explain that further investigation is warranted. It is appropriate to tell the woman that her baby may in fact be healthy and that the attempt to locate the fetal heartbeat may have failed because of the method of detection used. At this point, an immediate ultrasound evaluation of the fetus is imperative. Delaying this type of fetal evaluation any longer than absolutely necessary prolongs and heightens the patient's anxiety. It is unconscionable to dismiss the patient with the advice not to worry.

USE OF ULTRASOUND FOR DETECTING INTRAUTERINE FETAL DEATH

Confirmation of Death

Sonography is the definitive method of confirming intrauterine fetal death. Its use, however, often places ultrasound technicians or the ultrasonographer in the awkward position of knowing that the fetus is dead, yet not being designated as the one who is to tell the patient that this is so. Clearly, the patient's primary care provider should tell his or her patient that her baby is dead. This situation is complicated further by the patient's urgent concerns. The options for the ultrasound technician are three: (1) Tell the patient outright that her baby is dead. This may be the most honest approach, but it ignores the possibility that the sonogram may be in error. Moreover, most obstetricians do wish to tell their patients themselves when a fetus has died. (2) Tell the patient that the ultrasound pictures will be interpreted later by an ultrasonographer, who then will relay the results to the patient's physician. This approach is problematic, because most patients can tell if the baby is all right from the technician's facial expressions and manner during the ultrasound exam. Furthermore, quite often, the patient herself may be able to view the screen and so can draw her own conclusion, faulty or not. (3) Acknowledge that the baby's heart was not seen beating and that, although this might mean that fetal death has occurred, there have been occasions where even ultrasound has been incorrect. If this explanation is offered, a repeat ultrasound the next day is indicated. Although not applicable in all circumstances, this approach conveys honesty, while it allows the patient 24 hours to adjust to the very real possibility of fetal death. Furthermore, confirmation of an intrauterine fetal death by the second ultrasound scan establishes that the diagnosis was made only after serious consideration and was based on two separate determinations. Whatever explanation is provided, the ultrasonographer should contact the patient's obstetrical care provider with the information and direct the patient to see him or her immediately.

Honesty Is Important

Certain circumstances may lend themselves to any one of the courses of action suggested above. Nonetheless, most people realize that if the fetal heartbeat is not seen the baby is most likely dead. If a woman asks directly if this is the case, it is inconsistent for the ultrasound technician, a specialist who performs these studies routinely, to plead ignorance.

Transportation

It is important to ask the woman how she got to the doctor's office or the hospital for her ultrasound evaluation. She should not have to drive at such a time. Someone should have the woman wait while a relative is called to come to the ultrasound office to accompany the patient home or to the office or clinic she visits for her prenatal care. Allowing a woman to leave alone and unescorted after confirmation of an intrauterine fetal death is negligent. She is certain to be in shock to some degree. If she were to drive herself, the danger that she could become involved in an accident is very real.

THE OBSTETRICIAN'S FIRST RESPONSE

Once fetal death has been confirmed, most patients are overwhelmed immediately by questions—"Who should I tell?" "Where should I go?" "What should I do?" In part, patients will find answers to such questions based on their ability to resort to their own established patterns of problem solving—"I'll have to call a funeral home." "We can have a neighbor take care of the kids." Although these questions and problem-solving statements are appropriate, they often may be voiced in a rapid-fire manner that reveals the patient's state of panic and fear.

Removing the Burden from the Patient

The author has found it helpful to relieve the patient or couple of such tasks momentarily. Immediately after confirmation of intrauterine fetal death, the focus should be only on the loss itself. "Tonight (or today) you don't need to make decisions that will affect your care. We will help you by notifying anyone in your family you wish to be informed about this situation. We also will notify other care providers such as the chaplain or social worker who will help us examine your choices, one at a time, so that you can make the best decisions for your circumstances. We cannot take away your pain. But, we can help you organize your thoughts as you make necessary decisions during the next few days." Relieving parents of the decision-making process, even for a matter of hours, grants them time to grieve without immediate additional burdens.

ALTERNATIVES FOR MANAGEMENT

After intrauterine fetal death has been confirmed, the question is, "What are the alternatives for this patient?" Management of the pregnancy with an intrauterine fetal death may require either (1) induction of labor or (2) continued pregnancy observation while anticipating spontaneous onset of labor. The choice of management ultimately may be based on the woman's clinical or medical evaluation. Numerous factors have to be considered in managing the pregnancy terminating with intrauterine fetal death.

Quick Solutions versus Best Solutions

It is incorrect to assume that all people desire the most rapid method of delivery when intrauterine fetal death has occurred. For some, learning of the fetal death is the worst moment; carrying the dead fetus in utero still permits a closeness of mother and baby that will be lost once delivery occurs. Many, on the other hand, are anxious to proceed to the business of delivering the baby. A decision by the physician to induce labor, if made without consultation or input by the couple, may be misinterpreted as guilt or a quick solution. Discussing the facts and alternatives with the woman and her partner conveys compassion and understanding. In most cases, this helps to defuse feelings of anger, suspicion, and guilt, which are typically felt initially by all care providers and patients after such a disastrous finding.

IF LABOR IS NOT TO BE INDUCED

Patients who are not candidates for induction of labor or who elect to await spontaneous labor will return home and receive continued outpatient care. These patients should be seen twice weekly for medical and psychologic support. The woman's partner or a supportive relative or friend should accompany her on all of these visits. (For further discussion, see Chapter 10.)

MEDICAL ISSUES

Spontaneous Onset of Labor

The patient who carries a dead fetus in utero awaiting spontaneous onset of labor seldom encounters medical problems. In separate studies, 306 (1) and 165 (2) women with IUFDs were followed expectantly. Seventy-five and 90% experienced spontaneous onset of labor within 2 weeks, respectively; 89 and 93%, by 3 weeks.

Coagulopathy

The development of maternal coagulopathy following fetal death in utero is well recognized but seldom observed. The primary manifestation is that of a progressive fall in plasma fibrinogen often associated with increased clot fibrinolysis and decreased prothrombin and platelet count. Pritchard (3) evaluated the coagulation profile of 100 women with IUFDs. None exhibited fibrinogen levels of less than 150 mg/100 ml when the fetus was dead less than 5 weeks. Of 50 women followed for over 5 weeks, 26% developed hypofibrinogenemia (plasma fibrinogen of less than 150 mg/100 ml). In each case in which hypofibrinogenemia was noted, the decrease in plasma fibrinogen levels was progressive, averaging about 50 mg/100 ml per week. Based on these findings, weekly plasma fibrinogen determinations are currently recommended while the woman awaits spontaneous onset of labor. Weekly pelvic examinations should also be carried out to determine whether the cervix is inducible.

In a more recent report, Jiminez and Pritchard (4) used heparin to arrest the progressive course of hypofibrinogenemia associated with intrauterine fetal death while preparations for induction of labor were being made. In that series, plasma fibrinogen levels were noted to rise at a rate of 35–70 mg/100 ml per day in response to heparin infusions of 1200–2000 units per hour for 72 hours.

Preventing RHO(D) Isoimmunization

Risk of Fetal-Maternal Transfusion

Following detection of an intrauterine fetal death, the care provider must consider prevention of RHO(D) isoimmunization if the mother is RHO(D) negative and the father is RHO(D) positive. Several recent studies suggest that significant fetal-to-maternal transfusion may occur (1) spontaneously in the antepartum period leading to fetal death (5, 6), (2) in response to maternal trauma (7), or (3) at delivery (8). (See Chapter 13, "Value of the Perinatal Autopsy.") The author's recommendations for administering RHO(D) Immune Globulin (RHIG) to women with IUFD are:

Administration of RHIG

If IUFD is confirmed prior to onset of labor, perform a Kleihauer-Betke analysis of maternal blood to determine if fetal-to-maternal transfusion has occurred. If such a transfusion is documented, administer one 300-μg vial of RHIG for each 15 ml of fetal red blood cells detected by this method. If no fetal red blood cells are observed in the maternal blood, wait for delivery.

Once the stillborn fetus is delivered, administer one 300-μg vial of RHIG to the woman. If, however, placental abruption, placenta previa, cesarean section, or manual manipulation of the fetus or placenta occurs, additional fetal-to-maternal transfusion should be suspected. Kleihauer-Betke analysis of maternal blood should be carried out to determine the approximate number of 300-μg RHIG vials that must be administered postdelivery.

Counseling the Patient Awaiting Onset of Labor

The Angry Family

An immediate concern for couples awaiting spontaneous onset of labor is the reaction of family and friends when intrauterine fetal death has been confirmed and the woman is known to be carrying a dead fetus. Anger or guilt felt by family members may place the woman in the awkward position of having to explain why she was released from the hospital without being induced. The woman also may have to see friends and co-workers who are unaware of the fetal death. It is essential in the twice-weekly visits that the woman be (1) given suggestions as to how to respond to inevitable uncomfortable situations and (2) encouraged to discuss her own frustration over these encounters. One typical fear that many patients either feel themselves or are asked about by relatives and friends is that the baby will "poison" her—as if a fetus dead in utero could "rot" inside and introduce poisons into the mother's blood.

If Induction of Labor Is Chosen

How readily a patient will respond to induction of labor depends on an evaluation of her cervix and the method of inducing uterine contractions. Although several methods of evaluating inducibility of the cervix have been reported (9), that of Bishop (10) is best known. In Table 3.1, criteria for cervical evaluation are listed.

Methods of Induction of Labor

Using this method of cervical evaluation, Bishop found that patients with a score of 9 or greater experienced successful induction within an average of 4 hours. In contrast, patients with scores ≤4 had a 20% failed induction rate.

Several mechanical devices have been employed to improve inducibility of the cervix when a low Bishop score is encountered. In one series, Foley balloons placed in the extraovular space in the lower uterine segment rendered a more inducible cervix and a shorter induction-to-delivery period than those of

Table 3.1
Pelvic Scoring for Elective Induction of Labor*

	SCORE			
	0	1	2	3
Dilation (cm)	0	1–2	3–4	5–6
Effacement (%)	0–30	40–50	60–78	80
Fetal station	−3	−2	−1/0	+1/+2
Cervical consistency	Firm	Medium	Soft	—
Cervical position	Posterior	Middle	Anterior	—

* Reproduced from Bishop EH: Pelvic scoring for elective induction. *Obstet Gynecol* 24:266, 1964.

control patients not treated with a cervical balloon (11). In a more recent study, use of a cervical balloon was as effective as 5 mg of prostaglandin E_2 in vaginal gel for improving the status of the cervix prior to induction (12).

Laminaria

Laminaria (dried seaweed) offer a different method of changing the nature of the cervix prior to induction. In contact with moisture from cervical mucus, these devices swell over a 6- to 12-hour period, producing cervical dilatation and softening. Because laminaria are small hard sticks, and because several may be placed into the cervix at one time, there is the potential for rupture of the membranes, uterine bleeding, or infection after they have been placed into the endocervical canal. However, several studies have demonstrated the safety of this method (13, 14, 15).

Induction of Labor: Oxytocin or Prostaglandin?

Oxytocin

Oxytocin produces uterine contractions that are indistinguishable in intensity, duration, or frequency from those seen during spontaneous labor. The contractions are caused as the oxytocin stimulates neuralelectrical and contractile activity of uterine smooth muscle. For purposes of labor induction for fetal demise in midpregnancy, oxytocin has limited usefulness. Csapo (16) has shown that the very preterm uterus is resistant to oxytocin. Caldeyro-Barcia and Poseiro (17) demonstrated that the uterus exhibits an eight-fold increase in sensitivity to oxytocin between 20 and 39 weeks gestation. Most of the change in uterine sensitivity occurs during the last 8 weeks of gestation. Oxytocin has proven effective in midpregnancy when used in high concentrations. Liggins (18) reported 30 patients with missed abortions delivered with high dose syntocinon; all but two delivered with a mean induction-to-delivery time of 11 hours (18).

The antidiuretic properies of oxytocic agents become an issue when these drugs are used in high concentrations, because of risks of iatrogenic hyponatremia leading to seizure and death. Abdul-Karim and Assali (19) have shown that antidiuretic properties of oxytocin develop even before uterine contractile-stimulating properties are observed. In these cases, oxytocin acted directly on the kidneys to produce effects similar to those of pitressin. In doses above 45 milliunits/min, syntocinon does not seem to produce any additional antidiuretic effects on the kidneys; the effect quickly decreases once infusion of syntocinon is discontinued. Recommendations when oxytocin is being used for induction of labor are to limit the volume of solution in which the drug is administered and to restrict oral intake of fluid in order to avoid the potential hazards of hyponatremia.

Prostaglandin

For many clinicians, prostaglandins have replaced oxytocin as the drug of choice for inducing and augmenting labor contractions. In clinical trials, prostaglandin E_2 (PGE_2) has been given intravenously (20) or as a vaginal E_2 gel or suppository (21, 22). Local administration of PGE_2 as a vaginal suppository decreases gastrointestinal side effects (principally vomiting and diarrhea) which are prevalent when PGE_2 is given intravenously. Southern et al. (21), in a multicenter study, utilized 20-mg PGE_2 vaginal pessaries every 3 to 5 hours. Of 709 patients studied, 97% delivered successfully with a mean induction-to-delivery time of 10.7 hours. In this study, vomiting, diarrhea, and chills were reported by 56, 43, and 22% of the patients, respectively.

MacKenzie et al. (22) utilized 15-mg PGE_2 gel for women with intrauterine fetal deaths at less than 28 weeks gestation and 5-mg PGE_2 gel for those at greater than 29 weeks gestation. Of the 50 patients studied (28 primiparous, 22 multiparous), both groups responded similarly to this method of labor induction. Gastrointestinal side effects were reported by 15% of the patients, but only in those patients receiving the higher dosage gel. Average lengths of induction-to-delivery for patients at less than 28 weeks and greater than 28 weeks were 14.7 hours and 15.5 hours, respectively. Because prostaglandins were least effective for induction in very early pregnancies (that is, 11–13 weeks), suction aspiration was the method of choice for this group of patients (see Chapter 2, "Early Pregnancy Loss").

Despite increasing evidence of the effectiveness of vaginal prostaglandin treatment, reports of significant side effects have appeared in the literature. Sandler et al. (23) reported a single case of uterine rupture at 23 weeks gestation following vaginal PGE_2 suppositories in a woman with a history of prior cesarean section. Phelan et al. (24) observed fevers to 41°C (105°F), tachycardia, and hypotension in two women following administration of 20-mg PGE_2 suppositories. The authors commented on their difficulty in distinguishing these drug effects from endotoxic shock.

At the University of Cincinnati, the general guidelines that follow are used to select a method of delivery when intrauterine fetal death has been confirmed:

Suction Curettage

Pregnancies ≤16 Weeks. These patients are best managed by cervical dilatation and suction curettage. As many laminaria as possible (usually 2–5) are placed into the endocervical canal the night before the procedure and are removed the next morning just prior to suction aspiration. In many cases, further cervical dilatation at the time of suction curettage is not needed, because of the effectiveness of laminaria treatment. In certain cases, it may be important to alert the genetic laboratory that aspirated fetal tissue will be sent for chromosomal evaluation. All patients are to be advised regarding risks of excessive bleeding, uterine perforation, and the possible need for a hysterectomy if complications arise. The consent form describing the procedures and risks should be signed prior to placement of laminaria, *not* prior to suction curettage the next day. The potential risks of bleeding, infection, or artificial rupture of membranes during laminaria placement make this initial procedure an integral part of the suction curettage.

Showing the Removed Tissue to the Patient

Occasionally, patients may voice a desire to examine the aspirated tissue. In the author's experience, providing patients this opportunity establishes good communication and is not viewed as detrimental to the physician-patient relationship. In selected cases in which a patient with a missed abortion has been followed for several weeks, suction curettage may prove ineffective for evacuating all fetal tissue, due to fibrosis and tissue adherence. Sharp curettage should follow all suction curettages to assure complete tissue removal.

Preparation for Prostaglandin Induction

Pregnancies >16 Weeks with a Long, Firm Cervix. Although the safety of suction curettage has been demonstrated up to 24 weeks, the author and colleagues have chosen to place several laminaria into the cervix the night before and induce labor with PGE$_2$ suppositories the next morning. Prior to administering PGE$_2$ suppositories, the laminaria are removed and the patient is given the following: Tylenol, 650 mg by mouth every 4 hours to block the febrile reaction to prostaglandin; Lomotil, one tablet by mouth following each episode of diarrhea; and Phenergan, 20 mg intramuscular to control nausea and vomiting. Prostaglandin E$_2$ vaginal suppositories (20 mg) are placed every 4 hours as long as labor continues and the amniotic membranes are intact. Once the cervix reaches 4 cm, the amniotic membranes are ruptured and intravenous oxytocin is begun to augment the PGE$_2$ effect. Oxytocin is also administered if the amniotic membranes spontaneously rupture prior to adequate cervical dilatation.

Pregnancies with an Inducible Cervix. These patients respond as readily to oxytocin as to PGE$_2$ suppositories and usually are managed successfully with intravenous oxytocin. Amniotomy is performed once cervical dilatation has exceeded 3–4 cm.

What to Tell the Patient

Before any medical treatment is begun, patients should be fully counseled regarding the characteristics of different treatment alternatives. They should clearly understand the differences between an oxytocin- and a prostaglandin-induced labor. They should be aware that oxytocin produces a labor-like contraction pattern or that prostaglandin creates a sustained contraction that persists throughout the labor process.

Patients should also be given a reasonable estimate of the induction-to-delivery time. As important, especially with prostaglandin, the patient should be advised that her cervix may not change for several hours, but then may dilate rapidly just before delivery. It is helpful to point out that the cervix need not dilate as much to accommodate a midpregnancy delivery as must occur in a term delivery. This fact, coupled with the effects of laminaria insertion, means that according to most studies there is a mean induction-to-delivery time of about 12 hours, with a range of 4 to 24 hours.

Repeat Cesarean Section or Vaginal Birth after Cesarean Section

The Choice

If a woman has had a previous cesarean section, the option of this manner of delivery should be discussed seriously. It is quite possible that this patient planned to have her baby by a scheduled, repeat section. Or she may have wanted to attempt a vaginal birth after cesarean section. Now that the baby is known to be dead, cesarean section may be viewed by the mother as a desirable means of delivering the baby.

This may create a conflict for obstetricians who increasingly are favoring a trial of labor and vaginal birth after cesarean section. The patient sees a cesarean section as a quick way to get this terrible situation resolved. Her doctor, on the other hand, may raise as an issue the drawbacks of performing major surgery when the wellbeing of the fetus is no longer a consideration. Discouraging a patient from a quick-fix method of delivery may be difficult under these circumstances.

If labor is prolonged or complications arise, a cesarean section ultimately may become the means of delivery. Under these circumstances, a woman may become angry at what she perceives as poor or incompetent medical care, thus making her stillbirth experience that much more painful and difficult. Fortunately, vaginal birth after prior cesarean section is receiving increasing acceptance as a safe and effective mode of therapy (25). Ultimately, the woman may find that she appreciates having given birth vaginally, because of the easier recovery.

In agreeing to proceed with a cesarean delivery at the patient's request, the obstetrician should advise her as to the length of time she will need to recover. Also, the surgery's influence on the timing of a subsequent pregnancy should be raised. It is best to present a balanced review of pros and cons of both a vaginal birth after cesarean section and a repeat cesarean section, so that the woman can make a well-informed decision as to how she wants to deliver her dead baby.

MANAGEMENT OF LABOR AND DELIVERY

Proper care of the patient with an intrauterine fetal death during labor and delivery requires that the medical staff: (1) recognize unique aspects of labor resulting in delivery of a dead fetus, (2) be in attendance, and (3) be aware of professional resources in the hospital.

Anesthesia

Unlike labor resulting in delivery of a healthy baby, labor with an intrauterine fetal death offers no reward at the end. Consequently, concerns or fears that are often part of a normal labor process ("Will I tear?" "Will I embarrass myself?") are intensified by the knowledge that the labor process will only result in delivery of a dead fetus. Anesthesia for labor should be planned with two objectives: (1) to make the patient comfortable during labor and (2) to avoid heavy sedation that hinders efforts of medical personnel to address psychologic needs of the patient during this type of labor. Use of epidural anesthesia once labor is effectively established addresses both objectives. The patient may then labor in a generally pain-free state. As important, medical personnel can provide emotional support to the patient as labor progresses toward delivery. Providing sips of water or juice, making a radio or television available, and welcoming the companionship of family members help to relieve the sadness of this patient's tedious, unrewarding labor process.

Avoid Isolation

It is important during labor that care providers be attentive to the patient. Many women remember being isolated in a labor room and being left alone during labor with an intrauterine fetal death. Impressions left to the woman by this type of care include (1) "No one cares about me," (2) "This is so awful that even the medical staff are repelled by my labor," or (3) "I'm repulsive to the medical personnel because of my condition."

Professional Insecurities

Unfortunately, in many cases medical personnel *do* avoid the patient, but usually because they do not know what to say. They stay away because being physically removed from the patient is less threatening personally. The desire to run away from a patient because of personal insecurities about death is a natural and common response by the obstetrical community. It is difficult to sit at the bedside during this type of labor not knowing what to say or how to say it. Nonetheless, it is not appropriate to shy away from a patient because of such insecurities about confronting death. The patient is not asking for much—only that medical personnel not abandon her during her crisis. Merely remaining in the room provides comfort and companionship that will be remembered by the woman and her family long after the topics of conversation are forgotten. No one should be left alone and therefore lonely during labor for a stillbirth.

Conversation in the Labor Room

Occasionally, a patient may feel left out of any relaxed conversation and informal interaction between care providers and her family. It is common for conversations to involve her partner or relatives more than the patient herself, especially if active labor is in progress. There may be no way to resolve the conflict in the patient's mind of being lonely and sick by the labor while conversation goes on around her but does not include her. This conflict for the patient may be mentioned openly in the early part of labor as a means of educating the patient about emotional conflicts likely to surface, which are associated with labor following a fetal death.

ROLE OF THE CHAPLAIN OR SOCIAL WORKER

Utilizing Professional Care Providers

The chaplain and the social worker offer important resources for support during labor for an intrauterine fetal death. These professionals should be brought into the process as early as possible. Each offers unique skills that provide the foundation for sustained psychologic support. There is no way to remove from these laboring patients the sadness and sense of loss surrounding their clinical situation. Care providers must therefore focus on those emotions that can be mitigated as labor and delivery proceed.

Fear. With seemingly nothing to look forward to following delivery (that is, a healthy baby), the patient may lose her ability to judge labor as a normal physiologic process. Spontaneous or oxytocin-induced labors are characterized by periodic contractions and may be better tolerated by the patient than prostaglandin-induced contractions, which characteristically are sustained, tetanic contractions. Labor, by itself, may raise concerns for the patient about the possibility of damage to her reproductive organs.

Focusing Anxiety

A second source of fear may be based on the patient's expectations about her baby's appearance at delivery. Her idea of how a baby, dead in utero for days or weeks, may look at delivery almost always exaggerates the degree of change in physical appearance that a fetus undergoes following death. Some patients may even picture a process of decay, an image of death often depicted on television and in films. Fears about the physical appearance of the baby, if not countered by care givers, may negatively influence a couple's desire to see or hold their baby after delivery.

"Did I Cause This?"

Guilt.   Guilt is a common human emotion reflecting people's need to understand why a tragedy has occurred. The sense of absolute responsibility for fetal death is much more likely to be assumed by the woman than by her partner. "After all," she thinks, "was it not I who carried our baby in my uterus?" This sense of responsibility for the baby, experienced by most women during pregnancy, now may be translated into utter responsibility for the baby's death. She may irrationally evaluate physical activities, conflicts, sexual intercourse, arguments, or eating habits in an effort to assign blame. Although many of these "causes" involve other people, the sense of personal responsibility for the fetal death is a major obstacle for these patients.

Anger.   Another common emotion during labor is anger. Anger may surface as a protective shield. It enables the patient to ward off feelings of guilt or personal blame that may be present, but are too painful to acknowledge. Anger may, however, be directed either at obstetrical care, medical personnel, or other life events whose cause-and-effect role may be perceived by the patient. A well-informed patient is less likely to exhibit anger that is unwarranted by the circumstances. For the poorly informed patient, anger irrespective of its focus and logic may provide temporary insulation from her more frightening feelings of guilt or fear. In this case, anger is likely to interfere with the supportive efforts of care providers during her labor.

Fighting Loneliness

Loneliness and Isolation.   A sense of loneliness reflects the woman's feelings of isolation and fear of abandonment as she experiences fetal death. Often phrased as "Why me?" this feeling may be coupled with guilt, as the patient wonders if she has done something wrong and is now paying for it. Patients with strong religious beliefs may turn to their religion for an explanation. They may fear that their God has singled them out for some wrongdoing and is now punishing them. Others may interpret this tragedy as another sad event in a life filled with crises. The majority, however, are left to struggle with the unexplainable. They have a hollow sense that they alone have been deprived the rewards of their hopes and dreams.

MANAGEMENT OF DELIVERY OF A STILLBORN FETUS

The Issues

At delivery, care providers must balance the patient's perception of events with technical aspects of the procedure. All too often, stillborn fetuses are delivered into a pan or in the labor bed. Although these approaches may satisfy clinical standards for a stillbirth delivery, they can impart a very negative and uncaring attitude to the patient. It is difficult for care providers, be they physicians or nurses, to recognize how differently they and the patient perceive the dead fetus. Care providers may focus on problems with the patient's labor, concerns with bleeding, fears of uterine rupture, and postpartum infection. Under these circumstances, they may neglect such mundane issues as whether or not the dead fetus was delivered gently. Was the baby placed in a blanket? Was he or she traumatized at delivery? Naturally, these are issues of concern in the case of delivery of a live baby, but often they are entirely overlooked during delivery of a fetus known to be dead. Overlooked, that is, by all involved persons except the parents. To the mother of this baby, how the baby was handled, wrapped, and treated is often no less important now than if the baby had been born alive. Perhaps these issues become even more important in the case of stillbirth, when the patient struggles with feelings of guilt and the need to "do right by this baby" while still worrying about things she may not have done properly during her pregnancy.

Delivery in a Labor Bed

If the fetus is delivered in bed, he or she should be wrapped immediately in a blanket (not just covered with one). The umbilical cord should be clamped, and then the baby should be removed. At no time should the baby be left lying on the bed between the patient's legs while the placenta is delivered. Likewise, no baby should be delivered and placed into a pan or bucket. This image may linger with parents long after their baby has been buried. Once the baby is wrapped and separated from the placenta, he or she may be presented to the mother or retained in the blanket in a nearby room until the mother is ready to see her baby. Statements such as "You have a boy; there are no obvious abnormalities," may ease the initial tension of the moment. In a labor/delivery room, the patient may wish to watch the delivery itself. Requests such as this are very appropriate and should be granted. Watching her baby's delivery can help the mother begin the process of bonding that eventually can lead to a more satisfactory emotional recovery.

Delivery of a stillborn baby in the delivery room carries many of the same admonitions. No parent wants to think that her beloved but dead baby was delivered into a pan. The painful image of this manner of delivery is inappropriate for a human life now extinguished. Qualities that one attributes to living people are extrapolated by parents to their dead baby. Intellectually, they realize that life cannot be restored in their baby. Still, they expect their baby to be treated with the dignity accorded to all persons in death. The request that a loved yet dead baby be treated with respect and honor is simple to fulfill. To do so, delivery of the stillborn baby must be viewed through the parents' eyes. Care providers must remember during delivery that the patient is observing them as they handle her loved baby. Only when they have done this and have responded accordingly can they establish the foundations for subsequent care and counseling that are crucial for parents during the postpartum period.

SHOWING THE STILLBORN BABY TO PARENTS

Location

Once the placenta has been removed from the uterus, care providers may choose to present the baby to the mother and father in the delivery room. An alternative approach is to move parents to a quiet labor room or an isolated area in the recovery room where the couple can be with their baby. Occasionally, it is appropriate to show the baby to the father while the mother is being moved out of the delivery room to a quieter area. The advantage of presenting the baby first to the father is that he may then offer additional support if the mother is fearful of seeing her baby. Subsequently, the mother should be given the identical full explanation received by the father. This is important to note; it is unwise to expect the father to explain as well or even at all the information that was explained to him.

Timing

The mother should be awake and alert when she sees her baby. Make sure that any anesthesia has worn off, if the type of medication used can affect her ability to concentrate on her baby. It is a tragedy to hear a patient later bemoan the fact that she was too sleepy from the delivery medication to appreciate what was said to her or that she was too uncomfortable to enjoy holding her baby. When care providers examine the baby with the father and/or mother, they should realize that all people have a tendency to shy away from the dead. It is common to see a father standing nearby but unable to reach out and touch

Viewing and Holding the Baby

his stillborn baby. Some parents truly do not want to see or touch their baby. For many, however, this initial negative response reflects fears and misconceptions about death. Unfortunately, a mother who declines the offer to see and hold her baby often will regret this decision weeks or months later. Families may begin to question why care providers were not more helpful in advising and working with them during this period of fear and confusion. It is very important to tell parents explicitly that they may take their time, even if this means several hours.

Reducing Anxiety

To help a couple see their stillborn baby for the first time, there are several points that should be emphasized. Wrapping the baby in a colorful blanket is a helpful gesture which lends a semblance of normality. More important, parents should be prepared for changes in skin color and the skin desquamation that normally accompany death. These changes in integrity and color of fetal skin occur rapidly, often within 24 hours after death, and therefore are encountered as a matter of course during delivery of a stillborn baby. Presenting the baby wrapped in a blanket so that at first parents see only the face gives them a minute to adjust to their baby's lifeless body before they have to confront all the physical changes associated with death.

When the wrapped baby is presented to parents, certain mechanical maneuvers may enhance his or her appearance. Often, a stillborn baby has accumulated fluid in the scalp, thereby giving his or her skull a puffy, bloated appearance. When a hand is held up under the head, the baby's face and head can be made to appear more normal. This maneuver can also be used when the baby is being photographed. These gestures (wrapping, positioning the head) make the baby appear as normal as possible for parents.

Once parents have seen their baby, care providers may help them to overcome any initial hesitation to hold their baby by pointing out the normal appearance of impersonal parts of the baby's anatomy. Counting toes and fingers gives parents a moment to adjust subconsciously to the skin and other physical changes that can startle them or repel them from further contact with their baby's body.

Bringing Mother and Baby Together

If the mother is encouraged to examine more impersonal areas of her baby's body first, she is apt to be more relaxed once the face and head are fully exposed. At first, the presence of a care provider during the parents' initial examination often helps them overcome fears of touching a dead body. Parents should then be allowed to be alone with their baby. The care provider may step away from the bed, after initial physical contact has been observed. Generally, parents will continue to touch and handle their baby curiously and naturally.

Staff and Parents Do Not See the "Same" Baby

It is also important to note that, while medical professionals may view the disfigured head or body of a stillborn baby as an unattractive sight, a parent properly guided in the initial examination of a baby can begin to project his or her own perception of the "future child" into the stillborn baby. A couple does not see just the remains of their baby. Unlike proud parents of a healthy baby excited about their newborn's tiny fingernails, parents of a stillborn look beyond the baby's appearance to get a feeling for the person their baby would have become. They are viewing a projected image of what they wish their baby would have looked like. It is not uncommon to hear parents exchanging statements like, "She has my nose," or "He's got your jaw." This attention to details validates the "dream" psychologists describe that is lost following a pregnancy loss. Ultimately, most parents will remove the blanket entirely in order to see the whole of their dead baby.

Deformities

Even when a baby has obvious deformities, seeing him or her is very important for most parents. With sensitive preparation, care providers can facilitate this step. When the viewing is carried out in a considerate manner, most parents appreciate later having been able to see their deformed baby. Too often, otherwise, parents who hear about but never see their abnormal baby naturally try later on to picture in their minds how their baby looked. In the end, their image of what their deformed baby looked like is almost always worse than reality.

Time Alone with Their Baby

In all cases, parents must be given an opportunity to be completely alone with their baby. Care providers should explain that they are leaving so that the parents can have privacy. With experience, a care provider may be able to sense at what point couples will be comfortable enough to be left to themselves, but not feel abandoned. The length of time that the parents require with the baby differs among couples. Frequently, a couple who have said they have been with the baby long enough will express a need only minutes later to take more time. They should be told explicitly that it is acceptable to request more time with their baby. It is possible also that a woman will want her mother or another significant person to view the baby. Such a request should be granted if that person is present or can arrive within a reasonable amount of time. Only when both parents are completely satisfied with their experience should the staff remove the baby for subsequent management.

TAKING A PICTURE

It is extremely important that a picture be taken of the baby *wrapped in a blanket*. This is a gesture of respect for the person the parents see in their dead baby. Efforts should be made to make the picture appear as lifelike and normal as possible, since weeks or months later this picture will probably be the only permanent record of what the baby looked like. By moistening the skin and cradling the head with a hand, the physician or nurse can position the baby to look more lifelike. Esthetic consideration should be given to such aspects as whether the eyes and mouth look better open or closed. Taking the picture directly from the front gives a flat, two-dimensional appearance to the face; pictures taken slightly off center empha-

Emphasizing "Normalness"

size the shape of the nose, jaw line, and forehead and thereby allow the couple to identify family features.

Babies with severe anomalies can be made to appear more normal when a cap is placed over a skull deformity or the blanket is used to cover a defective extremity or other anomaly. Often, bringing a normal arm out in front of the blanket aids in exposing more of the "normal baby" and leaves a lasting impression of a normal appearance.

Many hospitals keep an instamatic camera in Labor and Delivery for these purposes. Some feel that instamatic pictures are best because the final picture is "softer" than a picture taken with a 35 mm camera, and it therefore does not emphasize blemishes in the skin occurring after death. However, this response may reflect more the reaction of medical staff taking the picture than the feelings of parents themselves. A strong argument for a clearer and more detailed picture can be made. It is sad when a mother pulls out a blurred picture months later and wishes it had been clearer and more vivid.

NAMING THE BABY

A Name Creates a Personality

It is very important to ask parents what they have named their daughter or son. Refer to the stillborn baby as a son or a daughter and, whenever possible, use the baby's given name. This courtesy transforms an otherwise lifeless "pathology specimen" into a human being and conveys an element of respect and dignity to the stillborn baby. The name that parents choose often reflects the significance of the moment. Some families have "saved" a previously selected name and have used instead a family name to memorialize the dead baby. As a consideration, parents may be advised to reconsider using the originally selected name. This gesture is helpful in acknowledging this baby as a person who did exist so that parents won't fuse another, later baby's identity with that of this dead one. Answers to a simple question such as, "Why did you choose that name for your son (or daughter)?" often provide insight as to the emotional significance that parents attach to this baby. This line of questioning encourages parents to speak frankly about their feelings for their baby and how they perceive him or her as part of their family lineage.

OBTAINING AN AUTOPSY

Among the most frequently asked questions months or years after delivery of a stillborn baby are "What happened?"

and "What went wrong?" Answers to these questions may be found when a carefully conducted autopsy has been performed. Requesting an autopsy immediately after delivery of a stillborn baby, however, can seem uncaring and callous. It is easy to understand why requests for this procedure often are refused by distraught patients and not pursued by care providers.

If an Autopsy Request Is Refused

Patients often deny autopsy requests because they lack understanding as to the value of the results and the nature of the procedure. When asked how they visualize an autopsy, many patients describe the procedure as a disfiguring, mutilating operation. It is not surprising then that many patients, even though they can appreciate the importance of findings, will oppose such a procedure for their baby.

Overcoming Misconceptions

When seeking autopsy permission, care providers must consider their timing of the request for an autopsy and for inquiring into the patient's concept of the procedure. It may be very useful to address the issue of autopsy in initial discussions following detection of intrauterine fetal death or at least in the early phases of labor. This approach familiarizes parents with concepts that may later be reinforced after delivery. It is often inappropriate to approach a patient with an autopsy request in the first hour or hours after delivery of her stillborn. The shock of the event may lead the mother to refuse the autopsy despite its predictive value. The error of approaching a patient too soon after delivery may be compounded if the care provider accepts as final her decision to forego an autopsy. Valuable information is lost forever. Later, the patient may come to understand how useful the information could have been, and she may greatly regret not having had the autopsy performed.

Timing the Request

The proper approach toward obtaining permission to perform an autopsy is to delay making the request until the patient has had some time to begin to assimilate the impact of the event. For some patients, this period may only be 1 or 2 hours; for others, 12 to 24 hours may be required. The baby, in the meantime, should be kept in the morgue. Once the patient is approachable, she should be informed as to the importance of information to be gained and asked her concept of an autopsy. Gross misconceptions often may be picked up in this type of counseling. Even if a mother refuses an autopsy for her baby, care providers should approach her again at a later time. It is a tragedy to lose the important data an autopsy can yield because the patient was approached too soon after delivery or refused because of her lack of understanding. When the autopsy is described as a surgical procedure that will not disfigure the baby but one that may give important information as to why the baby died, most patients readily grant permission. Reassurance that the baby may still be buried and granted the respect and love that parents wish to bestow on him or her diminishes many of the fears associated with an autopsy. (See Chapter 13, "Value of the Perinatal Autopsy.")

FROM LABOR AND DELIVERY TO THE WARD

Once a patient is ready to be moved from Labor and Delivery, care providers should ask her if she would prefer a room on a gynecologic (GYN) or an obstetrical (OB) floor. Many women will choose a GYN floor because it is isolated from crying babies and may protect them from the emotions these sounds can produce. Conversely, it is also understandable that a woman would prefer the OB floor because it is a means of beginning to cope, to face the reality that there are a lot of babies around. Surprisingly, certain patients who have been hospitalized prior to delivery of their stillborn baby may choose to return to the antepartum floor to be with other antepartum patients with whom they grew friendly before delivery. This is just a reminder to care providers that support for grieving patients during hospitalization often can come from people other than care providers themselves. Recognizing these resources can help considerably in early management of these patients.

CARE ON THE OB OR GYN FLOOR

Once a patient has been moved to her chosen floor, communication and cooperation among care providers are essential. The delivering physician should visit the patient at least twice daily. These visits are not only to express sympathy, but also to encourage the woman to begin the long process of seeking answers to "Why?" Although it may be helpful at this stage to review the hospital chart and antepartum events with the patient, the presence and attentiveness of concerned care providers in the first few days after delivery serve to establish a level of communication that will be important over the ensuing weeks or months of continued outpatient care.

Breast Engorgement   Breast engorgement is a specific postpartum occurrence that must be addressed. Before the patient leaves the hospital, her physician should be certain that she is aware that this normal postpartum response following delivery is likely to serve as an emotional and stressful reminder of her tragedy. Although it is customary for a nurse to instruct the maternity patient about breast management, this issue may be overlooked (or avoided) by nursing staff following fetal or neonatal death. Some physicians may elect to place their patients on Parlodel, 2.5 mg twice daily, for 2 weeks to hasten the decrease in breast engorgement. Even if this approach is selected, it is essential that the physician confirm the fact that the patient has received proper instruction regarding breast engorgement before she leaves the hospital.

AFTER DISCHARGE FROM THE HOSPITAL

During the woman's hospitalization, management of the couple experiencing delivery of a stillborn baby taxes the medical knowledge and caring attitudes of medical care providers at all levels. What is not universally appreciated by the medical community is the lasting impact that a stillbirth has on a couple. Care provided while the patient is in the hospital is only the beginning of the process of care and recovery that may extend over months or years. Chapters 10–14 describe in detail the long-term counseling methods and support network that should be an integral part of the recovery process.

REFERENCES

1. Dippel AL: Death of foetus in utero. *Bull Johns Hopkins Hosp* 54:24, 1934.
2. Tricomi V and Kohl SG: Fetal death in utero. *Am J Obstet Gynecol* 74:1092–1097, 1975.
3. Pritchard JH: Fetal death in utero. *Obstet Gynecol* 14:573–580, 1959.
4. Jiminez J and Pritchard JA: Pathogens and treatment of coagulation defects resulting from fetal death. *Obstet Gynecol* 32:449–459, 1968.
5. Laube RW and Schanberger CW: Fetomaternal bleeding as a cause of unexplained fetal death. *Obstet Gynecol* 60:649–651, 1982.
6. Fay RA: Feto-maternal hemorrhage as a cause of fetal morbidity and mortality. *Br J Obstet Gynecol* 90:443–446, 1983.
7. Rose PG, Strohm PL, Zuspan FP: Fetomaternal hemorrhage following trauma. *Am J Obstet Gynecol* 153:844, 1985.
8. Prevention of RHO(D) Isoimmunization. *ACOG Technical Bulletin* #79, Aug 1984.
9. Steiner AL and Creasy RK: Methods of cervical priming. *Clin Obstet Gynecol* 26:37–46, 1983.
10. Bishop EH: Pelvic scoring for elective induction. *Obstet Gynecol* 24:266, 1964.
11. Embrey MP and Mollison BG: The unfavourable cervix and induction of labor using a cervical balloon. *J Obstet Gynecol Br Comm* 74:44–48, 1967.
12. Ezimokhai M and Nwabinski JN: The use of Foley's catheter in ripening the unfavourable cervix prior to induction of labor. *Br J Obstet Gynecol* 87:281–286, 1980.
13. Lackritz R, Gibson M, Frigoletto FD: Pre-induction use of laminaria for the unripe cervix. *Am J Obstet Gynecol* 134:349, 1979.
14. Stubblefield PG, Naftolin F, Frigoletto FO, Ryan KJ: Laminaria augmentation of intra-amniotic prostaglandin F2α for mid-trimester pregnancy termination. *Prostaglandins* 10:413, 1975.

15. Cross WG and Pitkin RM: Laminaria as an adjunct in induction of labor. *Obstet Gynecol* 51:606, 1978.

16. Csapo A: Function and regulation of the myometrium. *Ann NY Acad Sci* 75:790–808, 1959.

17. Caldeyro-Barcia R and Poseiro JJ: Oxytocin and contractibility of the pregnant human uterus. *Ann NY Acad Sci* 75:813–830, 1959.

18. Liggins GC: The treatment of missed abortion by high dosage syntocinon intravenous infusion. *J Obstet Gynecol Br Comm* 69:277–281, 1962.

19. Abdul-Karim R and Assali N: Renal function in human pregnancy: V. Effects of oxytocin on renal haemodynamics and water and electrolyte excretion. *J Lab Clin Med* 57:522–532, 1961.

20. Gordon H and Pipe NGJ: Induction of labor after intrauterine fetal death. A comparison between prostaglandin E_2 and oxytocin. *Obstet Gynecol* 45:44–46, 1975.

21. Southern EM, Gutknecht GD, Mohberg NR, Edelman DA: Vaginal prostaglandin E_2 in the management of fetal intrauterine death. *Br J Obstet Gynecol* 85:437–441, 1978.

22. MacKenzie IZ, Davies AJ, Embry MP: Fetal death in utero managed with vaginal prostaglandin E_2 gel. *Br J Med* 1:1764–1765, 1979.

23. Sandler RZ, Knutzen VK, Milano CM, Gleicher N: Uterine rupture with the use of vaginal prostaglandin E_2 suppositories. *Am J Obstet Gynecol* 134:348–349, 1979.

24. Phelan JP, Meguiar RV, Matey D, Newman C: Dramatic pyrexia and cardiovascular response to intravaginal prostaglandin E_2. *Am J Obstet Gynecol* 132:28, 1978.

25. Lavin JP, Stephens RJ, Miodovnik M, Barden TP: Vaginal delivery in patients with a prior cesarean section. *Obstet Gynecol* 59:135–148, 1982.

Death of a Newborn: Merging Parental Expectations and Medical Reality

JAMES R. WOODS, Jr., M.D.

The pediatric medical community has been much more active and innovative than the obstetric community in its efforts to fulfill expectations of parents experiencing a pregnancy loss. There are several reasons why pediatricians have acted as a vanguard in this area of medicine:

1. Parents bring their living children to the pediatrician actually seeking to engage him or her in conversation about a pregnancy loss.

Inherent Sensitivity to Parents' Needs

2. Pediatricians have recognized for years the need to inform parents of their child's condition. A neonatal death naturally involves them in this form of dialogue with parents.

3. Pediatricians rely on parental support as a necessary element in the care of children with such conditions as leukemia and other lethal childhood cancers.

4. There is a blending of roles; the pediatrician is very likely a parent himself or herself and can relate to parents of young patients.

5. Public and medical attention paid to the Sudden Infant Death Syndrome (SIDS) has highlighted parents' grief reaction to a baby's death.

6. Pediatricians care for children through a range of ages. Their specialty means that they are accustomed to encountering death of a newborn, infant, or older child. In such cases, their interaction with parents in the period leading to the

child's death is likely to be extensive. Intense and continued contact in anticipation of the child's death may influence the professional in his or her approach to parents.

STILLBIRTH AND NEONATAL DEATH: WHAT ARE THE DIFFERENCES?

There are many similarities in care that parents experiencing a neonatal death and parents delivering a stillbirth should receive. These similarities, however, are confined exclusively to care provided to parents after the newborn has died and during the ensuing period of grief. The reader is referred to other sections of this text for a complete discussion of care plans that apply mutually to both groups of parents (see Figure 4.1).

Anticipating Grief; Viability

Despite many similarities that exist in care of parents experiencing a stillbirth or neonatal death, there are issues that are unique to the period following a live birth that concludes with the baby's death. Issues that are specifically (although not exclusively) characteristic for neonatal death are (1) anticipatory grief and (2) the differing interpretation of "viability" between parents and medical staff. To illustrate these important points, Chapter 4 presents four representative situations in order to point out issues common in the responses to a neonatal death.

CASE 1: *Delivery of a nonviable newborn who dies*

A 30-year-old gravida 1, para 0, white female in premature labor at 19 weeks gestation. Despite care during labor, vaginal delivery occurred in a labor bed, resulting in the birth of a 375-

Holding the baby (Chapter 3)

Pictures and mementos of the baby (Chapter 3)

Burial plans (Chapter 9)

Role of the chaplain or social worker (Chapters 7 and 8)

Role of the funeral director (Chapter 9)

Outpatient counseling: When and for how long? (Chapter 10)

The office nurse (Chapter 11)

Response of children or grandparents (Chapters 1 and 8)

Value of the perinatal autopsy (Chapter 13)

Genetic counseling between pregnancies (Chapter 12)

Reaction during a subsequent pregnancy (Chapter 15)

Format for a peer support network (Chapter 17)

Figure 4.1. Care offered parents after their baby's death.

gram male, with Apgar scores of 1 at 1 minute and 1 at 5 minutes. The only evidence of newborn activity was a heart rate of 60 beats per minute at both 1 and 5 minutes. The baby was taken immediately to the neonatal intensive care unit (NICU) and placed in an isolette. He was pronounced dead at 30 minutes. In this situation (common to tertiary centers), opportunities for failed communication between parent and medical staff are great. The following points concerning a case such as this illustrate those attitudes on the part of the medical community which may severely impede care for parents.

Nonviability and Parents' Response to Their Baby's Struggle

The intellectual and emotional definitions of "nonviable." In this case, medical personnel know that the fetus delivered at 19 weeks gestation is too young to survive. This knowledge is a product of nursery experience at the institution and of medical teaching in general, which documents repeatedly that newborns this young cannot survive. Unfortunately, this inevitability is not generally understood by the nonmedical community. Many parents assume that even the tiniest babies ought to live, with the help of modern technology. After all, to parents, a fetus of this age looks like a miniature term baby. Parents usually do not realize that nothing can sustain an incompletely developed, young baby's life outside the uterus. They must be informed about the realities of the situation. Still, even after they have comprehended that their baby cannot survive, parents justifiably may want something done for the baby while he or she does live, however briefly, after delivery. The 19-week newborn who, after delivery, makes some movement ought to be given oxygen and kept warm, as parents see the issue. The impression that the author has gained from talking with parents who have experienced this is that few of them can abandon hope that their baby will survive, even though they hear that survival is impossible by all medical and intellectual standards.

Figure 4.2 contrasts expectations of medical personnel and parents for the baby delivered at 19 weeks. Differences in expectations by both parties affect subsequent management decisions.

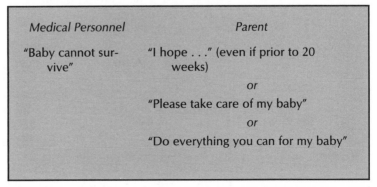

Medical Personnel	Parent
"Baby cannot survive"	"I hope . . ." (even if prior to 20 weeks)
	or
	"Please take care of my baby"
	or
	"Do everything you can for my baby"

Figure 4.2.   Differing expectations regarding the newborn delivered at 19 weeks gestation.

CREATING A UNIFIED CARE PLAN

Critical in the management of this situation is the need for obstetrician and pediatrician to meet jointly with parents in order to educate parents about realistic outcomes and present a unified plan of care.

Parent

Obstetrician ⌒ **Pediatrician**

Joint discussion with parents prior to delivery offers the following reassurances to the couple:

Accord between Obstetrician and Pediatrician

1. The obstetrician and pediatrician agree.
2. There will be a continuum of care, which affirms that obstetric and pediatric care are but two components of the same process.
3. Information that parents receive represents the product of two specialties in medicine, as if a second opinion had been obtained.

NEED TO DOCUMENT DECISIONS

Communicating Clearly through Shift Changes

It is essential that information given to parents before delivery be documented in the mother's chart. In many group obstetric practices, the physician responsible for care changes when change of shift occurs. Decisions made with parents, such as that no cesarean section will be performed if fetal distress develops or that resuscitation of the newborn will consist only of temperature support and oxygen by mask, may not be conveyed to new care providers. The same miscommunication may occur as pediatric faculty and nurses change. Truly, it can be a tragedy if the 19-week newborn's birth occurs after a shift change and a neonatologist bursts into the delivery room to embark on full resuscitation, unaware of decisions made beforehand by parents and admitting physicians. When time allows, parents may assume responsibility for communicating their personal desires and prior management decisions to uninformed new care providers. Unfortunately, the unpredictable nature of obstetrics often makes this type of anticipatory decision making difficult or impossible. In these instances, uninformed care providers may act reflexively, thereby selecting management techniques that are consistent with good medical care but that conflict with parents' wishes. In hospitals with obstetric or pediatric residency training programs, the danger that decisions will not be communicated to residents in subsequent shifts is even greater.

**Verbal and Written
Reports**

Clear documentation in the mother's chart decreases the possibility that conflicts arising out of poor communication will occur. It is not sufficient, however, to enter into the chart only the fact that the mother and her partner were counseled. Proper documentation requires:

A brief summary of the clinical situation;

A description of alternatives for patient management;

Input from parents;

Decisions made as to selection of care plan and response of parents to this choice.

Additionally, a verbal report should be provided new personnel when change of shift occurs. This type of communication, in addition to proper documentation in the chart, reduces the chance that a pediatrician, called to the delivery room before he or she has had time to review the records, will be uninformed about previously made care plans for the newborn.

WHAT IF THE COURSE OF ACTION IS UNCERTAIN?

**Verifying Unclear
Decisions**

Occasionally, discussions with parents prior to delivery fail to yield a concise plan of management for the newborn. For some, ethical or religious issues complicate formulation of care plans. More often, issues have not been presented to parents in a clear enough manner to allow them to participate in decision making. Medical students are taught that if they are unable to develop a definitive diagnosis following history taking and physical examination, then they should return to the patient and retake the patient's history. This approach should be extended to care of the newborn patient, whose parents are his or her advocate. When newborn care plans are inexact, care providers should go back to the parents and review pertinent issues. Only then can a clear plan of management be developed.

WHERE TO DELIVER? WHERE TO TAKE THE BABY?

When newborn survival is not an issue, medical personnel may see no harm in allowing a patient to deliver in a labor bed. This decision may be seen as unavoidable because of the unpredictable manner in which a tiny fetus passes through an incompletely dilated cervix. Unfortunately, the mother may view this decision in a very negative manner. Fear of abandonment is common among women in labor with a dead or nonviable fetus. The woman laboring alone in a labor room (or, even more unfortunately, in her bed on the ward), who delivers before someone gets back to her, can feel terribly isolated and rejected by the staff. Also, being left to deliver in a labor bed may contribute to the woman's sense of failure and feeling that she was not important enough to be taken to the delivery room and was left to soil herself and her bed. Worse is the more painful feeling, "My baby wasn't important enough to be given the care he or she needed." What is the difference in the manner in which medical personnel and parents perceive such a delivery? The difference is not in expected outcome. The 19-week newborn will die. The difference is in the perception of what can be done.

Professional Perceptions of the Event

The physician (or nurse) analyzes this event and knows, "We cannot do anything for this baby." Yet, when parents hear, "We cannot help your baby," withholding resuscitation may be linked in their interpretation by cause-and-effect to outcome. Whenever the message that the baby cannot be saved is conveyed to the parents, it should be clearly stated that no amount of resuscitation will allow this baby to survive. Medical staff may believe that if the outcome is predetermined, then resuscitation in any form is of no value. This premise leads to the clinical argument that the baby can be delivered in a labor bed. Since the baby is only of 19 weeks' gestation and will not survive, the staff will not transport him or her to the nursery, which would only increase the parents' medical bills unnecessarily. Moreover, taking the baby to the neonatal intensive care unit (NICU) might mean that the staff would have to attempt full resuscitation, including endotracheal tube placement, use of ventilators, and umbilical artery catheterization—all for what purpose?

Parents' Needs

Parents may view these events differently. They want everything possible done, as they cling to hope for a miracle that will save their baby, in spite of what they know to be inevitable. Despite the inevitable outcome, parents still have strong needs (see Figure 4.3). Parents often conceptualize their baby in adult terms: "If an adult only needs oxygen under these circumstances, then maybe that's all my baby needs." They do not want their baby to suffer any pain. It is these desires that can provide direction as medical personnel struggle to resolve the dilemma: "How can we 'do something' when our medical knowledge is clear on the outcome for this 19-week newborn?" The answer lies in distinguishing between "doing something for the baby" as a process by itself and "resuscitating" in order to attempt to save the baby's life.

Parents want to believe that their baby did not die alone or lonely.

They want to feel that "everything reasonable" was done to support their child as long as he or she survived.

Concern that their baby was abandoned by the medical staff or suffered with pain or cold before he or she died is extremely difficult to bear.

Most parents, if offered the opportunity, desperately want to be with and hold their baby before and, if possible, while he or she dies.

Figure 4.3. Concerns of parents whose baby is too young to survive.

WHAT ARE THE CHOICES?

There is no simple formula for managing delivery of a previable fetus. A fundamental question that must be examined early in the process is, "What are the parents' wishes?" An extension of this is, "Are these wishes realistic and soundly based on information given parents by the obstetric/pediatric team before delivery?" Two choices that reach some middle ground between parents' needs and medical (and financial) realities are as follow.

What Actions to Take Upon Delivery

1. *Let parents hold their baby in the delivery room.* If this choice is offered, parents must also be informed that their baby, because of his or her extreme immaturity, will die. The parents should be asked if they would prefer to hold their wrapped baby in the delivery room for the brief time before death occurs. Medical personnel should respect the meaning of this moment in the family's life and thus be aware of noise levels and activity in the delivery room. Any medical procedures that must be performed for the mother should be carried out with a minimum of interference in parents' time with their dying baby. Parents and baby may be moved to a quiet room to be together after their baby has died.

   It is important that a pediatrician be available in case questions suddenly arise in the minutes following delivery. There are three medical issues that must be considered. First, if the baby is larger or more advanced in gestation than expected, the pediatrician suddenly may need to change care plans and transfer the baby to the neonatal intensive care unit (NICU). Second, parents must be informed prior to the birth that their baby may make involuntary movements, gasp, or exhibit a slow heart rate for minutes or hours after delivery. This information is important for parents to know in advance so that they do not, in retrospect, come to believe that their decision to hold their baby in the delivery room prevented him or her from surviving, or even that their decision hastened their baby's death. Finally, some member of the medical team may need to decide if, after a given period of time (e.g., 20 minutes), the baby exhibits strong activity, whether he or she should be taken to the NICU even though death is inevitable. In this circumstance, care providers must understand, however, that the rationale to leave the baby with parents or to move him or her to the NICU must be based on relieving parental anxiety. This decision should not be made out of convenience to the medical staff or as a method of resolving personal anxieties of care providers. Allowing parents to be with their baby as he or she dies must be compassionately balanced with ensuring that parents know that their baby was not denied appropriate medical care.

2. *Take the baby to the neonatal intensive care unit (NICU).* Some parents may prefer that their baby be provided care in the NICU. In many ways, this parental response may effectively act out the plea, "Please do what you can for my baby." Unfortunately, this option can cause a rift between some neonatologists/pediatricians and parents, which could be avoided if medical personnel were to consider this issue through the parents' eyes. To physicians and nurses in the NICU, the issue creates its own crisis: the emphasis becomes one not of "whether" but "where" the baby will die. The medical team, accustomed to extensive, highly technologic resuscitative procedures, may be frustrated and made to feel inept by their role of merely placing a tiny baby in an isolette and only piping in oxygen by small tubing.

Parents' interpretation of what they perceive as "high tech" care may help to diminish the frustration experienced by medical personnel. Statements such as, "The pediatricians and nurses did everything they could," or "She [the baby] was a real fighter, right up to the end," underscore the parents' need to reassure themselves that they were not responsible for their baby's death and truly "did everything" to assist medical faculty to care for the baby. Other statements such as, "Several nurses were specially assigned to her crib," and even, "There were a lot of people in the delivery room I didn't recognize, but they were all very concerned for our Jamie," indicate how important the perception of events is to parents as they begin to confront their sadness, guilt, anger, and emptiness in the weeks and months afterward.

CASE 2: *Delivery of the potentially viable newborn who dies*

A 28-year-old gravida 2, para 1, black female in preterm labor with a breech presentation at 26 weeks gestation. Because of the failure of tocolytic drugs to inhibit labor, delivery by cesarean section was necessary, resulting in the birth of a 750-gram female with Apgar scores of 3, 4, and 7 at 1, 5, and 10 minutes, respectively. Appropriate resuscitation was carried out in the delivery room by neonatal personnel. The baby was stable in the NICU during the first day, but required ventilatory support. The next day, her condition deteriorated rapidly. Over a 4-hour period, it became increasingly difficult to maintain her heart rate and blood pressure. The decision to discontinue life support was ultimately made, and the baby expired.

Delivery of the very premature baby creates many new issues that do not exist when the baby is clearly nonviable.

WHEN TO STOP RESUSCITATION?

A troublesome question for pediatricians is when to stop resuscitating the baby who fails to respond to all efforts. The anticipated anxiety created by this concern evokes the questions, "Should we begin resuscitation at all?" and "If we begin to resuscitate, when should we stop?" This conflict is most often encountered when an extremely premature newborn of 500–750 grams delivers. It is complicated by the fact that survival rates of newborns weighing 500–750 grams continues to improve—the survival rates of such infants delivered at the University of Cincinnati increased from 14% in 1981 to 35% in 1984 (1).

Guidelines for Initiating Resuscitation

As a reasonable approach to this difficult issue, one may choose to begin resuscitation when in doubt about the baby's weight or when the baby is believed to be older than 24 weeks or larger than 600 grams. If the baby responds to resuscitation (improvement in heart rate, respiratory response, tone, activity, or color), he or she is stabilized and taken to the NICU for further care. If the baby is judged to be younger than 24 weeks or under 600 grams and resuscitation fails to elicit evidence of response, the most senior pediatrician on the resuscitation team at some point should discontinue resuscitation and declare the baby dead.

Under these circumstances, as parents helplessly observe the fruitless resuscitative measures, they must be informed that their baby may make involuntary movements or even gasp occasionally. If parents choose to hold their swaddled baby in the delivery room, a pediatrician should stay to assist them and to answer questions that commonly arise during this critical period. Occasionally, a baby will gasp or make involuntary movements for what seems to be a very long time, which distresses parents. A considerate gesture in such an instance may be to offer parents the option of transferring their baby to a warm isolette in the NICU.

IMPACT OF THE NICU—REASSURING OR FRIGHTENING?

Having a baby in the NICU for any reason is considerably stressful to parents. The medical community views the NICU as the acme of pediatric high technology. They must try, however, to see the unit through the eyes of uninformed, worried mothers and fathers. Parents whose baby's destiny will be determined in the NICU are both pulled toward and repelled by the elaborate and complex equipment and procedures in the NICU.

Within this strange technologic environment, parents confront a potential loss and a real loss. The possibility of their baby's dying may become more real as time passes and their understanding of their baby's condition increases. A more immediate and tangible loss is the loss of control over their own family, a sense that in this setting they are incapable of acting as parents. Parents are unable to reach across the barriers of plastic tubes, monitors, and intravenous lines to protect their baby from pain, isolation, and death.

Parents May Listen Selectively

Parents of a newborn in the NICU desperately want information about their baby's condition. This information must be provided clearly, concisely, and simply. As hospital staff attempt to keep parents informed of a newborn's condition, they often find that the stress of this situation may cause parents to listen selectively. The dedicated young resident approaches the parent whose newborn son has just been brought to the NICU and says, "*We* have never seen a baby that small survive." The parents hear instead, "We have *never* seen a baby that small survive." As parents enter the NICU to see their baby for the first time, the neonatologist warns them, "Your son is awfully small." They only hear the message, "Your son is *too* small." The nurse explains that the ventilator is designed to help the immature baby breathe. Parents think that the ventilator is a support system of final resort and that if it is turned off it heralds the end of their baby's life. Other ambiguous expressions that can convey alarming messages are, "Your baby is unstable," "is not looking good," "had a bad night," "is not as responsive," "has deteriorated," or "has gone downhill."

"HOW CLOSE SHOULD I GET TO MY BABY?"

Parents' Need to Protect Themselves versus Their Need to Create Memories

This is a question that parents frequently ask when their very premature newborn is in the NICU. The dilemma was encapsulated by one parent who said, "How close should I get to my baby, whom I do not yet know, but who may soon die?" This question illustrates an understandable struggle. To become emotionally involved with this new baby, parents have to open themselves up to their feelings. This can be very painful when it is either possible or, in fact, probable that their baby is going to die. Getting close to their baby means that parents are not trying to "protect" themselves, and so the sense of loss they would feel if their baby were to die is more personal. To withdraw from a baby whose prognosis is poor presumably protects parents' emotions. But, after the baby dies, parents realize that they missed a precious time that they cannot recover.

The same conflict exists universally in the case of a dying child or adult. What differentiates the situation in the NICU from any other type of anticipated death is that the new parent-child relationship has no past. In the NICU, even as parents try to create a bond with their baby, they see it disintegrating. This conflict, with which each parent must cope individually, can produce confusion, fear, anger, and frustration. The longer the newborn's condition remains unstable, the more complicated this struggle may become.

Helping Parents Bond With Their Baby

It is the author's opinion that all parents should be encouraged to spend as much time as possible with their baby in the NICU, to become as close as time and medical interventions permit. When parents are seen weeks or months after their baby has died, they express their appreciation for having had those moments together. No parent has ever said, "I wasted time by being with my son (or daughter) before he (or she) died." Parents who consciously pulled away from their baby before death as a means of protecting their own emotions may later regret this distancing. In the end, this attempt is pointless, and parents are disappointed and angry with the medical staff for "allowing" them to distance themselves from their son or daughter. NICU staff can accelerate parental efforts to bond to their baby by helping create a "personality" for the baby. Figure 4.4 lists means of achieving this bond. Even an hour or a day may be sufficient time to create a "past" on which parent and baby can bond. To fail to commit such time to this relationship leaves parents feeling empty, with the profound wish that they had done things differently.

Always refer to the baby by his or her name.

Provide parents information about unique aspects of the baby's behavior that they can perceive as "their baby's behavior." Examples of such observations are:

He likes to sleep on his side;

She seems to know when you [the mother or father] are here;

He sometimes gets cranky when we replace the endotracheal tube;

She's a real fighter.

These statements identify a baby as unique and uniquely personable to a parent desperate for evidence of family lineage.

Messages written on the isolette as if from newborn to parent provide information to parents as well as a sense that they have communicated with their baby. These messages may be as simple as, "Hi, I'm Sara," or "Dear Mom and Dad, a parents' support group is meeting next Tuesday evening to talk about babies like me and families like ours." Whatever their content, these messages convey a sense of family ties and common goals.

Figure 4.4.   Enhancing bonds between parent and baby in the NICU.

LEAVING WITHOUT THE BABY

Delivery of a very premature newborn mandates that the mother will be discharged from the hospital without her baby. In most cases, therefore, parents return to their home that they have made ready for their baby, fearing that their baby will never come home. Parents feel guilty when they have to leave their baby behind. They worry that their baby will not be cared for by people who love him or her as much as they do. Some guilt arises from the concern that, if their baby's condition deteriorates drastically, they will not have time to get to the hospital to be present when death occurs. Time becomes a focus of anxiety. A universal concern among parents is that their baby will be left alone or lonely. The medical community can ease this fear by explaining to parents the responsibilities of staff members caring for their baby.

ROLE OF THE NICU NURSE

In most NICUs, the number of nurses assigned to care for each newborn is limited. Thus, parents can rely on a few nurses who have primary responsibility for their baby's comfort and care. These nurses, because of their day-to-day, round-the-clock contact with the baby, become the unique common denominator in all interactions between baby and parent, baby and staff, and also parent and staff.

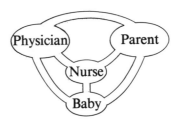

Nurse As Primary Advocate for the Baby and Parents

As constant care provider among the medical staff, the nurse may recognize early, subtle changes in a baby's condition. Does the baby exhibit bradycardia when he or she is touched or stimulated? Does he or she appear to be more stable in one position than in another? How does the baby tolerate oral or tracheal suctioning, reintubation, or tube feedings? By conveying changes in behavioral or response patterns to the physician, the nurse may be responsible for significant modifications in the baby's care plan, and therefore is best qualified to anticipate serious changes in the baby's condition.

As advocate for the parents, the nurse must search for cues from parents in order to anticipate their needs. The nurse must recognize these points:

Parents may be overwhelmed to see that their baby is much smaller than they expected he or she could be.

Parents may need assistance and encouragement to reach into an isolette and touch their tiny baby.

Parents may be intimidated by the wires and monitors connected to their baby.

Parents may be frustrated at their inability to pick up and hold their baby when he or she cries.

Toys placed in the isolette offer visual or tactile stimulation for the newborn. They also operate as a symbol of normal childhood activities, representing the parents' hope that their baby someday can leave the hospital nursery and go home to a healthy, normal childhood. Toys also soften the sterile, hospital appearance of the isolette specifically and the NICU in general.

Some parents wish to become familiar with medical terminology and procedures that relate to their baby. When this need is evidenced by parents, the nurse and physician should encourage all questions. They should explain events clearly to the parents, as a means of closing the gap between medical jargon and normal conversation.

Other parents may seek reassurance that their baby is improving, even if this reassurance must come in the form of technical terms such as pO_2, heart rate, blood pressure, or respirator settings. No component of medicine is so sophisticated that it cannot be described in simple and understandable terms. If these types of measurements are provided to parents as gauges of their baby's condition, they should be explained clearly, in a way that parents can understand. Even if medical jargon is difficult to translate into more understandable terms, no one should assume that parents will not be interested enough to warrant that effort on the part of the staff.

Some parents express a desire for information, but then are intimidated by too many facts. The care provider must exercise judgment in conferences with parents in which either lengthy care plans or complicated discussions of the baby's status are discussed. The risk of overwhelming parents with too much information can be reduced if in follow-up the parents are asked questions such as "Did you understand what was said?," "Did the discussion raise new questions?," or "Was anything said that you did not understand?" Following up on a formal discussion by meeting for a second informal session—say at the baby's isolette—puts parents at ease and encourages future communication.

Some parents do not know how to ask questions or even which questions they ought to ask of medical personnel. These are parents who are likely to be most confused or frightened about their baby's condition. They may be at highest risk of being traumatized by the NICU experience. Special attention should be paid to a parent who neither asks questions nor expresses his or her emotions. Passivity can be a warning signal that this parent is suffering overwhelming emotional damage and cannot cope with the situation.

Fathers generally prefer to visit a baby in the NICU for shorter periods of time than mothers, who often exhibit a desire to spend most of their time in the NICU. This difference in visiting patterns may in no way reflect the individual parent's love for his or her baby. Instead, the length and frequency of visits may be influenced by work schedules, family responsibilities, or individual preference. Nonetheless, differing needs and expectations can produce anger between parents if the duration and number of visits become equated with involvement with or commitment to the baby.

All parents hope that their baby recognizes them when they come to visit, even if the baby is extremely immature or if his or her health is severely compromised. They imagine that their baby's actions, such as grasping the parent's hand, turning his or her head, or making facial expressions subtly acnkowledge the parents' presence. It is immaterial if these actions are reflexive on the baby's part. If a mother perceives them as a sign of communication with her baby, then their meaning ought not to be depreciated by the medical staff. Rather, this form of communication between parent and baby should be strongly encouraged as a way of establishing a family bond that may at best be tenuous or incomplete.

After their baby has been in the NICU for more than a few days, parents become aware of and begin following the clinical course of newborns in adjacent isolettes. For many, the camaraderie among parents whose babies are next to each other can be beneficial. True adult friendships may emerge. Occasionally, even friendly competition between families develops, as daily weight gain, activity, and feeding habits become the indices of comparison. The positive effects that sharing and support have under these stressful circumstances need not be spelled out.

When a newborn's condition deteriorates, his or her parents' attitudes toward other babies' parents and the staff may change. Anger may surface when their own baby is doing worse than those in adjacent isolettes. Parents suddenly may resent the fact that other newborns (and their parents) are not experiencing similar problems. This response, by itself, can evoke guilt as the parent struggles with the issue, "What type of person am I to wish this on others?" Parents thus pull back from friendships that have been developing in the NICU. The other parents' support may diminish, too, because they feel threatened by what they see happening to the baby whose condition is worsening. Under these circumstances, it is more important than ever that communication between staff and parents remain intact. If rapid medical intervention has to be initiated and the parents are shoved aside, even if only momentarily, then they may feel that they are being excluded in medical decisions for their baby. Intellectually, they are aware of the need for immediate action, and they realize that they cannot assist in the effort.

NICU nurses must be aware of these dynamics and their impact on the parents of a baby in the nursery. They must anticipate parents' needs and respond by volunteering information, introducing a shy couple to other parents in the NICU, or showing parents how to make contact with their isolated baby. Nurses can identify potential problems and warning signs to help parents cope emotionally with whatever outcome they face for their baby. In time, a blending of responsibilities between parent and medical staff occurs, thereby diminishing parents' fears that "no one" will be with their baby if an emergency occurs. Making an effort to allow parent and care provider to gain trust in each other promotes a team concept of care.

ANTICIPATING THAT THE BABY MAY DIE

Anticipatory Grief

For some parents, there is a point of recognition in the course of their baby's care that death is probable. This awareness may be manifested by missed visits to the NICU. Other parents may exhibit fatigue, as if worn down by their hopeless vigil. Lindemann (2) first described this phenomenon in which a person pulls back emotionally from a dying loved one as protection from the impact of sudden death. Referred to as "anticipatory grief," the response as initially described represents an individual's efforts to confront his or her adjustment after a dying loved one's death by experiencing stages of grief before the death occurs. In this process, depression, preoccupation with the deceased and the death itself, and hope that a miraculous recovery is possible may precede the baby's death. When the baby does die, parents may experience less of an acute reaction. It is as though accepting the inevitable has allowed them to begin the transition from grief to recovery in a safe and predictable environment.

WISHING THAT THE BABY WOULD DIE

Sense of Hopelessness

Sometimes, parents deep within themselves begin to wish that their precious baby would die. They may or may not be capable of acknowledging this horrifying thought. But, when they begin to wonder if any of the drastic medical procedures undertaken for their baby will do any good, they may have to suppress the wish that it all could be over—for their own sake as well as for their baby's. If the baby's doctors make it sound as though the baby has little chance for a normal, healthy life, then this desire may intensify. Parents justifiably begin to acknowledge what it would mean to bring home a handicapped, unresponsive baby and to have to care for him or her in quite a different manner than they had anticipated. Yet parents feel terribly selfish and guilty about admitting, even if only to themselves, that they might be better off if their baby were to die. It is extremely painful for parents to recognize that this thought has invaded their consciousnesses, even if only fleetingly. When the baby does die, parents cannot help feeling guilty for having contemplated the death.

BREASTFEEDING

The issue of breastfeeding, seemingly so beneficial to the baby in the NICU, can create significant conflict for parents. It is common practice in NICUs for staff to encourage the mother to pump her breasts and provide milk for her baby. The reasoning is, "Since your baby is very small, he (or she) will need the nourishment and antibodies only your breastmilk can provide. We hope, for your baby's sake, that you will pump your breasts and bring us the milk, so that we can store it and give it to your baby when he or she needs it." This request clearly focuses on the baby's needs. How can it produce a conflict?

Breast engorgement in the postpartum period is a constant reminder that delivery has occurred. When delivery yields a healthy baby, breast engorgement is greeted as a physical sign of a positive event. When pregnancy results in a critically premature newborn who lies in the NICU close to death, breast engorgement may be viewed negatively or even with anger by the mother who is left with physical signs of the process, but without the desired product, a healthy baby. Indeed, a problem that the mother confronts is trying to believe that her baby will ever need the breastmilk. When the baby's prognosis is very poor, the mother may find it impossible to believe that there is a reason to pump her breasts, collect the milk, and store it properly until she transports it back to the NICU. Additionally, she may feel so despondent about her baby's situation that she cannot manage the strenuous effort necessary to do all of this.

Conflicting Demands on the Woman

A sense of guilt increases as requests for breastmilk complicate attempts by the couple to begin reestablishing their own sexual relationship. In itself, efforts to put normality back into their lives create conflict. Engaging anew in their sexual relations serves the future-oriented purpose of rebuilding the man-woman relationship. But sexual intercourse also is the cause by which a tiny baby now lies in an NICU with little chance for survival. Breast stimulation for many couples is a pleasurable component of their sexual activity. Thus, breast stimulation and breast engorgement may emerge as opposing processes. The woman is at the center of this conflict. To have to select one over the other may make her feel forced to choose between her baby and the father of the baby. She feels guilty because she "failed" her baby and partner by delivering prematurely. She also may feel guilty if her partner wants to resume their sexual relationship as soon as her doctor indicates that she has recovered sufficiently from her pregnancy and delivery. Many women have little desire for sex in the time immediately following delivery, particularly when the postpartum period is complicated by stress and depression that accompany premature delivery and a vigil at the baby's bedside in the NICU. Clearly, there is a large potential for guilt and confusion as parents strive to rebuild their personal lives without abandoning the needs of their baby in the NICU.

HOW FREQUENTLY TO VISIT

The unconscious desire to protect one's emotions from anticipation of the baby's death may manifest itself in the frequency with which parents visit the NICU. It is an understatement that visiting the NICU two or three times a day to be with a baby impacts heavily on other family activities or needs. The emotional drain and commitment to be at the hospital so often, especially over an extended period, exact their toll on the family as a whole and on individual family members. When a parent misses a visit, the seemingly harmless statement, "I noticed you didn't come in to see Johnny yesterday," can be interpreted as condemnation and criticism, as if confirming the idea, "You are less of a parent than you should be."

Certain circumstances may exaggerate these conflicts of guilt and responsibility. At times, a baby may need to be transported to a larger hospital for more extensive newborn care. In rural areas, this may mean several hours of travel between home and hospital. Physical separation, knowledge that unknown nurses and doctors now are involved in the baby's care, and the inherent difficulties in maintaining close communication between parent and medical staff create a major challenge for the healthcare system. The frequency of parental visits may decrease as parents attempt to deal with their situation. Care providers may misinterpret this phenomenon and begin to suspect that these parents do not care. Once this attitude begins to pervade the NICU environment, trust disappears rapidly, and an irreversible breakdown in communication between parents and medical staff can ensue. For the parent who unconsciously pulls away from a dying baby to protect his or her emotions, this sequence becomes a self-fulfilling prophecy. By talking months or years later with parents who experienced this problem, one can appreciate the resultant extraordinary sense of loss and separation. Their sadness and emptiness are complicated by anger directed at the medical community, who knew better but allowed these parents to use emotional defense mechanisms to try to insulate themselves against their baby's death.

Scheduling Visits to Reduce an Unrealistic Sense of Obligation

To relieve some of the burden associated with visiting the baby, care providers may choose to help parents establish a reasonable visiting schedule. When long-term newborn care is involved, the stresses involved with daily visitations soon are

An established visiting schedule permits parents, when they are at home, to concentrate their energies on such family issues as other children, household necessities, and the marital relationship.

When parents do visit their baby in the NICU, their attention can be focused entirely on the baby. The goal is to help diminish the sense of guilt that they should be at home doing other things.

When parents are at home, they should feel confident that their baby is in the care of familiar and trusted nurses and physicians. They need reassurance that any changes in the baby's condition would be relayed to them immediately.

Visiting schedules may vary depending on a baby's condition, the number of days or weeks since delivery, and the distance of the parents' home from the hospital.

Figure 4.5. Helping parents establish a schedule for visiting the NICU.

particularly strong. One cannot be in two places— physically or mentally—at the same time. Yet, the guilt caused by a parent reducing the number of hospital visits may overshadow this reality. The NICU nurse may be the first care provider to detect the conflicting demands imposed on parents by home and by hospital. Informal conversations between parent and nurse may verify the nature of this conflict. The nurse (or nurse and physician together) may acknowledge the stresses that home and hospital impose on parents and suggest that a more reasonable visiting schedule be established. Saying, "It's okay if you don't come every day. We'll keep you informed of everything that's happening," may remove a considerable burden from a family. Additional discussion may include advice on the points raised in Figure 4.5. For some parents, dropping one visit per week may be the most they can allow themselves to depart from their schedule of daily, twice-daily, or several visits per day. For others, depending on the circumstances, the expectation that they will visit two or three times per week allows them to restore some structure in their lives.

"HOW WILL I BE NOTIFIED IF SOMETHING HAPPENS?"

Consistent Phone Contact to Relieve Parents' Fears

An inevitable fear for parents is that they will receive a phone call from the hospital telling them that their baby has died. This fear is made worse by the common assumption among parents that "any news is bad news." To forestall this attitude, NICU nurses at the University of Cincinnati call parents on a regular basis to update them on their baby's progress. Knowing that a phone call from the hospial is likely to contain good news ("good activity today," "fed well," "seemed very alert") greatly reduces parents' anxieties when they hear the phone ring. In addition, offering parents the use of a toll-free number (when available) to call for specific information permits parents ready access at all times to the NICU staff. This form of ongoing phone contact decreases the emotional distance between home and hospital for parents who must make the trip several times a week from the outside world to the specialized world of the NICU.

HOW CAN PARENTS BE BETTER EDUCATED?

Many NICUs have established peer support groups for parents. In group sessions, usually held weekly or monthly, many problems that arise within the NICU are openly discussed. Topics that parents discuss with other parents and with medical staff are listed in Figure 4.6. At the University of Cincinnati, group meetings for parents with babies in the NICU are held twice monthly.

NICU Support-Group Meetings for Parents

At the first of these meetings, the month's attending neonatologist and an NICU nurse talk with and answers questions from parents. At the second meeting, held 2 weeks later, the hospital chaplain and/or social worker serve as moderators for conversations and expressions of concern among parents. A nurse from the NICU is present at every meeting, which brings

Stresses on the family with a baby in the NICU.

Fear that the baby will die.

Fear that the baby will survive handicapped.

Visiting the baby in the NICU—how often, how long?

Parental guilt—where does it come from?

How do the baby's brothers and sisters react to the NICU?

What are emotional conflicts felt by grandparents?

How does a parent maintain contact with a baby in the NICU and at the same time rebuild a life at home?

If the baby's condition changes rapidly, will parents have time to get to the hospital before he or she dies?

If the baby dies, will he or she die in pain?

Figure 4.6. Support group topics for parents whose baby is in the NICU.

continuity to the discussion. In most critical care nurseries, nurses are familiar with most of the babies' histories. This level of awareness on the part of nursing personnel gives parents the sense that each baby is important and cared for. At the second meeting, videotapes concerning parental reactions to the NICU experience are shown to encourage parents to express their own feelings. "A Joyful Tear" (Ross Laboratories) is one such videotape available commercially for this purpose.

The meetings are held in a room close to the NICU. When it is time for a meeting to begin, a general invitation is issued in the NICU to any parents who have time to join in the discussion. Many parents who might not travel from home to attend such a meeting will agree to join in because they are already at the hospital and because, as they view their baby in the NICU, the reality of their stressful situation is undeniable.

In addition to holding meetings to explore issues of concern to parents, many NICUs have created programs to teach parents skills, such as cardiopulmonary resuscitation (CPR), which might be needed if their baby ultimately is discharged from the nursery. Whether or not parents will actually need these skills, learning them makes parents feel more in control and more confident that they could assume responsibility for their baby. This form of education also serves to broaden parents' understanding of the activities within the NICU and to demystify procedures and methods of care provided the baby.

CARING FOR PARENTS AS A BABY DIES

Sudden Death.   There is little warning when a very premature baby's condition suddenly deteriorates and the baby dies. Because of the unpredictable nature of this event, parents often are not at the hospital when it occurs. In most intensive care nurseries, the nurse or physician will baptize the baby. This simple gesture, although easily overlooked in the commotion of the moment, is extremely important and appreciated by most parents months or years after the baby's death. The urgent primary task is to inform parents of their baby's death. The following recommendations are suggested:

Guidelines for Informing Parents

The pediatrician or neonatologist most involved in the baby's care should telephone the parents. In some centers, the NICU nurse, because of her long-standing relationship with the baby and family, may be the one who contacts parents directly. This action on the part of specific physicians or nurses precludes the possibility that parents will imagine that the phone call was made by mistake to the wrong parents.

It is wrong to tell parents over the telephone, "Your baby has taken a turn for the worse; I think you should come in now," if, in fact, the baby has already died in the NICU. Hearing this statement, parents will drive hastily to the hospital, hoping to get there before it is too late. Cases of car accidents resulting from parents' panic and sense of urgency underscore the dangers of this type of message. Moreover, parents who rush to the hospital—only to find that their baby died before the doctor or nurse called—will be angry, discounting entirely any good intentions of medical personnel. The physician or nurse speaking to parents by telephone should advise them to have a neighbor or friend drive them to the hospital, to reduce their risk of being involved in an auto accident.

Once parents have arrived at the hospital, they should be allowed time alone with their baby in a quiet room. (These principles have been discussed in detail in Chapter 3.)

Important messages that should be communicated to parents are (1) their baby did not die in pain and (2) nurses or other medical personnel were with the baby when he or she died. If they themselves are unable to be present at the time, all parents wish when their baby dies that he or she may be with people who care.

Imminent Death.   There are times in the NICU when a very premature newborn fails to respond to resuscitative measures and his or her death is imminent. This situation is difficult for everyone concerned. However, if managed properly, it represents medical care at its finest. The scenario is usually a variation of the following: Upon delivery, the baby's health may have been stabilized in response to ventilator support and IV therapy. At some point, however, the newborn's condition becomes unstable, and he or she may even require resuscitation once or repeatedly. The heart rate and blood pressure begin to fluctuate and then, despite stabilizing drugs, to decline. NICU personnel converge and agree that continued resuscitation will not reverse the process. They agree that death is expected.

Calling Parents before Baby Has Died

At this point, the most senior pediatrician, neonatologist, or NICU nurse should call the parents, if they are not in the hospital, and inform them of their baby's changing clinical course. In honest, firm, but considerate terms, parents should be told that their baby is likely to die soon and that they should come to the hospital. This information should be related in a concerned but not an alarming manner, in order not to exacerbate parents' apprehensions. The parents should be asked if a friend or neighbor can drive them to the hospital. In this interim period, every reasonable effort should be made to keep the baby alive until parents arrive at the hospital. The importance of parents' being able to hold their dying baby cannot be emphasized enough.

When the parents arrive at the hospital, they should be met by the baby's pediatrician and nurse as soon as possible. During this encounter, the baby's health and anticipated death should be discussed calmly and honestly. These points should be discussed thoroughly:

1. Additional resuscitation or other techniques or tests will not reverse the process. The baby's death is inevitable.
2. The baby is being attended to continuously by nursery personnel who know and care about him or her.

The parents should be taken to their baby's isolette. They should be permitted to see and touch their baby.

HOLDING THE BABY AS HE OR SHE DIES

Parents have to decide whether or not they wish to hold their baby while he or she dies. The complexity of this issue must be appreciated before it is presented to parents. In an isolette, the baby is separated physically from parents by respirator tubing, IV lines, and EKG or other wires. The emotional impact of these barriers is even greater at the time of death. Months later, parents will comment that equipment obstructed their ability to reach out to their baby. They feel terribly sad that they could not freely caress their baby in the last minutes of life.

WHEN TO REMOVE THE "EQUIPMENT BARRIER"

Offering the Choice to Remove Life-Support Equipment

When death is imminent, the physician and nurse should give parents an opportunity to hold their baby as the life-support equipment is withdrawn. This option should never be offered in such a manner as to suggest that the decision to withdraw life support rests with the baby's parents. Parents must not feel that they are responsible for their baby's death. Instead, the physician should make the statement that life-support equipment can no longer contribute to the baby's care. Therefore, the equipment may be removed if the parents choose, so that they may hold their baby at the moment of death. EKG leads and other lines should be gradually discontinued. The baby should then be taken off the respirator and ventilated by hand. These actions should not be done quickly, but should be carried out in a caring and compassionate manner. The baby should then be wrapped and placed in the arms of the mother or father. The family should be seated, preferably in a quiet area of the nursery. Finally, with the parents' consent, the endotracheal tube should be removed and the baby allowed to die. Intense emotions pervade the moments as the baby dies.

CASE 3: *The unexpected death of a newborn*

> *A 40-year-old gravida 2, para 1, black female at 43 weeks experienced an unremarkable labor, leading to vaginal delivery of a term 4380-gram male with Apgar scores at 1 and 5 minutes of 8 and 9, respectively.* The baby was moved to the normal nursery for routine care. That night, the baby deteriorated and died suddenly. The parents refused to have an autopsy performed.

One may choose to dismiss this type of newborn death as "unusual," "unique," or "very infrequent." It is similar, however, to a more common case, such as when the newborn dies shortly after birth from meconium aspiration, a cardiac anomaly, or placental abruption. Common to these events is the anguish and anger shared by parents and medical staff. This event is complicated further if general anesthesia has been given to the mother for an emergency cesarean section and the baby dies before she has awakened. It is even more frustrating and disturbing if the parents will not permit an autopsy. This type of case comes as a shock to medical personnel and parents alike. It does not necessarily bring them closer together. The unjustified nature of the baby's death evokes unpleasant and often distrustful feelings for both.

Shock, Guilt, and Anger

In the absence of any forewarning, the baby's death brings out in parents many of the emotions observed following detection of an intrauterine fetal death. In this case, however, the three most intense feelings that surface are disbelief and shock ("What do you mean, my baby died?"), guilt ("I did this to my baby"), and anger ("Term babies don't just die in our sophisticated medical atmosphere. Someone messed up." Or, "They have switched babies on me!").

Medical personnel, pediatric or obstetric, may struggle with the following doubts:

Inevitable Doubts of Medical Personnel

Did I do something wrong?

What could I have done differently?

How do I confront this couple?

What if the family is angry at me?

These questions may ultimately evoke feelings of anger or rationalization as a protective shield:

Why didn't the patient agree to an autopsy? Now we'll never know exactly what happened.

We probably wouldn't have been able to do anything anyhow.

It's better that the baby died. It would have been worse if she had survived handicapped.

In this shocking, disastrous series of events, it may be difficult at times to distinguish care provider from care requirer. Both parties experience guilt, feel deprived unjustifiably, and resent the loss of a "sure thing." The patient refuses an autopsy because "You [medical personnel] have done enough already." The physician responds with, "By refusing an autospy, you [the parents] are depriving me of important information I need." The emotions build, so that any possibility for meaningful communication is destroyed. And both parties add to their loss.

Professional Responsibilities Toward the Patient

It is incumbent on medical personnel to recognize how readily this type of conflict can develop under such dramatic circumstances. Moreover, medical personnel must acknowledge that it is their responsibility, not the family's, to intervene in order to prevent an emotional impasse from developing. In this regard, the relationship between care provider and patient is obligatory in one direction only. The patient has a responsibility only to her immediate family and to her dead newborn. In contrast, the care provider is committed to caring for the patient and her family, despite any emotions that surface between them. To reject this obligation is to reject the basic premise upon which medical care is based. The care provider can help the patient in the following ways:

The obstetrician and pediatrician should meet with the patient and her family. The NICU nurse who attended the baby or the OB nurse may also wish to participate in the discussion.

Obstetric management and pediatric care of the newborn should be reviewed clearly, honestly, and unemotionally.

It is appropriate to express sadness over the baby's death. Conveying this type of intense emotion is not tacit acknowledgment of guilt or poor medical judgment.

Subsequent meetings should be arranged as often as necessary, even daily, with the family. In these meetings, the same issues may need to be discussed repeatedly. Sometimes, new questions will arise in response to previous discussions, and parents may have other issues to raise as their numbness wears off.

CASE 4: *The sudden infant death syndrome (SIDS)*

> *A 30-year-old gravida 1, para 0, white female delivers prematurely at 28 weeks gestation and experiences an uneventful postpartum course.* The daughter remains in the NICU for 2 months and then is discharged home to her parents' care. Growth and development are unremarkable. One afternoon when the baby is 7 months old, the mother has a babysitter in while she goes shopping. The baby is napping. When the sitter checks her, she finds the baby limp, cyanotic, and unresponsive. The life squad responds quickly to the sitter's call, but resuscitation is unsuccessful. At autopsy no cause of death is determined.

The sudden and unexplained death of a seemingly healthy infant ranks among the most chilling and destructive experiences that parents could ever encounter. This condition, referred to historically as a "cot death" or "crib death," today is more appropriately called the Sudden Infant Death Syndrome (SIDS). A few facts are known about this condition (3):

What Is Known about SIDS

SIDS is the third largest cause of infant mortality, after perinatal conditions and congenital anomalies.

It strikes 1 in 500 infants between the ages of 8 days and 2 years.

The peak age is 3 to 4 months; the peak time of year is winter.

Males are affected more often than females.

Most do not appear to have struggled before they died. By their orientation in the crib or the displacement of a blanket, some babies appear to have been active in the final moments before death; but many have been found lying in the same position as when they fell asleep.

The autopsy usually fails to reveal a cause of death.

Many theories have been proposed to explain this event. At this time, no clear etiology for SIDS has been documented.

Problems Arising after a SIDS Loss

The impact of this event on young parents is devastating. The unexpected death of their healthy child is unthinkable, horrifying to contemplate, and devastating to confront. After their shock has diminished, parents naturally begin to experience extreme guilt. In the absence of an explanation for their baby's death, their feeling of total responsibility may be made more intense by probing questions of neighbors or relatives. Worse, the coroner, police, or other officials may ask questions that pointedly probe for indications that child abuse has been involved. Tormented in the midst of their grief for their baby, couples may become victims of marital conflicts, face difficulties with their surviving children, and experience intense anxiety about future pregnancies (3).

Parents' reactions to and recovery after a SIDS death have been the subjects of several recent studies. Bluglass (4) reported six cases in which parental psychiatric disorders were linked directly to SIDS deaths (summarized in Figure 4.7). Although a small group by number, their diversity emphasizes how insidious this terrible event can be on both the nuclear and the extended family. Woodward et al. (3) followed 14 families, 8 of them closely, for several months after a SIDS death (2). In this series, couples were offered intense counseling by social workers, pediatricians, general practitioners, and peer support groups. The authors concluded from their investigations and interventions that professional counselors must be included as an essential component of the medical support system to assist families recovering from a SIDS death.

Children's Response to a SIDS Loss

The intense grief felt by parents of a SIDS baby also is experienced by surviving siblings but with more confusion or misunderstanding. Williams (5) evaluated 49 children from 23 families within 9 months of a SIDS death. Thirty-one of the 49 children were under 6 years of age, 8 were 6 to 9 years, and 10 were over the age of 10 years. Because the majority of these children had been present when the baby was found dead, many recalled seeing their discolored and lifeless sibling. Two children in a related study blamed their fathers for killing the baby. Both had watched their fathers' unsuccessful resuscitation attempts (3). Children under the age of 6 exhibited a variety of initial

Case 1: A father was embittered by being excluded by the rest of the extended family, who focused all their attention on the mother of the baby.

Case 2: Parents experienced extreme anxiety about their surviving child, which led to many inappropriate visits to the pediatrician and the emergency room.

Case 3: Foster parents of a 14-year-old mother whose child died of SIDS experienced intense but unrecognized grief. The foster grandmother exhibited many psychosomatic complaints that were poorly understood by the woman herself or by her physician until the issue of the baby's death was brought out and addressed.

Case 4: A husband developed many hypochondriacal complaints in an unconscious effort to draw attention to himself and his grieving.

Case 5: A mother blocked her grief reaction initially. Her failure to grieve resulted in severe depression and led her to consider suicide.

Case 6: The surviving twin of a SIDS baby was blamed for the mother's psychiatric maladjustment following the baby's death.

Figure 4.7. Six cases of parental psychiatric disorders following loss of a baby due to SIDS. Adapted from Bluglass (3).

reactions, ranging from screaming or crying along with the parents to maintaining normal play activities. In the weeks following the event, many children experienced anxiety and insecurity, frequently asking questions about what the outcome would be when they got sick or went to sleep. Some asked, "Who killed him [the baby]?" and others revealed their notion that the little brother or sister would return, as if death were a place to visit. During the period of follow-up, death of a pet or relative permitted some surviving siblings to express more completely their reaction to the SIDS death.

Children 6 to 9 years of age were able to accept the finality of death. Some became very supportive of grieving parents; others exhibited their preoccupation with the death of the sibling through drawings or play behavior. The oldest group of children (over 10 years of age) exhibited behavior similar to that of an adult. The children felt intense anger and sadness, but they often refused to talk about the baby's death.

From extensive counseling data, Williams (5) concluded that:

The response of young children is heavily influenced by egocentricism, magical thinking, and their belief in spirits and demons.

The ability of children to discuss a sibling's death with parents is influenced by the level of communication that exists between child and parents prior to the SIDS experience.

Families with preexisting abnormal behavioral dynamics respond more poorly to the baby's death than a family with a more stable background of interaction.

Foundations such as the National Sudden Infant Death Syndrome Foundation in Landover, Maryland, have been instrumental in educating parents and medical professionals alike about SIDS (6). The questions parents ask reflect the confusion and guilt that surrounds the event:

Did my baby suffer? Did he or she suffocate?

Did my baby have some kind of infection? Are my other children at risk?

Would breastfeeding have prevented this?

Will future babies be at risk of SIDS?

It is apparent, from the growing body of literature on SIDS, that the medical community has a significant responsibility to parents and families who experience a SIDS loss. Regrettably, news that a SIDS death has occurred may not always be relayed to proper care providers. The obstetrician involved in the SIDS baby's delivery often is uninformed, or if informed, is uninvolved in subsequent care of the parents. If there are no surviving siblings, the role of the pediatrician as counselor may be curtailed. The NICU nurse, who supervised the baby's care for days or weeks during the neonatal period, may learn of the baby's death only through unofficial channels. Parents may be fortunate enough to be referred to a peer support group. Until recently, however, the concept of SIDS was so poorly accepted (or even acknowledged) that parents were excluded from traditional community support systems. Fortunately, recognition of the need for parental support following a SIDS loss is rapidly expanding throughout the medical community.

PARENTS CALL FOR HELP

Typical SIDS Experiences

In a small community, the infrequency of a SIDS crisis makes it difficult to establish and maintain a clear communication network upon which to call when such an event occurs. On discovering their baby, parents usually call the police or fire department. The police make a determination as to whether or not they believe that child abuse was involved. In the absence of evidence of abuse or trauma, they release the baby to the parents. From the home the child is usually taken directly to a funeral home, unless the coroner or parents request an autopsy. In this unstructured arrangement, opportunities for involvement by other community health providers is limited and may not be used at all.

In Cincinnati, a communication network has been established to help when parents discover that their baby has died at home of SIDS. The parents, having found their baby dead, typically notify the fire department or life squad. Because of greater availability of fire ambulance units than of paramedics, the fire department usually is first to arrive at the home. If the baby is resuscitated, he or she is brought immediately to Children's Hospital Emergency Room for continued care. Many times, unfortunately, the baby cannot be resuscitated.

ROLE OF THE POLICE

When the initial phone call by parents is made, the police are notified simultaneously. They usually arrive within moments of the fire or paramedic unit. If the baby clearly is dead, then police, using a special van, transport him or her to Children's Hospital Emergency Room where he or she is pronounced dead. Police have access to a citywide chaplaincy service (provided by the Counsel of Christian Communions), which has been a resource available to the Cincinnati Police Department since 1971. Individual officers may or may not call in a chaplain to come to the family's assistance in the case of a SIDS death.

EMERGENCY ROOM RESOURCES

At the point when a SIDS baby arrives at the emergency room, several resources are activated simultaneously:

The social services unit immediately becomes involved to assist parents. This group of individuals is skilled in caring for parents of SIDS babies and acts as advocate and advisor.

The coroner is contacted by the emergency room physician and may select one of two management approaches:

1. To perform an autopsy.

2. To release the body to a funeral home. (If this choice is selected, social workers help parents contact the funeral director who, in turn, will cooperate with the parents to decide on subsequent care of the baby and burial decisions.)

Guidelines for Providing Support

In this *community* network, opportunities for extended care of a SIDS baby's parents originate from personnel resources in the emergency room.

The social worker (or emergency room physician) should contact the baby's pediatrician. The pediatrician can then establish a time to meet the parents. He or she may also notify the obstetrician of the crisis. (Chapter 10, "Obstetrician As Outpatient Counselor," offers recommendations for continued, long-term outpatient care.)

If applicable, the social worker should also inform the NICU of the baby's death. During the days and weeks that the baby was in the NICU, attending nurses very likely had become friends, confidantes, and advocates for the parents. In this time of crisis, these relationships with the parents take on renewed importance.

The social worker can advise parents of peer support groups in the community. Perhaps more important, in the first few weeks after such an event, the social worker can notify a SIDS support group that these parents have experienced this crisis and should be contacted by the group at a later date.

In this structured program, healthcare resources of the community are utilized in a logical manner to promote improved care of parents during the immediate crisis and to establish opportunities for long-term follow-up.

Cain and Cain (7) described in general terms four components to appropriate mourning that can be applied to parents experiencing a SIDS death. Parents must:

1. Comprehend and accept their baby's death;
2. Resolve anger and irrational guilt related to the death;
3. Eventually withdraw emotional investment from their dead baby;
4. Redirect interest and involvement with the lost baby's environment toward other children or activities.

Only when healthcare professionals such as obstetricians, pediatricians, nurses, chaplains, social workers, and peer support group leaders become involved in the SIDS issue will parents be provided the level of care needed for them to recover from this devastating life crisis.

SUMMARY

In this chapter, the author has discussed many complex issues surrounding delivery and death of a nonviable newborn, a potentially viable newborn, a term newborn, and an infant with SIDS. Common to these seemingly unrelated events is the psychologic trauma that impacts on parents, extended family, nurses, physicians, and other care providers. Each situation, however, is uniquely characterized by ethical, medical, and emotional decisions that confront parents and the medical community. Moreover, parents' perceptions and expectations of their newborn baby's care may differ significantly from that which is understood or generally accepted as reality in a NICU environment. Appropriate care of parents prior to or following death of their newborn requires that care providers understand clearly the unique aspects of each clinical situation and the parents' expectations for their baby.

REFERENCES

1. Tsang RC: Personal communication, NICU Statistics at the University of Cincinnati Medical Center, 1985.

2. Lindemann E: Symptomalogy and management of acute grief. *Am J Psychiatry* 101:141–148, 1944.
3. Woodward S, Pope A, Robson WI, Hagan O: Bereavement counseling after sudden infant death. *Br J Med* 290:362–365, 1985.
4. Bluglass K: Psychiatric morbidity after cot death. *Practitioner* 224:533–539, 1980.
5. Williams ML: Sibling reaction to cot death. *Med J Aust* 2:227–231, 1981.
6. National Sudden Infant Death Syndrome Foundation, Landover, MD, 1979.
7. Cain AC and Cain BS: On replacing a child. *J Am Acad Child Psychiatry* 3:443–456, 1964.

Professional Responsibilities for Patient Care

PART

Care of the Patient during Hospitalization

Medical Training in Obstetrics: Are We Meeting Patient Expectations?

JAMES R. WOODS, Jr., M.D.

The relationship that a patient develops with her obstetrician during pregnancy is unlike that seen in any other medical specialty. The unique bond between patient and physician stems from the fact that pregnancy is the only medical condition for which a patient receives extended care and ultimately is hospitalized as she experiences a natural physiologic process. Consequently, the obstetrician attending the pregnant patient is viewed in a variety of roles simultaneously:

Coordinator—To oversee the process of pregnancy from the mother's initial prenatal visit through her delivery and afterward, in the postpartum period.

Supervisor—To observe the baby's development in order to identify any departure from normal progress.

Medical specialist—To intervene in the event of abnormal obstetrical developments to ensure the safety of both mother and fetus. Also, to recognize nonobstetric medical complications and obtain proper medical care or consultation for the patient.

Confidant—To act as advisor and friend, sensitive to the psychologic changes and perceptions that may surface during pregnancy.

Delivery Signals the End of the Process

This unique relationship is tested when a pregnancy loss occurs. From the patient's point of view, her relationship with the obstetrician is more important than ever. Her doctor is the expert source of information on whom she has depended during her pregnancy. It is a natural extension of this relationship that she expects in the period following her pregnancy loss. From the obstetrician's point of view, in an unfortunate number of cases, the pregnancy's conclusion—regardless of outcome—signals the end of the medical professional's responsibility to the patient. A routine 6-week follow-up examination is classically the final duty that the obstetrician performs for a patient, except for annual gynecologic examinations. In the majority of cases with successful obstetric outcomes, the severing of the physician-patient relationship is mutually satisfactory. When a pregnancy ends in failure, however, severing the relationship at this point may be the obstetrician's way of avoiding true responsibilities still required for the bereaved patient.

Pregnancy Loss Is an Obstetric Responsibility

The major theme that pervades this book is that pregnancy loss is an obstetric responsibility. The obstetrician must coordinate short- and long-term care for patients when their babies have died. When these responsibilities are disregarded, a woman may be victimized by fragmented care or ignored completely, left to rebuild her life without the information or guidance that could help her and her family assimilate the experience.

FAILURE TO REMAIN INVOLVED

It is disheartening to observe the confusion that exists within the medical community when professional roles with respect to pregnancy loss are poorly defined. I was invited once to speak on the subject of pregnancy loss in a small, midwestern city. The invitation originated from pediatricians who were frustrated by a deficiency of obstetric involvement following a fetal or neonatal death. When these cases occurred, pediatricians often found themselves explaining (or having to justify) the obstetric care for a stillbirth during an office visit for another child in the family. At other times, failed obstetric management resulting in delivery and death of a very premature baby was not addressed by the obstetrician and was relegated to pediatric interpretation.

My visit stimulated a fruitful exchange of ideas and discussion of methods. The sincerity and concern of the pediatric community and other allied healthcare professionals were apparent. But the reaction of the obstetric community? Despite good advance publicity, not one obstetrician attended the half-day-long conference. Possibly, their busy schedules made it impossible for any of them to attend. Unfortunately, it is more likely that obstetricians in that community did not attend the meeting because they (and obstetricians in general) do not see themselves as primary and principal care providers for patients after pregnancy loss. In the void that this failure to assume responsibility creates, other professionals—pediatricians, clergy, social workers—rush to fill in the gaps in patient care overlooked or avoided by the obstetrician. In assuming such a burden, these professionals and patients are frustrated, angry, and confused about the obstetrician's role in patient care following pregnancy loss.

**Parents'
Disappointed
Expectations**

Patients are often disappointed in their obstetrician's lack of involvement after a pregnancy has failed. They would like to receive more compassionate care after a loss, but actually may not expect to receive it from their obstetrician. Recently, I met for the first time with a young woman to counsel her after she had experienced a stillbirth at 30 weeks. After we had discussed certain medical issues, we focused on her emotional reactions to the event, and the following exchange occurred:

PATIENT: Are you a psychologist?
ME: No, I'm an obstetrician. Why do you ask?
PATIENT: Because you are asking me all these questions about my feelings.
ME: Why does it surprise you that I would ask you these questions?
PATIENT: Because I thought all obstetricians just came in, did their thing, and went about their business.

This conversation, if somewhat humorous, provides a sobering insight as to how the public perceives the obstetrician's role following pregnancy loss.

The belief that obstetricians are not or cannot be concerned with the whole patient is reinforced when the patient returns for a postpartum examination following her pregnancy loss. As a rule, this visit at 6 weeks is the first contact she has had with her obstetrician since discharge from the hospital. During those 6 weeks, the woman and her partner have struggled unaided and uninstructed through the most difficult period of recovery. What has been happening, most often, is that they have been grieving for their baby. At the 6-week examination, the initial exchange in the 15 minutes usually allotted for the postpartum examination may take place in awkward and intimidating circumstances. In many busy practices, the patient may have been asked to undress and drape for her examination before the obstetrician enters the room.

OBSTETRICIAN: Hello, Mrs. _____. How are you doing today?

PATIENT: (*Feeling the actual or assumed pressures of the short time interval set aside for the office visit and the authoritative posture of the busy obstetrician*) I'm fine.

OBSTETRICIAN: (*Immediately focusing on medical issues*) Have your menstrual periods resumed yet (*even though resumption of menses may serve as a painful reminder of the failed pregnancy*)? And what do you want to use for contraception?

PATIENT: (*The patient gives brief answers to these questions.*) (*The nurse enters; the patient is examined; and then the obstetrician steps out while patient dresses.*)

OBSTETRICIAN: If you have any questions (*may not even state questions about what*), I want you to be sure to ask them.

PATIENT: (*May ask some trivial question in response to the obstetrician's question; otherwise smiles and says little.*)

In this oversimplified scenario, obstetrician and patient both have failed to address the true issues. The patient has not expressed her sadness, concerns, questions, or fears. The obstetrician (perhaps unconsciously) has relied heavily on medical issues to use up any time allotted for discussion. He or she has managed the postpartum visit routinely, in spite of the patient's abnormal outcome. No effort has been made to put the patient at ease so that she might feel comfortable enough to discuss the painful feelings that have been dominating her life in the aftermath of her pregnancy loss. In the end, both parties have avoided the real reason for the visit. This example illustrates the following points, which exacerbate problems caused by unskilled or insensitive obstetricians for their patients following pregnancy loss:

Steps for Improving Care and Communication

1. No contact until 6-weeks postpartum creates a major break in continuity of care. *Solution*: See the patient and her partner in the office within 1 week after discharge for counseling only. One visit or several weekly visits may be necessary to address the couple's needs. Defer physical examination until 6-weeks postpartum.

2. One 15-minute appointment for the postpartum physical examination is inadequate to provide appropriate care after a pregnancy loss. *Solution*: The initial office visit in the first week postpartum should be at least 30 minutes (and perhaps as much as 1 hour) long. It should be devoted entirely to reviewing medical issues about and discussing emotional reactions to the pregnancy loss. These topics may need to be addressed more than once. The patient also should be given more time during her 6-week postpartum follow-up visit, so that she may have time to discuss any remaining concerns with her obstetrician.

3. Failure on the obstetrician's part to address the subject of the loss usually intimidates the patient, who interprets this

as a cue that she may not mention her failed pregnancy. *Solution*: The obstetrician must initiate (if necessary) a discussion about what happened and must be specific and directive in his or her questions, in order to encourage good physician-patient communication. (See Chapter 10, "Obstetrician As Outpatient Counselor" for a discussion of the obstetrician's counseling approach.)

WHY SHOULD THE OBSTETRICIAN BECOME INVOLVED IN COUNSELING FOLLOWING A PREGNANCY LOSS?

Enhancing the Professional Image of the Obstetrician

Active physician involvement in pregnancy loss clearly offers personal satisfaction and community benefits. The caring obstetrician, deeply involved in the extended care of a patient with a failed obstetrical outcome, expands his or her professional roles as friend, confidant, and healer, which have developed during the pregnancy. This positive professional image contributes to the building of larger obstetric practices by inspiring referrals from patients and medical colleagues. Additionally, the hospital benefits by being able to represent itself as an institution that endorses compassionate and understanding care. Obstetrics is becoming a highly competitive service, and such an institutional philosophy contributes significantly in attracting patients to use their obstetric resources. Finally—and this is not to be dismissed—a caring attitude by obstetrician and hospital will reduce malpractice claims.

REASONS WHY OBSTETRICIANS FAIL TO BECOME INVOLVED

Despite obvious benefits, many obstetricians have not actively assumed responsibility for follow-up care of patients with pregnancy loss. In fact, they have contributed significantly toward increasing the perceived distance between physician and patient. Where in the development of attitudes and learning skills have obstetricians failed to acquire a perception of death as a natural extension of life? Perhaps the lack of skill in dealing with death and dying is founded in the very process of medical education, of which physicians are a product.

Death Is a Professional Failure

Knapp and Peppers (1) suggest that medical education is oriented toward curative therapy and technique. Traditionally, what the first-year medical student remembers best is dissection of the cadaver, a "patient" to whom no name or past is attributed. Medical education in the second year focuses on histopathology. In this orientation, disease becomes paramount; any potential emotional involvement with the patient becomes secondary to the pursuit of diagnosis. The curriculum during the third and fourth medical-school years moves the medical student from classroom to clinical arena, but still fails to establish the patient as the central theme. Instead, according to Knapp and Peppers (1), death becomes the enemy to be avoided and opposed at all costs. For students cultivating this attitude, death symbolizes medical failure. It is not recognized (or accepted) as the endpoint of a natural physical process. Thus, in this life-oriented environment, the medical student may graduate without conceptualizing life and death as part of an acceptable whole.

Limitations of Residency Education

Obstetric and gynecologic residencies, perhaps more than those in any other specialty, perpetuate this flaw of medical school education. Obstetrics in particular may enable the resident to avoid confronting issues concerning death because of its unique focus on the beginning of life. Furthermore, Knapp and Peppers (1) observe that the Ob/Gyn resident, involved in a high-volume service, seldom establishes long-term contact with any patient. In this environment of rapid turnover, inevitably there is a lack of patient accountability. Why should the resident become involved today in a patient's life and family problems when she will be someone else's responsibility tomorrow? In response to this short-term involvement, the educational emphasis of medical training shifts to medical techniques and a rapidly expanding body of technical knowledge about obstetric disease processes and therapeutic modalities. Small wonder that, in this setting, the patient becomes an abruptio placentae; the patient's fear for her baby becomes a cesarean section; and her baby's death becomes a nonissue. To refocus on the emotional impact of a baby's death forces the resident to strip away the insulation of medical technology and jargon to confront human sorrow, heart-wrenching sadness, and emotional emptiness.

DEFENSE MECHANISMS THAT INTERFERE WITH SYMPATHETIC CARE

Dissociation

Stack (2) describes a series of protective emotional responses by obstetricians to distance themselves from a patient's pregnancy loss. Some completely dissociate themselves from the event and the patient, as if physical and mental separation exempt them from responsibility for confronting the many questions that should be addressed. Instructing a patient with a pregnancy loss to return for her first postpartum office visit 6 weeks after hospital discharge evinces this impulse.

Intellectualization

Others intellectualize the pregnancy experience, especially, as Stack (2) states, when a patient's care is one's particular responsibility. Toward this end, the obstetrician may justify adverse results based on the disease entity encountered. "The placenta was so fibrosed, the fetus never would have survived." "Her hypertension was so severe, it was a wonder the patient survived, even if her baby died." "We were carrying out antenatal testing for fetal wellbeing every week. It just goes to show you that no test is perfect."

Projection

Other physicians resort to projection as a reaction to pregnancy loss. By this approach, the patient is held accountable for the negative outcome. "If only you had come in a few days earlier, when you first noticed that your baby wasn't moving . . ." "I don't recall your telling me about your family history of diabetes mellitus." "Why didn't you call me when you first had vaginal bleeding?" Unfortunately, most patients already do feel responsible for the baby's death. The obstetrician must not aggravate that burden for the patient simply to alleviate his or her own feelings of inadequacy.

Denial

Some obstetricians utilize denial as a protective shield. Failing to show the stillborn baby to the mother reinforces the suggestion that this death is a nonissue. It conveniently precludes a direct physical confrontation between dead baby, physician, and parents. Strangely, some medical care providers would label this decision protective, when, in fact, confrontation by itself could establish honesty and defuse suspicion.

Inappropriate Humor

Humor is occasionally a weak crutch that obstetricians use to ease tensions and anxieties between care provider and patient. However, this tactic is seldom effective from either party's point of view. On the contrary, it actually widens the gap in communication between physician and patient. Figure 5.1 lists clichés often used inappropriately to provide the obstetrician relief from the stress of direct communication with the patient. A statement such as, "Go drink some wine and get this off your mind [actually said to one patient by her former obstetrician]," is likely to send the patient directly from her obstetrician's office to a lawyer's office. It is not clear why someone would resort to inappropriate humor to dodge a topic that stirs up his or her own insecurities (2). The obstetrician counseling a patient suffering from pregnancy loss must be cautious of this human weakness.

"Therapeutic Listening"

In a study of 100 couples interviewed by Knapp and Peppers (1) following pregnancy loss, over 50% described their obstetricians as insensitive. The significance of this observation was underscored by findings that the most intense emotional need experienced by these 200 mothers and fathers was the desire to talk to someone about their baby's death. The obste-

It's for the best—the baby wouldn't have been right.

It's nature's way of getting rid of something bad.

It's not as if you were far enough along to feel the baby move. At least you didn't know the child.

You can always have another baby. You'll probably be pregnant again in no time.

At least you have other kids at home.

It's God's will. You have a little angel up there.

You should have taken better care of yourself.

The best thing to do is forget about it and get on with your life.

Pull yourself together—you have to be strong for the rest of the family. Don't let the kids see you this way.

At least you are okay . . . you didn't die.

It was just a blighted ovum.

Dispose of the remains.

Abortion.

The baby is sleeping.

Vanishing twin.

Figure 5.1. Common clichés and phrases to avoid.

trician clearly is a logical choice to whom parents would want to turn. Bergman (3) described the skill that the obstetrician needs as "the art of therapeutic listening." By offering this type of needed counseling, the obstetrician communicates to the patient 2 important types of information. First, uncompromised attention, at the patient's bedside and later in the office, conveys interest, attentiveness, and compassion. Although it is not verbalized, this message reassures the patient that she will not be abandoned to struggle alone with her baby's death. Second, the obstetrician may, over several sessions, address facts essential to the patient's understanding of and recovery from her pregnancy loss. This level of care also should be extended to patients during a subsequent pregnancy.

The author hopes that the skills of counseling and therapeutic listening, so important in the care of pregnancy-loss patients, will achieve parity soon with ultrasound, amniocentesis, and other technical procedures in the educational background and practices of obstetricians. Only then will patients with pregnancy loss be accepted as high risk, will obstetricians hold themselves accountable as primary care providers, will counseling be recognized as a necessary technical obstetrical skill, and will the continuity of care for patients with pregnancy loss become an obstetrical responsibility.

REFERENCES

1. Knapp RJ and Peppers LG: Doctor-patient relationship in fetal-infant death encounters. *J Med Educ* 54:775–780, 1979.
2. Stack JM: Reproductive casualties. *Perinatal Press*, Mar 1982, p 31.
3. Bergman AB: Psychological aspects of sudden unexpected death in infants and children. *Ped Cl Med* 21:115–125, 1974.

Role of the Nurse during a Pregnancy Loss

BEVERLY MALONE, R.N., Ph.D.
CATHERINE L. McELWAIN, R.N.

Three concepts direct the nurse's role during a patient's pregnancy loss: (1) advocacy, (2) continuity of care, and (3) professional sensitivity. *Advocacy* is the process of supporting the right of the patient and her family to receive quality care. *Continuity of care* involves progressive and predictable quality care from the time the woman enters the hospital until she returns to her community. In terms of this discussion, continuity of care specifically includes the patient's movement from preadmission to the labor and delivery area, to the recovery room, and finally to the postpartum, gynecologic, or other area where she will remain until her discharge from the hospital. Continuity of care requires coordinated efforts by a variety of nurses (day, evening, and night shifts; labor, delivery, and postpartum) and all other staff who provide care to the patient. *Professional sensitivity* is the nurse's response to her own emotions, as well as to those of others, derived both from nursing theory and experience.

The death of a baby never becomes a routine event to which the nurse is inured. A miscarriage, an ectopic pregnancy, an intrauterine fetal death, or delivery of a premature, critically ill newborn all make different demands on the nurse. To help people who are experiencing the devastating loss of their baby, the nurse has to call on her nursing skills, sensitivity, and insight gained on the job. The nurse is the primary source of professional care and comfort to the family at the moment when their pregnancy loss becomes a reality.

ADVOCACY

The nurse has 24-hour responsibility for patient care. Frequently, she is the one who cushions parents as they begin to cope with their loss. The nurse acts as primary negotiator for the patient. She provides the mother with a place to stay and with appropriate food and clothing, and orchestrates the mother's hospital experience. The nurse must be prepared to serve as the mother's advocate as the hospital system begins to affect her.

Communication with Other Hospital Support Services

The nurse must have well-established communication between nursing and other hospital support services, such as dietary and housekeeping. Good relationships with staff in these areas are essential. A perinatal grief checklist, such as the one developed by Beckey et al. (1), organizes and lists means of individualizing care for each patient and her family. Flagging a grieving patient's chart and room is an example of action taken that prepares the hospital environment and staff to be receptive to grieving parents. Such steps are an important part of the nurse's serving as an advocate.

The goal is for the nurse to provide space and support for grieving. The hospital itself may become a major obstacle in accomplishing these goals. Hospitals and the professionals who operate them are oriented toward life-sustaining activities. Grieving is a "time-out", a slowing-down process that a busy hospital usually fails to support. The nurse as advocate must create a more consistently positive institutional response to grieving mothers and their families.

Nurses sometimes say that hospital protocols and necessary medical procedures interfere with the special attention that they should extend to the couple who have lost a baby. It is true that the system may not support an individual nurse's efforts to provide special care to parents who are in the midst of their pregnancy loss. Too often, a labor and delivery unit or gynecologic floor may be understaffed or overburdened with patients. However, a troublesome question can be raised. Does this situation impede the nurse from providing the kind of care that a couple needs during a loss, or does it act as a buffer that allows the nurse to justify not exerting extra effort?

Over the years, individual nurses have adapted their own methods of caring for patients undergoing pregnancy loss. The profession is composed largely of women. Through their own first-hand experience, they may understand the impact of pregnancy itself and, if they also have experienced one, the impact of a pregnancy loss. It is the nurse who comforts and consoles patients and their families as the loss occurs. Many nurses think that their efforts in these cases are blocked or undermined by unsupportive physicians and fellow nurses, who regard pregnancy loss as a professional failure and who consequently ignore the patient's needs as a means of denying the "failure."

Need for Consistent Responses by Nurses

The ways in which the individual nurse can help pregnancy loss patients are many, and they vary according to the type of loss taking place. If nurses respond consistently and assertively to the special needs of patients with pregnancy loss, they can achieve two critical goals. First, they can provide the individual and her family with the care and support they urgently need. Second, nurses can influence attitudes of hospital staff and—of paramount importance—direct the attention of physicians to issues of concern for their patients with pregnancy loss. If nurses' methods of caring for these patients gain acceptance, then the general level of care offered by the institution will improve dramatically.

For the woman admitted to labor and delivery with an impending pregnancy loss, there are considerations common to all types of losses that may be addressed uniformly. These common issues are:

Need for continuity of care;

The family's extreme vulnerability;

The family's and patient's right for privacy within labor and delivery and the postpartum setting.

CONTINUITY OF CARE

Nurse as Primary Care Provider

Whenever possible, the nurse responsible for the woman undergoing a pregnancy loss should emerge as the primary care provider. The patient should perceive the nurse as "her" nurse. The importance of individualized attention increases over the period of time that the patient remains in the hospital. She and her husband or other family members can grow more comfortable in the nurse's presence as time passes and the event proceeds. This process encourages a patient to ask questions and take in information. It also enables both the patient and her family to express intense emotions they feel. When they begin to see the nurse as an individual, rather than as a stranger and one of many professionals involved with the woman's care, they all can relax their guard and benefit from the help and explanations that the nurse is prepared to offer.

Change-of-Shift

Change-of-shift necessarily interrupts this process. But the nurse who is going off duty can make an effort to see that the nurse taking over is provided with any pertinent information that will help her approach this family with sensitivity. It is helpful if the nurse who has established a relationship with these people can be present, if only for a moment, when the new nurse arrives. This eases the transition for the patient's sake.

Change of Location in Hospital

Continuity of care is an issue of particular concern when a patient is moved from labor and delivery to the gynecologic or postpartum area. Nursing staffs change from one unit to the other, and the rules and routines of each unit are different. Family members may be expected by staff to recognize and respect differing visiting policies and procedures in different units. This is often an unfair expectation for any family, but particularly for the grieving family. In addition to moving from labor and delivery to an entirely different atmosphere on the postpartum or gynecologic floor, the patient has to cope with the phenomenon of changing shifts. The day shift has a very different routine and ambience than afternoon and night shifts. The model of patient care delivery that incorporates all these variables is *primary nursing.*

PRIMARY NURSING

24-Hour Accountability

Primary nursing is a 24-hour model of nurse accountability for patient care. It is intended to minimize communication obstacles between changes of shift and the varying effectiveness of different nurse care providers for a given patient. Consistency of nursing accountability is particularly helpful for a grieving patient. Inherent in the primary nurse's role definition is patient advocacy. In each nursing area, the patient is assigned a primary nurse who has 24-hour accountability for care delivered to this particular patient and her family. At change-of-shift, this primary nurse signs off to an associate who continues to provide care consistent with nursing goals developed by the primary nurse. The patient is able to identify her primary nurse by name, and the unfamiliar setting in which her pregnancy loss has occurred becomes more manageable.

The primary nurse, under leadership of her nursing supervisor, manages the healing environment for the grieving patient following pregnancy loss. Many professional and nonprofessional support services are involved in the care of the patient, such as pharmacy, dietary, laboratory, and housekeeping. The primary nurse coordinates activities of the support services and provides information to facilitate a safe and supportive healing milieu.

Concern for Patient's Short- and Long-Term Adjustment

The primary nurse designs the overall framework of the hour-to-hour care provided to her patient. Any interstaff conflicts about which nursing strategy to pursue must be negotiated. Creative support tactics must be implemented. All resources must be focused on the psychologic and physical healing of the patient. This is the role of the primary nurse. The primary nurse, furthermore, must look beyond the patient's hospital experience, because the patient's adjustment back into the community without her baby is even more stressful than the immediate hospital experience. The primary nurse must work closely with the patient's physician, chaplain, psychologist, and social worker to ease the patient's transition out of the hospital and back home.

Assessing Individual Needs

The advocacy role cannot be effectively managed unless the nurse knows the situation, personality, wants, and needs of the mother within the context of her family structure. Therefore, at the same time that primary nursing tasks must be accomplished, an assessment of the psychosocial dynamics of the mother and family must also be conducted. "What does the loss of this baby mean to the mother, her husband and/or others? Where was this baby going to "fit" in terms of this family's life goals? What were the dreams and fantasies for this baby?" By answering these questions, the nurse can organize information necessary to serve the needs of the individual patient. Actual nursing intervention based on assessment is directed by the nurse's professional judgment and by grieving parents' receptivity to intervention at any particular time. Intervention should be timed according to the appropriateness of the setting and to the mother's emotional state. The nurse can scale her intervention up or down. The following are examples of scaling interventions up and down.

Scaling Up

NURSE: How are you feeling today?
PATIENT: Not very good. How do you expect me to feel?
NURSE: My expectations are not important. How you are feeling is the only important issue.
PATIENT: I feel horrible. (*Pause*) I wonder if I killed my baby. You know, I didn't stop smoking while I was pregnant. I even took a drink several times. (*Patient is crying.*)
NURSE: (*She provides tissues for the patient and moves closer to her.*) When you lose a baby, it's natural to wonder if it was your fault. The most important thing is to be able to talk about your feelings, both good and bad. Talking it out will help. . . .

Scaling Down

PATIENT: I don't want to see anyone. Your hospital is terrible. Terrible things happen here. People don't care. . . .
NURSE: I care. Losing your baby is a terrible thing. Is there something I can do to help?
PATIENT: No, no one can help me.
NURSE: I'm here if you need me. I'll be back in a half hour to check on you. If you need someone before then, just press your light.

Scaling up opens communication and intensifies nurse-patient interchanges. *Scaling down* acknowledges the grieving mother's right to close off communication. The nurse makes it clear that she will remain available and indicates that she is prepared to talk if the patient wishes to do so at some later time.

PITFALLS OF ADVOCACY

Overidentification

The nurse's role as patient advocate may best be understood by the issues involved in carrying out this responsibility. First, it is the nurse, physician, social worker, and chaplain who act as a patient's advocate. No individual should behave as if he or she were the patient's only true advocate. There is a self-righteous component of the advocate role that can be abused by any care provider. A self-righteous nurse advocate is usually one who overidentifies with a particular family. She is at the point where, for some reason, this pregnancy loss has become her own personal loss. Overidentification can lead to ineffective interventions with fellow care providers as well as with grieving parents. Any person can fall victim to the self-righteous theme. Frequently, other care providers can alert the self-righteous advocate that he or she has strayed from a professional advocacy role.

Acquiring Confrontational Skills

Second, advocacy is not an adversarial activity, but rather is facilitative. The nurse advocate is the bridge between parents and hospital. At times, the advocate also may be the bridge between grieving mother and father. Bridging any gap as an advocate may involve the use of confrontational skills. If the nurse is not proficient and comfortable with skills of confrontation, then appropriate education and practical application situations should be provided by the institution. Confrontation used appropriately by care providers can help ensure that parents with a pregnancy loss focus on their initial grief in an understanding and facilitative environment. With any advocacy process, there may be conflicts for parents that interfere with interventions. The goal of the advocate is to simplify parents' confusion and intervene in any problems that may unnecessarily complicate the family's experience. Parents may feel that their world is falling apart because of the pregnancy loss. The compassionate advocate helps restore some form of order.

Identifying Pathologic Responses

An assumption for any loss is that, "I have done something wrong to deserve this loss." Women with a pregnancy loss often think that there must be something inherently wrong with them that has made this happen. The nurse may be first to notice signs of self-destructive thoughts or behavior in a patient. She must anticipate the possibility of such reactions and, working from a team approach, have practical strategies available to address any pathologic or potentially life-threatening grief response. Strategies may include the following:

Alerting all care providers to the extent of a patient's depression;

Recommending a psychologic consult to the grieving parent;

Communicating to associate nurses and other staff the intensity of the crisis that this patient is experiencing.

In communicating to fellow staff on all shifts, the nurse must make both written and verbal reports, spelling out any special precautions as deemed necessary. These precautions may involve having a family member sit at all times with the patient. Depending on the patient's condition, transfer to a psychiatric unit where a safe environment can be managed more routinely may be appropriate. It is never safe to take for granted how any mother will respond to the loss of her baby. The nurse must be prepared equally for an extreme as well as the more expected grief reaction.

PATIENT AND FAMILY'S STATE OF VULNERABILITY

Couples' State of Physical and Emotional Exhaustion

In all cases of pregnancy loss, the patient and her partner are in a vulnerable condition emotionally. Chances are that they are overtired from worry and lack of sleep. If the woman has been bleeding for hours or for several days, or if she has spent several nights trying to make her unresponsive baby move, then she will be physically exhausted. Another source of stress and exhaustion exists for the woman who has been in preterm labor of some duration. She may have been in and out of the hospital as efforts are made to halt her labor, and she is probably anxious about her condition and that of her baby. In all cases, her partner is likely to be in a similar state. They both are distressed and therefore less tolerant than usual of everything.

The woman's partner may be particularly conscious of his helplessness, as he is often treated as nothing more than an observer. This is frustrating to accept when, more than at almost any other time, he wants to protect his partner. As the staff works around him, he feels useless and as if he were in the way. The couple may appreciate it if the nurse intervenes to show the man ways to help his partner. In a late-gestation pregnancy loss involving a prolonged labor, the nurse can teach him to rub the woman's back or legs to soothe some of the woman's pain.

It is of value to note that many couples with preterm labor or with an intrauterine fetal death in the third trimester already will have been enrolled in a prepared childbirth course. If the nurse learns that the couple has begun attending classes, she can remind them of suggestions taught there to help the patient with her labor. Possibly, they already will have established their own routines that they have practiced at home. Such a couple may use these techniques in an attempt to retain some vestige of the normal labor and delivery they had hoped for, and they deserve support in this effort.

BENDING THE RULES

As necessary, nursing staff should be prepared to bend rules for the couple undergoing a pregnancy loss. This decision may involve allowing more than two people to be present in the mother's private labor room or birthing room. A husband and wife may desire to stay together during D & C. A patient may want her partner to be permitted to remain with her while she is being examined.

Another example of how the nurse can modify the rules to help a woman in prolonged induced labor is to offer her a drink of water or juice occasionally, with the attending physician's permission. Any reasonable flexibility that can promote the physical or emotional comfort of the patient and her family is justified and should be allowed by the staff. It is the primary nurse's responsibility to perceive a family's needs and to pursue the means of addressing those needs.

NEED FOR PRIVACY

One of the most difficult aspects of the hospital experience is the presence of so many other women and their healthy babies. The atmosphere in a labor and delivery unit is unavoidably imbued with striking reminders that this is a place where many families experience the joyful birth of a baby. It is unfortunate that a couple must confront the anguish of pregnancy loss in such surroundings.

Privacy within the Labor and Delivery Unit

When a patient whose baby has died is admitted to labor and delivery, she should be placed in a private room. This room should serve to insulate the family from sounds of fetal monitors, laboring mothers, and the cries of newborns. Many women view it as a necessary evil that they must undergo their pregnancy loss in this environment, and they appreciate consideration extended to them to buffer them from other people's happier circumstances. This courtesy may also be extended to the patient's family. The nurse may find it helpful to allow family members to gather in some other room than the common waiting room. Whenever possible, the patient should be returned to her private labor room following delivery, particularly in a labor and delivery setting in which all postpartum patients recover together in a general recovery room. The private room is also much better suited for parents to see their stillborn baby after delivery.

PROFESSIONAL SENSITIVITY

The final concept whose importance the nurse must recognize is professional sensitivity. Nurses, like anyone else, may be uncomfortable personally with issues of death and acute grief. Caring for patients and families confronting a death can be stressful and disturbing. Other staff, nurses and physicians alike, may share these feelings. To protect their own feelings, the staff may ignore the real emotional needs of people suffering a pregnancy loss. It is asking a great deal of all staff members to suspend their professional detachment and to become involved with fellow humans in deep emotional pain. However, the nurturing approach to care is fundamental in the nursing profession. So, perhaps there is no better place than within the labor and delivery nursing staff to introduce new attitudes toward helping patients in crisis who require a great deal more care than they have received in the past from the hospital community.

Acquiring Professional Sensitivity

Professional sensitivity is an acquired skill. Nurses may be poorly prepared academically and emotionally to deal effectively with patients' feelings of loss, in the face of their own responses. The fact is that the majority of nurses today are women. This means that there is great potential for nurses' overidentification with patients concerning issues of pregnancy, infertility, elective abortions, or pregnancy loss. Furthermore, the average age of the nurse in a hospital setting is 23. Thus, many nurses involved in care of pregnancy loss patients may not yet have confronted the issue of death. Emotionally, then, the staff nurse may be poorly prepared to support and facilitate a mother's grief.

Academic nursing education may impose an obstacle for the nurse who is seeking to learn behavioral skills that can help her intervene successfully with a grieving mother. In earlier years, baccalaureate nursing education was focused on a "wellness" model. This model diminished the importance of some course content and nursing practicums that could have served as a basis for the nursing student's clearer theoretical and practical understanding of death and dying. It was possible for a nursing student to complete 4 years of collegiate nursing education and experiential training and yet never encounter a dying patient or a patient with a pregnancy loss.

Experiencing Personal Emotional Upheaval

The topics of death and dying usually are discussed during the nursing student's psychiatric rotation. Examples and case studies typically involve suicidal patients. Thus, emphasis may be on abnormal responses to these issues. The nursing graduate, therefore, may be poorly prepared for normal emotional upheaval associated with loss. Quickly plunged into the demands of her first nursing job, the young nurse may be overwhelmed by the need to provide professional support while she is just becoming aware of her own emotional state and the necessity of communicating with her associate nurses. Dealing with patients' emotional pain may become a more complex task than she is ready to manage. The nurse has to develop her own set of responses to help herself and her patients.

Nurse's Self-Awareness

In order to develop professional sensitivity to families experiencing a pregnancy loss, the nurse must explore her feelings about children, death, and any losses she has experienced in her own life. Her exploration of these issues needs to be thorough and honest. This task can be accomplished in a small group setting with a skilled group facilitator or by one-to-one discussion with a trusted colleague. The important step is for the nurse to begin to examine her own feelings. If the idea of revealing her own experiences and weaknesses in front of a group or a colleague is too threatening, the nurse may choose to undergo self-exploration or individual counseling. It is crucial for the nurse to understand her own perspective of the losses that she has experienced. Self-analysis prepares the nurse for feelings of identification, blame, and anger that may pervade and interfere with care she provides patients and their families. An awareness of personal feelings helps the nurse empathize with a family's pain, even as she acts in a professional role to manage their situation more objectively than they themselves could. Also, understanding herself better more easily enables her to recognize these feelings in other care providers as well as in parents. Professional sensitivity allows the nurse to cry with grieving parents and yet be able to move beyond her tears to the problem solving essential to nursing care.

Lack of academic preparation challenges nursing colleagues and hospitals to upgrade their curricula to include systematic study of the pregnancy loss experience. On-the-job training can be traumatic and ineffective for healthcare provider and grieving parent alike.

SPECIAL CONSIDERATIONS FOR THE LABOR AND DELIVERY NURSE

The primary nurse is a vital link in the chain of the perinatal support service. She provides the immediate cushion for parents coping with pregnancy loss, reinforces the physician's explanations concerning the baby's death, encourages open communication among family members and with healthcare providers, and continues follow-up through phone calls and care plans. The primary nurse accomplishes these objectives through defined actions such as the following:

Providing support as parents are informed of their baby's death in a quiet, private atmosphere; sitting—not standing—preferably with both parents (or alternate significant others) present.

Offering to contact a chaplain for the family.

Contacting a social worker.

Providing the opportunity for the parents to see, hold, and touch their dead baby in a quiet and private atmosphere; preventing whenever necessary a nurse's or any other care provider's interference with a family's right to grieve.

Encouraging the family to name their baby; using the baby's name in conversation.

Providing a picture of the baby and/or locks of the baby's hair, obtained prior to the baby's death if at all possible.

Reinforcing the chaplain's or funeral director's explanations of available options for disposing of the baby's body; encouraging the family to hold a memorial service in the chapel or funeral home, and to procure, if economically feasible, a small gravesite for the baby.

Preparing parents for reactions they will experience after their baby's death; telling them about stages of grief, physiologic imagings, and avoidance of inappropriate guilt.

Assessing the mother's preference for a gynecologic or postpartum room assignment and conveying the information to the appropriate personnel.

Encouraging the father to show appropriate emotion (crying, grief, anger).

PRIMARY NURSE'S ROLE

The nurse's advocacy role and continuity of care process are enhanced by a nurse's professional sensitivity. These three overall concepts—advocacy, continuity of care, and professional sensitivity—are important to the prominence of the nurse's role during a patient's pregnancy loss. The nurse must regard herself as the round-the-clock professional on whom daily management of a family's pregnancy loss experience is largely dependent.

The primary nurse is frequently the watchdog for the perinatal support service. She is the negotiator who sees that hospital support services are delivered in a sensitive manner and is boundary keeper for family members, managing outsiders' access to grieving parents. The primary nurse guides a bereaved family through a tragedy that may appear hopeless. She is the coordinator of communication among team members through written and verbal exchanges. The nurse must be the parents' advocate, the facilitator of continuity of care, and the provider of professional sensitivity.

REFERENCE

1. Beckey RD, Price RA, Okerson M, Riley KW: Development of a perinatal grief checklist. *JOGNN* 14(3):194–199, 1985.

SUGGESTED READINGS

Carr D and Knupp SF: Grief and perinatal loss: A community hospital approach to support. *JOGNN* 14(2):130–139, 1985.

Estok P and Lehman A: Perinatal death: Grief support for families. *Birth* 10:1 1985.

Furlong RM and Hobbins JC: After office hours. *Obstet Gynecol* 10:207, 1970.

Johnson J, Johnson M, Cunningham J, Ewing S, Hatcher D, Dannen C: *Newborn Death*. Omaha, Centering Corporation, 1982.

Kennell JH, Slyter H, Klaus MH: The mourning response of parents to the death of a newborn infant. *N Eng J Med* 283(7):344–349, 1970.

Knapp RJ and Peppers LG: Doctor-patient relationships in fetal/infant death encounters. *J Med Educ* 54:775–780, 1979.

Kowalski K: Managing perinatal loss. *Clin Obstet Gynecol* 23(4):1113–1123, 1980.

LaFerla JJ and Good RS: Helping patients cope with pregnancy loss. *Contemp Obstet Gynecol*, 25(1):107–115, Apr 1985.

Lovell A: Women's reactions to late miscarriage, stillbirth, and perinatal death. *Health Visitor* 56(9):325–327, 1983.

Peppers LG and Knapp RJ: Maternal reactions to involuntary fetal/infant death. *Psychiatry*, 43:155–159, 1980.

CHAPTER

Chaplain's Ministry When a Baby Dies

REV. BERT A. KLEIN

From a religious perspective, experiences in life have meaning and significance, reason and purpose. The Judeo-Christian faiths provide a system of belief and values, a structure that helps people of these faiths to understand and deal with life's experiences. Whatever one's religious perspective may be, it is severely tested in the face of a baby's death. Faith in God is tried because it is believed that babies ought not die.

Source of Comfort to Bereaved Family

Therefore, how can a representative of God come into this terrible experience and attempt to give answers to unanswerable questions, to comfort when nothing but having the baby's life back would be enough, and to make sense out of something that is senseless? The chaplain dares to do so humbly. The very perception of a baby's death as unfair, unjust, and wrong invites the chaplain into the dilemma. Who is better qualified to enter the sacred arena of life-and-death issues than the clergy? There clearly is a role from the outset for the chaplain. In the hospital, that role includes the chaplain's being present as a nonmedical, religious, and personal source of comfort and support to the bereaved couple.

Too often, parents whose baby has died in a miscarriage, as a stillbirth, or after only a few hours of life are not "allowed" to mourn. Their loss, anger, and pain remain buried inside; in many instances their baby is not even buried. A chaplain's ministry is to enable the couple to talk about their loss, to listen

132

to them express anger, to acknowledge the couple's pain, and to offer comfort and hope.

This chapter discusses from the chaplain's perspective the shock, guilt, anger, fear, and crisis of faith that many individuals experience following a pregnancy loss. The chaplain's acts of pastoral care can be sustaining to families in crisis. Chaplains enter the scene as representatives of God, and as compassionate human beings. Acts of pastoral care begin with the initial visit and continue as the chaplain addresses parents' need for information and understanding. The chaplain is there to touch and hold bereaved parents, to clarify their comments, to acknowledge their shattered hopes and dreams, to explore their view of God, and to conduct a memorial or funeral service.

CHAPLAIN AS A NONMEDICAL FRIEND AND COMPANION

Bridging the Gap in Communication

The chaplain can help a grieving couple by being their friend. In the strange land of the medical center, medical jargon may seem elusive and evasive to the couple. It can create a barrier between care provider and patient so imposing that the woman and her partner may feel isolated. A friend who understands the language can be a companion who helps the couple communicate with others around them. The chaplain is perceived by parents as different from medical staff. The difference in perspective is apparent from the chaplain's choice of words. "Perinatal," "fetus," or "products of conception" are translated into the simple statement, "Your baby died." The hospital chaplain who is familar with doctors and staff and who enters as a friend to parents can serve to bridge a gap between professional and patient.

HELPING THE FAMILY DEFINE FAITH

Giving "Permission" to Grieve

Sometimes, religious individuals may adopt the attitude that strong faith makes one immune from feeling a loss. This notion can inhibit them from expressing very normal feelings of guilt, anger, depression, and fear. At the time of a pregnancy loss, a parent may believe that she or he should not grieve or question why God has taken the baby. Family members, too, may impose this attitude on grieving parents. They may try to suppress a woman or man's healthy grief, thus reinforcing the idea that it is "wrong" to grieve. The chaplain is well-suited to address this issue and give parents permission to grieve. Their loss, which is significant, needs to be recognized and acknowledged. Parents need to understand that their grief is the natural consequence of love and that it is all right to cry, to be upset, and to question. Biblical examples of people of faith who struggled with life's tragedies may help a couple overcome their idea that "God's will" means that the loss must not be mourned.

The chaplain's presence implies that, in some way, God will work things out. As parents are experiencing the immediacy of their pregnancy loss, they feel that nothing good, helpful, or positive could ever come of this event. It would be a travesty for the chaplain to suggest otherwise. Yet, the chaplain enters into the tragedy implicitly representing the hope that God will rescue and save these people even in their intense suffering and pain.

Chaplains should avoid ostensibly religious comfort about their baby being "with God" or "in heaven." Such comments imply that parents should be "happy" or "glad" for their baby. Parents want their baby with them now, not a promise of "reunion" in heaven in the future. At the same time, the chaplain can offer hope in a special way. Hope can come in words spoken with conviction regarding a life hereafter. But, it is important to stress that life will continue for parents after their baby's death. Reminders that God hears our cries, knows our sufferings, and shares our pains can be helpful. Again, both the exodus theme and the crucifixion account emphasize that death is not the final word and that God's word is not an abstraction, but rather speaks for actions which occur in our lives.

Allow the Couple to Express Negative Feelings

Parents often feel they are being punished and that God is vindictive. They need to be reassured that God is not "up there taking babies away from parents." The chaplain cannot let such a claim go without response. Difficult as it is to assert otherwise, the belief that this death is an act of retribution for the couple must be contradicted. Nevertheless, the couples' feelings, especially their negative ones, deserve to be explored and tested. The chaplain should explore, for example, parents' responses to the question, "Are you angry with [scared of] God?" He or she should agree with them that this is both a frightening and a frustrating time. Renewal comes by working together with parents during this crisis. Couples at first may want to deny the reality of their loss, to withdraw. But when they feel acceptance and support, they begin to deal with the loss. They discover that they can endure and that their lives will go on.

CHAPLAIN'S RELIGIOUS ROLE

Clergy may attempt unconsciously to distance themselves from these people in pain by using the tools of the trade, words from the "black book," in a perfunctory manner. Religious rituals, prayers, and readings are intended to address religious concerns and questions. Unfortunately, they can be used in such depersonalized ways that they fail to help grieving parents.

Religious Rites Dignify the Baby's Existence

Clergy need to individualize religious rites as part of pastoral care. For many grieving parents, baptism or a special blessing provides a measure of comfort and hope at this time. To deny parents such comfort evades their needs and isolates suffering people from a religious means of coming to terms with their loss. Clergy should willingly perform baptism or a blessing for a family who desires it and attempt to personalize such ceremonies for the circumstances. By talking with the patient's nurse beforehand, the chaplain may learn that parents have mentioned special characteristics about or dreams they had for their baby. It is important to have the family present at the ceremony and to make reference to these personal observations. If baptism is performed, a baptismal certificate is a meaningful memento to present to the parents. A special blessing over the baby is helpful for times when baptism would be inappropriate. The blessing acknowledges that this baby, loved by his or her parents, is entrusted to God's love. During the baptism or blessing, when the baby and parents are together, the chaplain should touch and hold the baby and be sure to call the baby by name. If the parents have not named their baby, the chaplain should use the personal pronoun "he" or "she."

Prayers that mention parents' grief and their confusion, anger, and pain evoke feelings that parents may find difficult to voice. Acknowledging these feelings and presenting them to God brings people who are experiencing sadness and loss to God's consoling spirit and to the process of healing. Familiar and brief sections of scripture can be helpful. Some suggestions are:

Psalm 23: The Good Shepherd walks with us.
Psalm 42: A cry of agony and despair can be a cry of faith.
Psalm 139: God knows your feelings, and God knows your baby.
John 11:35: Jesus cried, so can we.
Romans 8:39: Nothing can separate us from the love of God.

Role of Hospital Clergy

Pastoral ministry is often carried out by the hospital chaplain because of the urgency of the situation. Whenever possible, the family's own clergy should perform the rites that are part of their faith. Hospital clergy should assist and facilitate the family's own ministry, sharing information and regarding such consultation as part of the hospital chaplain's role. Offering resources such as books and pamphlets, together with the names and telephone numbers of support groups in the community, is also helpful.

The chaplain should be viewed as caring, nonjudgmental, and open. He or she should be perceived as someone who cannot give all the answers, but who will listen to parents and permit them to ask difficult questions. Clergy need not hide their own feelings of sadness and may express them openly with parents. The chaplain can spend time with parents while they are feeling confused or overwhelmed and can cry with parents as they cry. This response does not imply weakness or an inability to deal with the crisis. A genuine expression of sorrow shows parents that their grief is legitimate and that their baby is worthy of mourning.

ACTS OF PASTORAL CARE

Initial Visit

Encouraging Families to Talk about the Baby

The first visit often occurs following delivery. The woman usually will be physically tired and emotionally exhausted. If this is the case, the chaplain's first visit should be brief. The chaplain should briefly introduce him- or herself, and state that he or she has come to offer comfort. The chaplain can continue by focusing on the shock, numbness, and weariness, acknowledging and accepting these feelings as normal. Then he or she should ask about the baby. Even if this may seem intrusive, many women are often willing and eager to talk. A simple inquiry may be all that is necessary for a woman to begin to open up about her experience. The chaplain might ask, "Did you see your baby? Is it a boy or a girl?" At many hospitals, pictures are taken routinely, and often people show their pictures to the chaplain at this time. The chaplain may then ask, "Who does he look like?" and "Did you get to hold him?" Sometimes it is helpful to say, "People tell me that it is hard, but important for them to see their baby. In the past when a woman didn't see and hold her baby, she would later wonder who he looked like, and what features he had. Seeing him hurts, but it also helps."

Brief Visits Can Be Effective

Visits of 10 to 15 minutes can accomplish a great deal. They touch upon but do not invade feelings that are tender and frightening. Offering to say a prayer at the end of the visit is appropriate and will usually be appreciated. The chaplain should make it clear that he or she would like to visit again, and the woman will most likely indicate that a follow-up visit would be welcomed. During subsequent visits, the chaplain can explore other issues and concerns, allowing the woman or her partner to take the lead.

Some women are not ready to see their babies at the time of delivery. Frequently, though, a few hours or the day following delivery, their attitudes may change. If a woman has not yet held her baby, a subsequent visit can be used to discuss the subject with her and to assist in making arrangements for the baby to be brought to her. Some women never come to the point of being able to see their baby during their hospitalization; pictures should be taken and kept for them in the event that they will want them at a later time.

Information and Understanding

As parents attempt to cope with their pregnancy loss, they seek answers to questions about why it happened. Their struggle to survive and endure this tragedy comes out in reason-seeking questions and comments. It is fitting to assist parents while they acquire as much information and as many medical facts as possible. The chaplain should encourage them to verbalize the medical questions they have. What is also needed by parents is understanding. To go through this experience is terrible; to experience it alone is unnecessary. The chaplain is like the Good Shepherd who walks with his people as they go through the valley of the shadow of death.

The Isolation of a Pregnancy Loss

Many times, there is a sense (particularly among women) of being untouchable. Women may feel that the pregnancy loss has proved them to be a physical failure, an inadequate person. An arm on the shoulder, an embrace, a squeeze of the hand, and holding the woman's hand in prayer are small but significant ways of conveying acceptability, warmth, and the care that cannot be expressed in words. "A good hug without a lot of foolish talk helped me more than anything else," one grieving parent commented. The need and desire to be held may not be expressed, but a loving touch often meets that need and is appreciated.

RECURRENT PARENTAL ISSUES

Shock

Crisis produces a state of shock. Families' lives are turned upside down when a baby dies—the event is beyond their control and their world is thrown out of balance. Denial and numbness are two of the first responses. When I meet parents, I say, "This is like a bad dream, isn't it?," to which they frequently reply, "It's a nightmare." The reality of their baby's death is difficult to absorb. So, at first, parents often deny that it could be possible. They are feeling, if not saying, "This isn't really happening to me. My baby didn't die. It's a mistake." This is why it is so important for parents, if at all possible, to see, touch, and hold their baby. Such interaction begins the process of healing grief. When a woman holds her baby and says, "She's really gone, isn't she?" she is saying, "Yes, this *is* happening to me."

Chaplain's Directive Approach

Because of their shock, and because parents don't know what to expect or how to feel and react, it is helpful for the chaplain to be somewhat directive. A nondirective passive approach can lead parents to perceive the chaplain as someone who does not know what to say, and who is overwhelmed. Sharing with parents how others have reacted to a baby's death and mentioning feelings they may experience convey the understanding that the chaplain has attained a level of competence derived from previous encounters of this type. This assurance helps them trust the chaplain as a guide while they begin to accept their loss and deal with their emotions.

Guilt

Guilt is often of foremost concern to couples and it needs to be addressed by the chaplain. The normal and natural feelings of ambivalence that often come with being pregnant can easily erode into guilt. A woman may recall that she was not overjoyed when she first learned she was pregnant and now she cries, "Is that why God took my baby?" A woman who fears that she made her baby an idol experiences an equivalent sense of guilt. She fears that God is punishing her because she wanted her baby "too much." Thoughts are not always logical when grieving parents try to understand what has happened to them. They want to make some sense out of the trauma they are suffering.

Anger

Often, behind the question "Why?" is anger. This anger has no focus. Parents are angry at everything and everyone; at the same time, they realize that no one and nothing can be blamed. How frustrating this is! Sometimes, parents are able to express anger at God. They ask, "Why, when there are so many people out there who mistreat children, does God allow them to have babies, and yet He stops us from having this child we wanted so much?" For them, at this particular time, a God who is supposed to be loving is a vengeful God of hate. There is no answer to their angry questions. It may be helpful if the chaplain simply can acknowledge the pain behind their anger. Acceptance of such anger is reaffirming grace in action.

Fear

Reassurance That Grief Is Normal

Parents' fears become apparent by their anxious statements. "I wake up, certain that I hear my baby crying. Am I going crazy?" "I want to see and hold my dead baby. Is that normal?" "I have dreams about my baby. Is that natural?" Loss of a baby is bad enough, but fear of losing one's mind is overwhelming. The chaplain should reassure parents that their reactions and feelings are normal and natural.

After delivery, a woman's body goes through hormonal and physical readjustments. Sometimes, a woman imagines that she feels her baby moving. When her mind plays such a trick, a woman fears that she may be going crazy. The chaplain may mention that such feelings and reactions do occur. Letting parents know what they may experience after a pregnancy loss relieves them of their anxiety of losing control over their emotions.

CLARIFY WHAT IS BEING SAID

"God's will! It was God's will," a young mother once said. The chaplain's first reaction to this comment may be to contradict such a belief. God does not will the death of babies. The chaplain cannot understand, explain, or justify a baby's death. But the chaplain can say that God does not decide who is to die in any such premeditated manner. However, by pausing before "correcting" this idea, the chaplain may ask the woman what she means and in this way learn again the importance of clarifying what people say.

This young single woman believed that she was not responsible for her baby's death—God was. When she learned that she was pregnant, she considered having an elective abortion. Some friends advised her to terminate her pregnancy. But she finally decided to continue with the pregnancy, even though it was unplanned. She assumed responsibility for going to the prenatal clinic and for taking care of herself. Then the baby died. In the midst of her grief, this woman felt no guilt. She did not take her baby's life; God did. She was sad and did not understand it all, but she said, "God knew what He was doing."

This experience emphasizes the importance of confirming what people mean when they use particular words. What is the meaning of these words for this person and in this context? Clarification is always a task for the chaplain and others to work on. God's will continues to be an issue for dialogue, but establishing the meaning of words in the specific and personal conversation is paramount.

ACKNOWLEDGING PARENTS' HOPES AND DREAMS

Loss of Self-Image

The chaplain can help parents acknowledge their hopes, dreams, and desires they had for their baby, in order to help them see why they are grieving. Some parents are surprised at how deep their sorrow is over the loss of a baby who has not been part of their lives for very long. But they will recall that they have lost a baby who would have . . . , a sentence that they have completed numerous times with many ideas and plans. They have lost the opportunity to be parents of this baby. In a sense, they are grieving both for themselves and for their baby. They experience loss of self-image, of the goal to have this baby, and of the status of being parents to this baby. They leave the hospital with empty arms and with unfulfilled love.

When parents say, "No one can understand our grief; no one knows our heartache," they are right. The chaplain should not claim otherwise. No one else can know their unique pain. The chaplain should not attempt to take away their grief, but should help parents come to grips with that grief and assist them in the healing process of working through it. Enabling them to talk about their baby facilitates parents' grief and helps them to understand why they are grieving.

EXPLORING PARENTS' VIEW OF GOD

It is appropriate for clergy to probe parents' concepts of God, particularly how they view God in this situation. Is God far away or close by? Is He helpless or helping, punishing or comforting? Concepts of God that can be helpful are of God as hearer of our cries; God as accepting of our feelings, even of anger; God as fellow-sufferer, who shares our pain, knows our sorrow, and speaks to us from our midst. The biblical themes of the exodus and crucifixion are very applicable illustrations of these images. The chaplain must offer them with sensitivity and compassion.

OFFERING TO CONDUCT A MEMORIAL SERVICE

Clearly, the grief of pregnancy loss may have a religious component that needs to be addressed. There are a variety of ways in which clergy may speak about the issues and concerns that such a loss brings. One of these is to offer to conduct a memorial service for the baby. The service is not an isolated, individual act of pastoral care. Rather, it is preceded by several pastoral visits and is one part of pastoral ministry. During visits with grieving parents, a relationship of care and compassion is established. The chaplain becomes aware of a family's particular problems as well as their religious values and beliefs. Throughout the pastoral relationship, the chaplain supports the woman and her family, acknowledging and listening to their religious questions and concerns.

Funeral and Burial Are Preferable But May Not Be Possible

A memorial service may be suggested as an option for the family to consider. It is most frequently used when parents have agreed to allow the hospital to take care of disposition of their baby, so that there will be no funeral or burial in a cemetery. A funeral and burial are preferable, but not always possible. When they are not possible or desirable, often families still want to commemorate the existence of their baby through a religious service of love and respect. The memorial service offers the family a positive means of saying good-bye to their baby and represents an opportunity for the family to draw on the support of their faith. The service should take place in the hospital chapel before or when the woman is discharged from the hospital.

PERSONALIZED SERVICE

Family's Input Is Valuable

To get an idea of how best to handle the memorial service for a particular family, the chaplain should discuss the service with the parents. Sometimes, parents have ideas and suggestions regarding the service, such as special scripture, readings, and poems that are meaningful to them. Including their ideas and personalizing the service is very appropriate. However, many parents do not have or are not able to make suggestions regarding the content of the service. They are not yet thinking clearly or in an organized way. The chaplain then may draw on insight gained from previous visits for organizing the service. He or she should also invite family and friends to attend, if the parents wish, and refer to the baby by name.

A TIME TO ADDRESS PASTORAL ISSUES

A memorial service offers an opportunity to address issues important to parents and family. It can help them recognize that their love for their baby will never be fulfilled and that with their baby's death comes the death of some of their dreams. The memorial service gives a family permission to grieve. With the death of an unborn baby, too often parents and family do not think they should grieve in the same way that they would grieve the loss of an older family member. The service can be a time for friends and members of the extended family to hear that grief over a pregnancy loss is normal and needs to be expressed and accepted. It can help break the conspiracy of silence (1) that is often present among family—the unspoken belief that if you do not talk about the baby you will not think about the baby, and if you do not think about the baby you will forget. But parents *do* remember and *do* think about their baby. They will need to talk about their baby, and other family members and friends need to be aware of this. They should be encouraged to listen to and accept the parents' tears. The memorial service, attended by family and friends, commands respect for the dead baby and introduces the event to outsiders as a tragedy that must be dealt with.

WHAT SHOULD BE SAID?

What should the chaplain say during a memorial service to include all these concerns? The following is part of a service for James and Lori after the stillbirth of their son, John.

Who understands all that life brings? No one. We seek reasons and ask "Why?" But, sometimes, we get no answers; at least, not complete and final answers to all our questions.

I do not know why John had no life here on earth, but we cannot ignore the fact that John was part of your life. You, James and Lori, had hopes, dreams, and desires for him. We must not deny them.

There is a real sadness and sorrow over his death. We cannot, should not, forget him. We are here to show your love and respect for John through this memorial service.

In the midst of your grief, not knowing "why," we come to God for comfort and strength. Feeling hurt and angry, confused and alone, we seek the assurance of God's love.

In our grief and hope, we need to reach out to one another with care and compassion, to hold and listen to each other, to embrace and support one another. It is through our arms and hands that God will hold us, and draw us closer to one another. He will sustain and strengthen us.

A memorial service is for memory and mourning, for baby and parents, for death and life, for here and hereafter. It can be a significant component of pastoral care that seeks hope and renewal. The memorial service helps to change negative feelings to positive ones as it acknowledges, confronts, and moves beyond the reality of death.

Parents begin to accept that their baby is dead when they make a comment such as, "This is really happening to me." Their statements and feelings move from "No, my baby did not die. I cannot go on living," to "Yes, my baby did die, and it's hard to go on without her."

REFERENCE

1. Lewis E: Mourning by the family after a stillbirth or neonatal death. *Arch Dis Child* 54:303–306, 1979.

SUGGESTED READINGS

Birch BC: Loss of Children. *Christian Century*, Oct 26, 1983, pp 965–967.
Borg S and Lasker J: *When Pregnancy Fails*. Boston, Beacon Press, 1981.
Church M, Chazin H, Ewald F: *When a Baby Dies*. Oak Brook, IL, The Compassionate Friends, Inc., 1981.
Cowan, M: Mourning is a healing of heart. *Hum Devel* 3(2):31–35, 1982.
Kirkley-Best E, Kellener K, Gould S, Donnelly W: On stillbirth: an open letter to the clergy. *Journal of Pastoral Care* 36(1):17–20, 1982.
Kushner H: *When Bad Things Happen to Good People*. New York, Avon Books, 1981.
Mitchell K and Anderson H: *All Our Losses, All Our Griefs*. Philadelphia, The Westminister Press, 1983.
Morse H: Religious Perspective. In Marshall R, Kasman C, Cape L (eds): *Coping with Caring for Sick Newborns*. Philadelphia, WB Saunders Company, 1982.
Schiff HS: *The Bereaved Parent*. New York, Penguin Books, 1982.

CHAPTER

Social Worker: Hospital Advocate for the Immediate and Extended Family

ANDREA MATTHEWS, M.S.W.

Defining the Social Worker's Responsibilities

After a pregnancy loss has occurred, the social worker assumes responsibility for enhancing the problem-solving and coping capabilities of the individual and her family. The social worker acts as the family's and the patient's advocate and, as such, becomes their facilitator, coordinator, and supervisor in the face of a complex series of events. These events, thus differentiated, may then be managed more specifically by the physician, nurse, and chaplain. It is in this facilitator's role that the social worker offers networking skills important in the care of patients with pregnancy loss. This responsibility is broad but not unfocused.

As advocate for the patient, the social worker is the link between the individual and the systems—both medical and nonmedical—that provide resources and opportunities for recovery and healing. In this sense, the social worker supervises the "team approach" to patient care. He or she serves as the nonmedical liaison between patient and hospital system, capable of offering the medical staff insight into a family's dynamics that might influence patient care.

As advocate for the patient's immediate family, the social worker maintains contact with and communication among family members. Soricelli and Utech (1) evaluated 220 families experiencing the death of a child at Children's Memorial Hospital, Chicago, Illinois. Poor psychologic adjustment following a child's death was observed most frequently in those parents

Assessing a Family's Dynamics after a Pregnancy Loss

> With whom does the patient live?
>
> With whom is she close? Does the baby's father know about the pregnancy loss and how is he responding?
>
> Does she have a psychiatric history?
>
> Does she use drugs or alcohol?
>
> How are other family members reacting to her pregnancy loss?
>
> Does she have other children? If so, do they know about the loss? How did they respond to the baby's death?
>
> Does the patient have prior loss experiences? If so, what were the circumstances and how did she react?

Figure 8.1.   Assessing a patient's personal and family profile after a pregnancy loss.

with preexisting psychiatric problems, substance abuse, marital or family conflicts, financial crises, or previous losses. Questions whose answers may contribute to assessing the patient's reaction to her pregnancy loss are listed in Figure 8.1. Answers to these questions profile the family and make it easier for other primary care providers to interpret the appropriateness of the patient's and her family's responses to what has happened. Too often, medical professionals directly involved in the care of a pregnancy loss patient focus only on the event and its immediate consequences. The social worker must broaden the medical community's perspective of this loss for the patient, defining it as a significant event along the continuum of her life experiences.

The responses of extended family members after a pregnancy loss often are overlooked in a busy obstetric practice. Grandparents, aunts, or uncles may have their own hopes and dreams for the child-to-be. But, usually, their shattered expectations after the pregnancy loss are ignored completely. The feelings of members of a patient's extended family are significant and deserving of consideration. This was recently illustrated in the case of a patient who delivered a son at 26 weeks. Her baby died during his second day in the nursery. The complexity of the family network became apparent when, on the third day, the family revealed that the newborn had been named for a cousin's son who had died in adolescence. One can only imagine the rekindled feelings within the family when the newborn namesake also died.

RESPONSIBILITY FOR DOCUMENTATION AND DISPOSITION—CUTTING THROUGH THE RED TAPE

Responding to Individual Needs

In addition to providing other services, the social worker must assure that all proper documents are completed during the patient's hospitalization. Birth and death certificates or a stillbirth certificate are required by law in all states. Sometimes, however, statutory definitions of fetal death can raise an emotional issue for parents. A state law may require that birth certificates be issued only for liveborn babies after 20 weeks gestation. But a mother may want a birth certificate for her liveborn 17-week-old fetus. A similar, although unofficial, hospital birth certificate usually satisfies the family's desire for a record of their baby's delivery. Another unusual situation is dealing with the request of a patient who wishes to bury the remains of her miscarriage formally. The hospital system must be prepared to respond to such uncommon requests. The tragedy of a fetal death is significant enough for a patient without its being complicated by inflexible care providers or medical systems. It is under circumstances such as these that the social worker must recognize and make use of flexibility within the medical system.

Finally, the social worker should follow up all fetal or neonatal deaths to assure that the baby's remains are disposed of properly and satisfactorily. Unfortunately, in a busy obstetric practice it is not unusual to have confusion arise as to where a stillborn or a dead neonate was taken. If the baby was presumed to have been sent to the morgue for funeral arrangements but instead was sent to surgical pathology, confusion about a "lost baby" causes parents additional pain. Delay in locating a baby's remains usually is momentary; frequently, it is a matter of checking the paperwork on the baby, and it causes no great concern for anyone, except the baby's parents. "What do you mean, you lost our baby?" is a justified and explosive response to the honest admission, "We are not exactly sure where your baby has been taken, but I'm sure we will find him." When parents are attempting to gather a few threads of memory and mementos from their baby's brief life, the slightest confusion in the handling of their baby's remains can easily lead to suspicion, distrust, and lawsuits.

SOCIAL SERVICE INTERACTION WITH THE FAMILY AFTER HOSPITAL DISCHARGE

Outpatient Care as an Extension of In-Hospital Services

Of the various professionals who are involved in caring for patients with a pregnancy loss, social workers have been among the most active in bridging the gap between in-hospital care and extended outpatient care. Some have established a routine of telephone contact with parents in the weeks following discharge as a means for providing advice, extending concern, and measuring recovery, and as a resource for parents to direct questions, clear up misunderstandings, and express fears. Other social workers have developed or participated in community peer support groups for parents with pregnancy losses, in an effort to educate the public and discredit myths that abound about the impact or perceived lack of impact of a pregnancy loss. Space does not permit a complete listing of the many activities that have emerged from active participation by social service workers acting as care providers for patients with a pregnancy loss. The reader is referred to Figure 8.2 for a listing of chapters that offer a complete description of techniques and principles applicable to a wide range of care providers. The remainder of this chapter will concentrate on 2 important groups often overlooked unintentionally in the grieving process following pregnancy loss: the siblings and grandparents of a dead baby.

CHILDREN

The response of sibling children to a pregnancy loss has only recently become a subject of consideration. Although once dismissed as uninvolved and unaffected by the death of a fetal or newborn sibling, children now are understood to be made vulnerable by this type of life crisis. (The reader is referred to Chapter 1, "Pregnancy Loss and the Grief Process," for a detailed description of children's developmental stages in understanding the meaning of death.) Children's behavior patterns are observed to be affected by what has happened to the family. Parental responses to living children in the family may also be affected significantly following a pregnancy loss.

Parents unintentionally may alter their behavior toward their living children in response to a pregnancy loss (2). The child may suddenly be perceived as more vulnerable to death, prompting parents to become overprotective or, worse, causing them to smother their child with "protection." The child may

Chapter 10 Outpatient counseling techniques

Chapter 14 Information about the value of the peer support
group network

Chapter 15 Issues of importance during a subsequent pregnancy

Figure 8.2.   References to other chapters in this text.

no longer be allowed to walk home from school, and now must always be driven home. Neighborhood wanderings of children after dinner may be curtailed. By redefining (and narrowing) boundaries and limiting their children's previous level of independence, parents may strive (consciously or unconsciously) to "hang on" to that which has been deprived them through the death of their baby.

Children's Needs in the Event of Pregnancy Loss

In part, the medical community has contributed to and perpetuated misconceptions that children have of a sibling's death (2). Children are seldom shown or allowed to touch the dead fetus or newborn. For children under 2 to 3 years of age, not showing them the baby is justifiable, because children this young are unable to grasp the significance of the event. For older children, however, this omission may be interpreted as punishment, as if the child's unspoken feelings toward the pregnancy caused the baby to die. Indeed, children under the age of 12 as a rule are not permitted beyond the lobby of many hospitals. However, many labor and delivery units now offer sibling visitation hours to families experiencing a normal birth. Perhaps such institutions would be receptive to showing the older child his or her stillborn sibling, if such an action were deemed helpful for the child who understands that a baby brother or sister has died. Further pain may be caused if a child is restricted from memorial or funeral ceremonies. The child may feel abandoned and unloved by his or her parents who are so preoccupied with the baby's death.

Cain et al. (3) analyzed the responses of children to their mothers' miscarriages. In this study, 62 clinic patients and 25 nonclinic (private) patients were evaluated. Following are some of the many responses that they observed:

The child perceives the parents' anxiety but cannot understand the underlying causes and is puzzled.

Children who are too young to understand miscarriage may relate the event to their own play activities. They believe that the baby was killed or murdered, as they perceive such acts of violence portrayed on television.

The child may blame him or herself for the baby's death, fearing that his or her actions (for example, being too noisy or jumping on the mother's abdomen) killed the baby.

The child may sulk, reflecting disappointment or sadness. This response evidences the child's sense of the loss of a potential playmate.

The child may suffer from a sense of inadequacy, feeling that he or she is not good enough and that the parents were having another baby to make up for this child's shortcomings.

The authors have interviewed a number of children during the early weeks following a pregnancy loss and can add the following observations:

Children may fear that the parent will die also, leaving them abandoned.

Children may become protective of a parent. Examples: (1) At the funeral of a stillborn baby, the mother's 2 daughters pushed between their mother and her boyfriend, the father of the baby. In this case the boyfriend, who lived out of state, had shown no interest in the pregnancy and had returned to the city only upon learning of the stillbirth. (2) A child began to treat his mother as if he were her parent, criticizing her manner of dressing and her lack of energy following the pregnancy loss.

Children who accompany their parents during postpartum counseling sessions at the University of Cincinnati Perinatal Support Service have been encouraged to draw pictures illustrating their concepts of the baby's death. In one instance, the stillborn baby was depicted as being carried up in the sky on a white blanket with 4 balloons attached at the corners. Actually, the only time that this child saw his stillborn sister—at the baby's memorial service—she was wrapped in a white satin blanket.

Talking with Children

Bergman (4) encourages the use of "third-person technique" when talking with children about death. As modified from Gould and Rothenberg (5), dialogue with the child might proceed as follows: "When a baby dies, some kids worry that they might have caused it, even if they don't talk about it. Does that make sense to you?" There are 3 types of responses that the child may make to this question: 1) "No!," (2) "Yes, I suppose so; but I'm not one of them," and (3) "Yes, I'm glad to hear that because that is what I've been thinking also." The care provider must be sensitive to the child's feelings of fear, anger, guilt, and sadness (4). These responses, in fact, represent the 4 major emotions encountered by most children, adults, and healthcare professionals.

GRANDPARENTS

Although far less attention has been paid to the grief reaction of grandparents than to that of other members of the family, the authors feel that empathizing with the needs of these extended family members is instrumental in the long-term recovery of the grieving couple. It is an understatement that the needs of grandparents of the dead fetus or the newborn often are overlooked in the postpartum period. In fact, grandparents experience a significant sense of loss when their children suffer a pregnancy loss. It is an error to claim that only the couple and perhaps their living children grieve for the unborn or newborn lost baby. One grandmother decribed it, "The loss of a baby 2 generations 'down' from oneself is not just the loss of another baby in this world. Not when it is your baby's baby-to-be." Many expectant grandparents express a strong desire to be with their daughter or daughter-in-law during the labor process when an intrauterine fetal death has occurred. In some cases this urge may reflect an anxiety that their child is more vulnerable to death because the baby has died. For others, the need to be present may reflect a parental desire to protect their own child, as a natural extension of the family dynamics in force when the laboring patient was younger. Many labor and delivery units restrict family members from visiting a woman during a normal labor, to provide the patient peace and quiet. Although in the case of a pregnancy loss this guideline may benefit some patients, for others the compassionate attention of their own parents may offer comfort and may help to ward off feelings of isolation and loneliness, which commonly surface in the midst of a pregnancy loss.

Helping Grandparents during a Pregnancy Loss

Many grandparents have a strong desire to see or hold their dead or dying grandchild after delivery. This desire often is unstated by the grandparents and seldom is initiated by care providers. For many hospital personnel, the thought of encouraging the parents themselves to see or touch the dead child is disturbing enough. Involving the grandparents in this healing gesture may be additionally distressing. Or staff members simply may not think to offer this opportunity to grandparents because of the erroneous notion that the loss does not affect them. What is disregarded by this attitude is that grandparents have their own plans and dreams for a time when they and the grandchild can develop their own relationship exclusive of the child's parents. In this fantasy, the grandparents and child have a whole future ahead of them as special friends and companions. When the baby's death occurs, these dreams are destroyed as completely as are those of the baby's parents. An example of the special meaning attached by grandparents to their expected grandchild involves a male infant who died at 2 days of age due to extreme prematurity. In this baby's extended family, only female grandchildren had preceded his birth. He was the sole grandson, graced with the responsibility of extending the family's name. The grandfather, present at the baby's death, grieved the loss of hopes and dreams for his only grandson as well as the end of the family name.

**Responses of
Grandparents after a
Pregnancy Loss**

Given the dynamic interactions that exist between children, their parents, and their parent's parents, the underlying emotions of grandparents take these forms:

Guilt

Grandparents of the dead baby may have wished and even expressed aloud the wish that the baby would be born dead or retarded. This irrational statement may reflect anger at their daughter in the case of an unplanned pregnancy, for example. When the wished-for outcome becomes a terrible reality, the grandparents' guilt surfaces.

Isolation from Their Daughter

The patient's parents may feel a need to protect their daughter, fearing for her health. If they are asked to wait outside the labor room, or even are asked to wait in another part the hospital, they may feel cut off and isolated.

Feelings of Their Own Loss

Grandparents may have plans and hopes for their own relationship with the child-to-be. These hopes are destroyed when the fetus (or newborn) dies but may not be addressed by medical care providers.

Grieving in a Vacuum

After the pregnancy loss, most or all attention is focused on parents of the baby. Seldom does a care provider take time to sit with grandparents and allow them to express their own personal grief.

A grandmother reflecting on her daughter's stillbirth experience wrote,

> The sad part is that, after everything is over, the world has missed that baby, that girl, that woman. It will make a difference in the future. Some boy will miss meeting that girl and marrying her. Their babies won't be born. That saddens me for I shall have to miss her growing up, and she might have done something wonderful for the world. But at the very least, it deprives me of future generations.

The social worker, then, has an important opportunity following a pregnancy loss, to utilize his or her understanding of family dynamics to aid patients and their families in the process of bereavement. All family members grieve the death of a baby; each grieves in a uniquely personal way. The social worker, by recognizing and sympathizing with the individual needs of each member of the immediate and extended family, may assist the medical staff in addressing these needs.

REFERENCES

1. Soricelli BA and Utech CL: Mourning the death of a child: the family and group process. *Social Work* 30(5):429–434, Sept/Oct 1985.
2. Friedman SB: Psychological aspects of sudden and unexpected death in infants and children. *Ped Cl North Am* 21(1):103–111, Feb 1974.
3. Cain AC, Erickson ME, Fast I, Vaughan RA: Children's disturbed reactions to their mother's miscarriage. *Psychosom Med* 26:58–66, 1964.
4. Bergman AB: Psychological aspects of sudden unexpected death in infants and children—Review and commentary. *Pediatr Clin North Am* 21(1):115–121, 1974.
5. Gould RK and Rothenberg MB: The chronically ill child facing death—how can the pediatrician help? *Clin Pediatr* (Phila) 12:447–449, July 1973.

Funeral Director

RONALD TROYER

When a death occurs in our society, a funeral home is usually selected by the family to assist in final disposition of the body. For a family experiencing fetal or newborn death, the involvement of the funeral director can have a powerful impact on the family's (especially the parents') ability to resolve and adjust to their loss. It is the purpose of this chapter to discuss positive ways in which funeral directors can assist the family in dealing with the nightmare of burying their baby. Much of this book stands as recognition that there are a number of professional and nonprofessional careproviders in the community who can assist bereaved parents in a meaningful way. The funeral director is an integral component of this team approach.

DEFINITION AND PURPOSE OF THE FUNERAL

Creating a Moment for Acknowledging Grief

Lamers (1) has developed a definition of the funeral that is widely used and quoted. He describes the funeral as an organized, purposeful, time-limited, flexible, group-centered response to death. For parents of a dead baby, the funeral becomes an opportunity to express deep feelings of loss in a socially significant manner. Through the funeral ceremony, parents become the center of attention for social support. This extension of sympathy tends to give rise to a sense of comfort and social acceptability (2). In addition, the funeral ceremony and setting provide a time in which parents, grandparents, family, and close friends publicly express feelings that are not acceptable in most everyday settings. For example, parents may appear disheveled

153

and may be in tears much of the time. Statements made by well-meaning friends may evoke emotional responses of crying and tears. These same statements, if made in another setting (for example, the grocery store), would be upsetting and not socially or emotionally acceptable.

"High-Grief" Loss

The funeral gives parents the means to set aside the general societal perception of and response to a baby's death as a "nonevent" (3). It also recognizes a *person* (the baby) as having lived and shared in a love relationship rather than the general societal definition of a dead baby as a "nonperson" (4). The sudden, unexpected death of a baby is often perceived as unfair and unjust, and/or may be denied or resented by parents. Such a death can be termed a "high-grief loss" (5). Societal and emotional needs of family, friends, and community in such instances are greater and the potential problems of parents more extensive than in the case of what has been termed a "low-grief loss" (A low-grief loss for some would be the death of an elderly relative. Little notice to the death would be given, and duration and intensity of grief experienced would be minimal.) Focusing our attention on the death (event) and the baby's life (person) through a funeral ceremony is now recognized as therapeutic and helpful in most cases (6).

The value for surviving family members of having a funeral ceremony for the baby has been documented and discussed by physicians for nearly 20 years. Grunebaum (7) writes of a woman whose baby died during delivery. The mother was helpless during delivery, not allowed to see the baby after delivery, and encouraged to sign an autopsy form and burial permit for a mass grave. Eventually, this woman sought psychiatric help, and Grunebaum questions what positive effect seeing her baby and participating in the funeral would have had on her grieving process.

FUNERAL DIRECTOR'S EDUCATION AND AWARENESS OF THE COUNSELOR'S ROLE

Facilitative versus Functional Role

In the early 1970s, there was a growing awareness within the funeral service profession of the special needs and considerations surrounding infant death. Numerous articles appeared in funeral service journals on neonatal death and parents' need to participate actively in their baby's funeral service. Many funeral directors became increasingly aware of their role as facilitators versus the role of functionaries, which they had performed for many years previously (8). In the mid-1970s, the American Board of Funeral Service Education (the accreditation agency for all mortuary science colleges) mandated that a social science curriculum be taught in all accredited schools. This curriculum included material on infant death. Licensed funeral directors, through continuing education programs, were also learning of the growing body of knowledge on pregnancy loss. Dr. D. Gary Benfield (9), a neonatologist, presented a program to Ohio funeral directors in 1980 on "Caring for Bereaved Parents: The Intersection of Funeral Service and Newborn Medicine." A great deal of effort has been made by national and state funeral director associations to provide programming and printed and audio-visual material on the subject matter.

Not all funeral directors practice the methods and procedures examined in this chapter, but fortunately there are many who do. The latter are enlightened and progressive funeral directors who recognize their role and appreciate their opportunity to share this prominent moment in parents' lives. Funeral directors are constantly involved with crisis situations and crisis counseling (10). Most funeral directors agree with Dr. Edgar Jackson (11), a pastoral psychologist, who says, "Funeral directors do not choose as to whether or not they will be counselors. Their only choice is will they be a good or bad counselor" (p. iii). The crisis created by pregnancy loss occurs not only to married women but also to young unmarried women who want their baby, and more and more to older single women who want children but who also want to remain unmarried. These less conventional situations require a sensitive and compassionate counselor, and it has often been the funeral director who finds him or herself serving in this role by default.

NOTIFICATION OF DEATH

Involving the Mother in Funeral Arrangements

The initial notification of death to the funeral home is usually made within the first 8 hours following the delivery/death. The call may come from the father, grandparents, other family members, hospital chaplain, family clergy, or hospital employees (social worker, nurse, or admitting office clerk). The point is that the funeral home sometimes receives a death call from persons not closely affected by the death. Thus, the funeral director frequently is caught in the middle by "helpful persons" who attempt to be protective, certain that they know what is "best" for the bereaved mother. This type of initial notification almost always comes before the woman is discharged from the hospital. The woman's health is of primary concern to the immediate family; they think that they are doing the right thing by making the call to the funeral home, believing that final disposition of the baby must take place before the woman is released from the hospital. Funeral directors find that a common misconception exists: that final disposition must be made within 24–48 hours following death.

This misconception and others are a good reason why the funeral director should try to meet with the father or grandparents as soon as possible after the telephone notification. There is a need to sit down and discuss facts before misconceptions and feelings of protection isolate the woman completely from the funeral process.

The funeral director should explain that, although there is a time frame in which the funeral must take place, there is no rush. It is possible and highly desirable to wait until the mother can be part of the arrangements conference. The mother's participation and presence in the funeral process should be encouraged as a positive means of helping her cope with the feelings of loss that she will experience. The author often says, "We cannot take away your pain, but we can share it. We cannot prevent your suffering, but we can prevent you from suffering for the wrong reasons." Describing the possibility of a mother's experiencing a "second layer of grief" because of her exclusion from the funeral process is a useful means of demonstrating how important the funeral process is for both the mother and the father (9).

Purpose of the Directive Approach

Some professionals feel that advising the family in this manner is too directive. However, this approach is *meant* to be directive. There is a wealth of information on pregnancy loss available now, which indicates that an initial nondirective approach by healthcare or other professionals in advising a family can cause serious and unnecessary problems for them later on. The author's personal experience with fathers and other family members is that they often need directive counseling to understand the mother's needs and desires.

The booklet *When Hello Means Goodbye* (12) is well suited to give to parents during the initial meeting. This 32-page guide for parents whose baby has died at birth or shortly after is sensitive and informative. It is brief enough so that families are able to read through it quickly and gather information that reinforces the counseling of the funeral director, physician, nurse, or clergy. All persons who have contact with women experiencing pregnancy loss are encouraged to read this booklet.

ARRANGEMENTS CONFERENCE

Conference Held in Private with Both Parents

The funeral director should schedule a time when the parents can meet with him or her in order to plan the funeral service and final disposition. The importance of this meeting is underscored by LaMore (13), who describes the making of arrangements as "the superbly therapeutic first social, economic[,] and religious decisions one has to make to acknowledge the loss and initiate a new beginning" (p.10). Often, because of the mother's confinement in the hospital, the arrangements conference occurs in the hospital. Ideally, then, this meeting should take place privately in a small, comfortable room. If the family wants to wait until the mother is discharged, the conference can be held in the family's home or at the funeral home.

Providing Choices   The place, time, and officiant of the service are discussed. Information for the death certificate and the obituary is obtained. Beyond these routine procedures for a funeral director, the conference should lead to a thorough discussion of the choices that parents have in planning their baby's service. Parents should be told that they can take pictures if they choose to. These personal photographs supplement ones taken at the hospital and later can become very important as the parents' way of remembering their baby. The funeral director can offer to obtain a lock of the baby's hair or to make a set of footprints, if this was not done at the hospital. Parents are informed of their right to dress and hold their baby. Dressing and holding the baby are acts of parenting that are meaningful to some mothers and fathers. Not all parents will choose to do this but all should be given such a choice, with time to think about their decision. It seems that mothers are more likely to want to hold the baby, while fathers are less likely. However, experience has shown that fathers will help place the baby in the casket, if offered the opportunity.

Additional decisions regarding appropriate floral tributes, memorial folders, and music selections are made. Use of poetry, prose, or written family statements or letters for use during the service is discussed and often encouraged. The funeral director should mention that personal items, such as toys, pictures, letters, or religious items, may be placed in the baby's casket.

Decisions on final disposition of the body are made. If burial is chosen, usually there is discussion about where in the cemetery is best for the family—in a "baby land" section or in a family plot, or sometimes in a grave already occupied by a family member. For those families choosing cremation, a discussion of what they will do with the cremated remains is necessary. Often, it is best for parents to wait a few weeks before acting on a decision to scatter cremated remains; personal experience has shown that parents frequently regret this decision at a later date, since there is no final resting place for them to visit in the future. Some cemeteries allow family members to dig open the grave for the casket or urn. Although not all fathers will choose to do this, it can be an important act for some, if they are given the choice. Many fathers will want to carry their baby's casket to the grave if given the opportunity. The arrangements conference is a time to let parents know about the variety of ways in which they can participate in their baby's funeral and burial. Some will do a lot and some will do little, but they all should be given the choice to act in a parenting role as they see fit.

SELECTION OF CASKET, VAULT, URN

During the arrangements conference, the family and the funeral director discuss selection of a casket and related items. Most families are given several choices of caskets, made of different materials. Parents usually decide which is best for them after considering design, material used, and cost.

Funeral directors who have spoken with (and listened to) parents sometime after the complete service have learned that there are some important issues for parents concerning a baby's casket. These issues are discussed over and over in parent support groups. One issue is the type of material that is used to make the casket. For a number of years, funeral directors have made available a casket/vault combination. It is made of a polyurethane material that is usually white in color and lightweight. It is a highly durable and strong casket that can be sealed with an epoxy sealant. The problem in the past has been that parents are not always told about the durability and strength factors; commonly they select these caskets from a picture catalog. Without complete information, some parents respond negatively to caskets when they do see them, because of their color and weight. Parents will often say that such a casket looks like a "pop cooler" or "beer cooler." Some parents will seem to be haunted later on by having buried their baby in such a container. The same problem arises for other parents who chose metal caskets, which have been referred to as a "mailbox." To avoid this misunderstanding and confusion, parents should be given complete information (verbally and in writing) about the casket. They may be asked to look at, ask questions about, and carefully examine the casket before their baby is placed in it.

Selection of a casket and related items should be made by both parents. Funeral directors have reported receiving telephone calls from mothers on rainy days wanting to know if the baby would be "dry and warm" in this weather. Often, mothers with such anxieties were uninformed and not present during the casket selection. Experience has shown that the casket is viewed very subjectively and is of genuine concern to most parents. A perceptive funeral director will provide objective information, at the same time recognizing that the selection of the casket is an important part of the total experience that parents are trying to assimilate and understand.

FINANCIAL CONSIDERATIONS

During the arrangements conference, parents should be informed by the funeral director about financial obligations for which the family will be responsible. Rules mandated by the Federal Trade Commission in 1984 require the funeral director to provide a general price list showing the charge for professional services, facilities, and automobile equipment. This itemized list should be given to the family at the beginning of the discussion about funeral home charges. Charges for an infant service are, in general, significantly less than the charges for an adult service.

The "No-Charge" Service: Pros and Cons

Because of the relatively small number of infant services that a funeral home will conduct in a year, revenue thereby generated usually is not a budgeted item. Funeral directors should be acutely aware of the medical and incidental expenses that pregnancy loss can incur. They therefore should try to keep funeral home charges as reasonable as possible. Some funeral homes provide their services at no cost, as a community service. Interestingly, this "no-charge service" has in some cases caused more hurt than help to parents. Parents may perceive the no-charge service as confirmation that the baby's life and funeral service are of no value (monetarily). In a materialistic society, the amount of money spent is often equated with the amount of love. Funeral directors who have observed this often itemize their complete charges, then offer a generous discount, leaving a small balance for the family to pay.

There are expenses involved with most infant services that the funeral director has no direct control over. These include honoraria, cemetery charges, newspaper notices, and flowers. If the funeral home assumes payment of these charges, it is noted as a cash advance. During the arrangements conference, the funeral director prepares the purchase agreement, which itemizes all funeral home charges, merchandise selections, and cash advances. The purchase agreement is signed, and a copy is given to the family.

EMBALMING PROCEDURES, DRESSING, AND CASKETING

In most cases, it is possible for infant embalming to take place if the parent(s) give permission. The value of having the baby present for holding and viewing during the funeral process is now recognized by healthcare professionals as beneficial in the grief process (14, 15). In instances when the baby's delivery was very difficult for the woman, the embalming procedure allows additional time for her physical recovery before she participates in funeral activities. Parents who see their baby after proper embalming tend to be less anxious and seem to be more accepting of the situation. The reality of how the baby looks physically is much less frightening than the image imagined by many women who are not allowed to see their babies. Parents will see things in their baby's features that are very difficult for others to see. Thus, embalming can project some "normalcy" into an otherwise abnormal situation for parents.

Over the years, several embalming techniques for babies have been developed and put into practice with varying degrees of success. A recent technique, developed by Miley and written about by Doty (16), uses an angiocath and hypodermic syringe for injection. An angiocath is a small-diameter flexible catheter or tube with a hypodermic needle that fits inside. A 16-gauge, 3–1/4-inch combination is recommended. This technique is providing very successful results in preservation, skin texture, skin coloration, positioning, and general overall appearance. Funeral directors using this procedure can embalm very small babies with better results than were achieved with earlier common procedures.

Communicating with Pathologists to Preserve Integrity of the Body

When an autopsy has been performed, the success of the embalming operation is determined by the care that the pathologist has taken to leave vessels exposed and accessible. Funeral directors who have problems because of this are urged to meet with the pathologist to resolve the difficulty. Parents who give permission for an autopsy often ask the funeral director about the procedure. The funeral director should be positive, assuring parents that they have made the right decision in granting consent for this procedure. Later on, the autopsy report can be very important in helping parents understand their loss. The funeral director should encourage parents to meet with their physician to review the autopsy report. (Chapter 13, "Value of the Perinatal Autopsy," provides full discussion of the benefits of an autopsy.)

Guiding Parents as They Dress and Hold Their Baby

During the arrangements conference, parents have been given the option to dress and hold their baby. If they choose to do so, the funeral director should try to describe what they can expect to see and how they may respond. It is helpful for parents to be better prepared in this way before they enter the room. Before parents see their baby at the funeral home, the funeral director may dress the baby in a tee shirt and diaper (provided by the family) to cover incisions. A bonnet or hat usually is used when a cranial autopsy has been performed. The baby should be wrapped in a blanket and placed on a couch or low table so that parents can sit or kneel by their baby. Parents should be told to expect the baby's body temperature to be the same as room temperature. This 20°F+ difference between room temperature and normal body temperature surprises some parents unpleasantly, and it can leave them with a negative and painful impression of their baby as "cold." Parents often comment on the incisions, referring to them as "scars." The implication of this terminology is that the baby is healing and okay. The author never has chosen to dispute these comments, which are heard repeatedly. Some parents appreciate the funeral director's assistance in dressing their baby, although some do not want or need any help. The funeral director should ask what assistance the parents need and if they wish to be alone with their baby at this time. Most parents do want such private time. The funeral director can excuse him or herself from the room after telling the parents where he or she can be found if needed.

Many funeral homes provide a rocking chair for the mother to sit in if she wants to hold her baby. This can be very therapeutic and should be encouraged. Fathers generally are more reluctant to participate in dressing and holding a dead baby. After parents are satisfied with these actions, the baby may be placed in the casket, along with any personal items that parents have decided to bury with their baby.

VISITATION

Some parents choose to have a visitation or wake during the evening before or on the day of their baby's funeral. This period of time is set aside for family members and friends, work associates, and community members to visit with parents to express concern and love. Viewing the baby's body during this time generally allows those in attendance to see a "normal" baby. This visual reality usually reduces the number of questions about the baby's appearance that the parents may face from others later on.

Responses of the Extended Family

The author has observed family interactions at visitations for a number of years. Several comments are of interest. During the visitation for a baby, the grandparents of the mother and father often seem most comfortable with the situation and adept at comforting the baby's parents (their own grandchildren). As a rule, the parents of the baby's mother and father tend to be very protective and more reserved. Probably, this is because of the pain they feel in seeing their own children hurting over their loss. It is likely that grandparents, because of their age (60–70), have already experienced significant first-hand losses. Grand-parents seem more objective and open in discussing the loss. Also, people in this age group grew up in a period of time in our society when pregnancy loss was more common. Many grandmothers of women who experience pregnancy loss today may reveal for the first time that they, too, had a similar loss. This phenomenon may have a significant impact on a grand-daughter's resolution of her own pregnancy loss. Perhaps a study conducted on this relationship might yield data to this effect.

FUNERAL SERVICE

The style of the funeral ceremony or service that takes place often is predicated on the officiant's (clergy's) personal and doctrinal responses to pregnancy loss. A wide range of response to this type of loss by clergy has been observed. Some clergy prefer only to participate in a quickly arranged graveside service or memorial service, although others are more willing to officiate at a service in the church, temple, or funeral home with the baby's body present. Families who depend heavily on their clergy for advice and consolation most often accept with-out question the type of service their clergy recommends. Some-times, the funeral director finds him or herself caught between a family's desire or need for a more meaningful service and the officiant's desire to "keep it simple." "Simple" usually means quickly arranged and without the mother present at the service. Fortunately, this conflict occurs less often now that more infor-mation on the impact of pregnancy loss is available.

Assembling to Share the Family's Sorrow

The funeral is an opportunity for the community to assem-ble, express love, and share in parents' sorrow. In the past, it seems that professionals who cared for the woman during her pregnancy and after its unexpected outcome generally remained absent from this important service for the family. The funeral is the beginning of a process, the process of grieving over the death of a wished-for baby and the loss of the inherent dreams for that child. Healthcare providers have seemed to regard a baby's funeral as the end of a process and to have rationalized that their presence at the funeral would be unnecessary, intru-sive, and undesirable. Interestingly, to the contrary, families comment very positively about the presence of their physicians, nurses, and social workers when these professionals do attend

Meaning of Care Providers' Attendance at the Funeral

funeral services. It makes parents feel less isolated and alone in the aftermath of their loss. Although time and work demands cannot always allow professionals an opportunity to attend services, more consideration should be given to their attending whenever possible because of the positive effect that this gesture has on parents. Professionals who attend a funeral service also may benefit from having had an opportunity to express their personal feelings over the family's loss. Healthcare professionals are human, too, and they need to express rather than suppress normal feelings that can occur (1). Most of the "burnout" that occurs in the healthcare professions is death related (17). Expression of normal and natural feelings in a timely and organized fashion can do much to increase the effectiveness of the healthcare professional in subsequent similar situations.

POSTFUNERAL RECEPTION

Following the funeral service and committal service, many families gather together for a meal and time of fellowship. Funeral directors have observed the benefits of this gathering. During the arrangements conference, they should encourage families to plan this type of activity. Offering a meal allows neighbors, friends, and the religious congregation to be involved by preparing and serving the food. The extended family who has gathered together for the baby's funeral has an opportunity to strengthen and renew family bonds in an emotionally less-intense atmosphere. This sharing and open recognition of one of life's most painful experiences can assist in reducing the conspiracy of silence (18) that parents may feel at future family and social gatherings.

EXTENDED CARE FOR THE FAMILY

Many funeral homes offer to parents experiencing pregnancy loss information about additional resources that are available following the funeral, as their grief follows its course. This extended-care program is based on a knowledge that the impact of pregnancy loss on the survivor(s) is not felt or experienced completely within the time frame of the funeral. The most intense feelings about the loss may come several months later. It is then that couples may expect to lean on each other "but find [that they] cannot lean on something bent double from its own burden" (19). Couples expecting great closeness may instead experience disappointment and resentment.

Supplementing Support Offered by Primary Care Providers

The funeral director's involvement in this extended care will depend to some degree on the level of involvement that parents have with primary healthcare professionals after their baby's death. As greater knowledge of the impact that pregnancy loss has on parents and families is gained, more extended-care programs are being made available to parents by primary health-care providers. The funeral director's involvement then is to supplement rather than to initiate any such programs. Funeral directors who have organized and/or participated with bereavement support groups know the value of talking with someone who has had a similar life experience (20). The funeral director may provide parents with a list of pregnancy loss support groups and the contact person for each. The funeral director should follow up with a phone call to the mother four to eight weeks after the funeral service in order to determine if contact has been made with a group. If the mother has not contacted anyone, the funeral director may encourage her and her partner to do so.

Resources for the Well-Informed Funeral Director

Funeral directors can provide reprints of specific articles regarding pregnancy loss that are helpful to most parents. The Compassionate Friends is a national support group for parents who have suffered the death of a child, and their newsletters frequently contain articles specifically concerned with pregnancy loss, such as those by Church, Chazin, and McBeath (21), and McLaughlin (22). Funeral directors who subscribe to this newsletter can thereby obtain an ongoing source of helpful information appropriate to offer to parents bereaved by pregnancy loss. Funeral directors also can make available a list of books about pregnancy loss that parents can borrow from the funeral home library, public library, or support-group library. Borg and Lasker (23) and Peppers and Knapp (6) have written books that provide excellent bibliotherapy for many parents. A more recent publication by Schatz (24) deals specifically with healing a father's grief. It is a direct and well-written addition to the pregnancy-loss literature that is already available. Additionally, parents who have surviving children usually are interested in articles and books concerning how children respond to the death of a sibling.

The funeral director can also provide written information on ways in which parents may choose to memorialize a baby's brief life. Some parents purchase a monument or marker to place on the baby's grave. Parents are encouraged to give careful thought to the design and wording on the monument. They may need additional time for this, and they should not feel rushed in making this decision. One form of memorialization that parents find suitable is an engraved wall plaque. Again, wording on the plaque should be carefully considered. This type of memorialization may be beneficial and meaningful when there is no gravesite available to visit and when parents have a strong desire to remember and recognize their baby's life.

CONCLUSIONS

And let us not grow weary in well-doing; for in due season
we shall reap, if we do not lose heart.
—GALATIANS 6:9

Over the years, many professionals trying to console and help parents suffering from pregnancy loss have found themselves discouraged over the lack of support and understanding from their fellow professionals. This is changing, fortunately, thanks to a number of persistent women who have lived through this painful experience. When we deal with pregnancy loss and its emotional impact on the family, it is precisely what we do not know that can hurt us and those whom we serve the most. Worse, on several occasions, the author has encountered professionals whose treatment is influenced by something more harmful than ignorance, that is "knowing" something that isn't so. Fortunately, the width and depth of knowledge on pregnancy loss is growing rapidly.

What funeral directors most need is to share this information and experience with each other. This is not a new or original idea (15). Physicians, nurses, social workers, and funeral directors need to spend more time discussing how they can operate as a team to serve those who need support and understanding. Lastly, all members of this team need to listen closely to those who have been through the experience of pregnancy loss. They know only too painfully the reality of a dream's being shattered, of hope turning to despair, of meaning becoming absurdity, of life shifting suddenly to death. They can be the greatest teachers. They rightfully deserve admiration and respect.

REFERENCES

1. Lamers WM, Jr.: Funerals are good for people—M.D.'s included. *Med Econ* 46:4, 1969.
2. Pine V: *Social Meanings of the Funeral*. New York, Foundation of Thanatology, Columbia University, 1974, pp 12–13.
3. Bowlby J: *Attachment and Loss: Vol. III: Loss*. New York, Basic Books, 1980.
4. Lewis E: The mangement of stillbirth—coping with an unreality. *Lancet* 2:619–620, 1976.
5. Fulton R: Death, grief, and the funeral in contemporary society. *The Director*, 1976–1977, p 9 (Reprint).
6. Peppers L and Knapp R: *Motherhood and Mourning*. Philadelphia, Praeger Publishers, 1980, p 126.
7. Grunebaum H: Grief. *Psychiat Opinion* 5:38–43, 1968.
8. Nichols RJ: Funerals: a time for grief and growth. In Kübler-Ross E (ed):

Death: The Final Stage of Growth. New York, Prentice-Hall, 1975, pp 87–96.

9. Benfield G and Nichols J: *Caring for Bereaved Parents: The Intersection of Funeral Service and Newborn Medicine.* Presentation, Ohio Funeral Directors Association, Midwinter Institute, Feb 1980.
10. Snow L: The application of invitation theory to professional death and bereavement counseling. *Thanatos* 9:9–11, 1984.
11. Raether H and Slater R: *The Funeral Director and His Role as a Counselor.* Milwaukee, National Funeral Directors Association, 1975, p iii.
12. Schwiebert P and Kirk P: *When Hello Means Goodbye.* Portland, OR, University of Oregon Health Sciences Center, 1981.
13. LaMore GE, Jr: The art of dying. *The Director* 15(8):10–11, 1985.
14. Davidson G: Death of the wished-for child: a case study. *Death Education Quarterly,* Fall, 1977.
15. Benfield G and Nichols J: Living with newborn death: the challenge of upstream caring. *Dodge Magazine* 73:5–29, 1981.
16. Doty K: Infant embalming: A new approach. *The Director* 15(4):11–46, 1985.
17. Osterweis M, Solomon F, Green M: *Bereavement: Reactions, Consequences, and Care.* Washington, DC, National Academy Press, 1984.
18. Lewis E: Mourning by the family after a stillbirth or neonatal death. *Arch Dis Child* 54:303–306, 1979.
19. Schiff HS: *The Bereaved Parent.* New York, Penguin Books, 1982, p 58.
20. Troyer R: Living and loving more: enhancing support group outreach to the bereaved. *The Director* 15(4):16–49, 1985.
21. Church M, Chazin H, McBeath K: *When a Baby Dies.* Oak Brook, IL, The Compassionate Friends, 1980.
22. McLaughlin C: *An Oddyssey for Bereaved Parents.* Oak Brook, IL, The Compassionate Friends, 1982.
23. Borg S and Lasker J: *When Pregnancy Fails.* Boston, Beacon Press, 1981.
24. Schatz W: *Healing a Father's Grief.* Redmond, WA, Medic Publishing, 1984.

SUGGESTED READINGS

Benfield G, Leig, S, Vollman J: Grief response of parents to neonatal death and parent participation in deciding care. *Pediatrics* 62:171–177, 1978.

Brammer L: *The Helping Relationship.* Englewood Cliffs, NJ, Prentice-Hall, 1979.

DeSpelder L and Strickland A: *The Last Dance: Encountering Death and Dying.* Palo Alto, CA, Mayfield Publishing, 1983.

Feifel H: *New Meanings of Death.* New York, McGraw-Hill, 1977.

Jensen A: *Healing Grief.* Redmond, WA, Medic Publishing, 1980.

Lane M: Unexpected outcomes. *Christ Hospital Serving Cincinnati* 14:11–13, Summer, 1984.

Moffet MJ: *In the Midst of Winter: Selections from the Literature of Mourning.* New York, Random House, 1982.

Raether H: The place of the funeral: the role of the funeral director in contemporary America. *Omega,* 2:136–149, 1971.

Shaw CT: Grief over fetal loss. *Family Practice Recertification* 5:129–145, 1983.

PART

Care of the Patient after Discharge from the Hospital

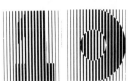

Obstetrician As Outpatient Counselor

JAMES R. WOODS, Jr., M.D.

DEFINING THE PATIENT'S NEEDS

Patients experiencing a pregnancy loss ultimately seek answers to 3 questions: What happened? Why did it happen? Will it happen again? Historically, these patients upon discharge from the hospital were offered virtually no insight as to the emotional consequences of a pregnancy loss. They were sent home to recover without support, lacking any consistent guidance or reassurance that they were suffering healthy grief. Confusion was complicated in many cases by a lack of information about medical events leading to the pregnancy loss. Burdened by confusion and anger, grieving patients were expected to function normally in a society that was itself unable to understand or to cope with this critical type of personal, family, and marital crisis.

The Need for Facts
Patients only begin to resolve their emotional conflicts when they can understand the events and issues concerning their pregnancy loss. When obstetricians arrange for only one follow-up visit at 6 weeks postpartum to make a physical examination, patients are left to their own devices to suffer through a most critical and painful period in their lives. If their care providers fail to give emotional support and to inform them about how they are likely to respond, patients will have no way of knowing what to expect during the first several weeks

after a pregnancy loss. Lack of information breeds confusion. Confusion breeds anger. And anger becomes suspicion as the patient attempts to rationalize or justify the events that led to the death of her baby.

Outpatient Counseling 1 Week Postpartum Is Important

The obstetrician possesses a unique opportunity to assist in a family's understanding and early resolution of the complicated experience following a pregnancy loss. Encouraging the patient to return for outpatient counseling within the first week after discharge after a loss is warranted for the following reasons:

1. The patient or couple, because of their unusual circumstances, should be pulled out of the mainstream of obstetric care and designated as unique, requiring specialized medical attention.
2. The patient desperately needs support and information. When she and her family receive such care from her physician, this individual attention is perceived as evidence that medical care providers are equipped to confront this most sensitive of issues.
3. Anger, confusion, or suspicion, which the patient may be inclined to focus on the medical community, is minimized when care providers demonstrate a willingness to confront difficult issues by explaining medical decisions and procedures and by examining the pregnancy outcome in a straightforward and honest manner.

Patients have multiple reasons for requiring outpatient counseling. They seek answers to their questions concerning the pregnancy loss itself, and they need information and support that will help them recover emotionally from the experience.

MEDICAL QUESTIONS

Need for Additional Explanations

"Why did my baby die?" Despite adequate counseling while a woman is in the hospital, she begins afterward to raise the same as well as new questions about events leading to the death of her baby. After she has had time to adjust to the reality of her loss, the woman begins to think more clearly about what has happened. Also, although questions may have been answered sufficiently while she was still hospitalized, she may have been too overwhelmed to comprehend any explanations given her. She needs to return for outpatient counseling to review questions and answers about her pregnancy loss.

Some patients merely seek a more complete discussion of medical events. "What is an abruptio placentae?" "Why did my blood pressure become so high in the last part of my pregnancy?" "Why did my baby's umbilical cord deliver into the vagina after my membranes were broken?" Others question why action was not taken, or they may challenge decisions that were made before the baby died. "Why didn't the doctor believe me when I told him my baby was not moving?" "Shouldn't the doctor have seen me in his office the first day I had vaginal spotting?" "Aren't there tests to tell if the baby is all right?" "Couldn't the doctor have controlled my diabetes in the last part of my pregnancy?"

Many such questions are legitimate; and the answers may be difficult for healthcare professionals to acknowledge, especially if alternate medical or obstetric management might have resulted in a different outcome. Regardless of how "uncomfortable" professionals may feel in a given case, all issues should be presented openly and fairly. Meeting the patient in the first week after hospital discharge with an accepting and understanding attitude diffuses the normal anger that exists behind these questions and which, if left unchecked, often results in malpractice suits.

EMOTIONAL NEEDS

Guidance for Parents Recovering from Pregnancy Loss

"How should I act now that my baby is dead?" All patients discharged from the hospital following a pregnancy loss must face bewildered, uninformed relatives, friends, and acquaintances. These people, with perhaps the best of intentions, raise questions about the pregnancy loss that can further distress everyone concerned. Patients and their partners ought to be provided advice as to the emotional consequences of these encounters. No one is prepared for or can predict how he or she will respond to the death of a baby. It is incumbent on the medical community to provide guidance and to maintain an ongoing relationship with couples as they begin their long process of recovery and healing. Questions, often unstated, that must be addressed are: "How should I deal with family members?" "How will I discuss the death of my baby with friends?" "How will I respond if my partner exhibits personality traits that I'm not familiar with when we discuss the baby's death?" When, in response to a pregnancy loss, the assertive patient becomes unassertive, the caring becomes selfish, or the energetic becomes easily fatigued and fears that she will never recover, the need for early and intensive outpatient counseling becomes clear.

WHAT ARE THE ISSUES AND WHEN SHOULD THEY BE ADDRESSED?

Immediate Concerns

During the past 3 years, professionals at the University of Cincinnati Perinatal Support Service have formatted pregnancy loss counseling sessions to meet patients' immediate needs. The focus is on events and activities that patients perceive as major stumbling blocks once they return home from the hospital. People progress one day at a time through the first few weeks after a pregnancy loss. A woman who normally organizes home, children, and work now must concentrate just to prepare a meal. Taking a walk may be too taxing. Disorganization and an inability to function as normal are in themselves stressful, both to the grieving individual and to the entire family.

Adjusting the Counseling to Meet the Couple's Needs

In the very early stage of acute grief, a person functions best when activities, tasks, and responsibilities are approached in single fashion. The obstetrician must adapt his or her methods of outpatient counseling to mirror the events and thought patterns of the patient at this point. In the first phase of outpatient counseling, to issue advice about the next pregnancy when the patient is wondering how she will manage to endure the next few days only widens the gap between patient and care provider. The effective counselor is sensitive to the patient's emotional state and calibrates the intensity of the counseling according to the grieving patient's needs. Advice at any session should be limited to helping the patient cope with stressful events that she is encountering at the moment. In general, issues related to a subsequent pregnancy or long-term coping skills should be discussed at much later outpatient visits, unless the patient chooses to discuss them.

WHAT STYLE OF COUNSELING SHOULD BE ADOPTED?

In the first few outpatient counseling sessions, the directive and instructional approach to patient counseling serves several purposes.

Benefits of the Directive Approach

1) The overall tone of the counseling sessions is one of informing the patient about events that led up to her pregnancy loss. This instructional form of counseling fulfills important early needs of the patient to have facts. It sets the tone for a more in-depth discussion of the emotional consequences of pregnancy loss. Many patients are made uneasy if, as the sole purpose of the outpatient counseling session, they feel obligated to share their emotional response to this life crisis at a time in their recovery when they probably are not yet able to engage in

this type of intimacy. Counseling sessions may be offered as an opportunity for the patient to talk openly if she desires. The invitation to talk may or may not be acted upon and the counselor responds accordingly.

2) The directive, instructional approach allows the physician to reinforce and support the concept that the patient is exhibiting an appropriate response to her crisis. The purpose of initial outpatient visits should not be to probe for deep-seated neurotic or psychotic tendencies to serve as an explanation for the patient's response to her pregnancy loss. In most cases, the patients seen in these sessions are normal people recovering from a terrible experience. Their method of recovery follows no guidelines or rules. They have to learn for themselves how to carry on with their lives. The physician can contribute greatly to their recovery by providing understanding and helpful advice that can simplify this process.

3) This approach utilizes experience and ideas gained from counseling former patients and therefore conveys the message that "You are not alone in your response." The author often uses the expression "This may not pertain to you, but I have had other patients tell me. . . ."

FIRST VISIT FOLLOWING DISCHARGE FROM HOSPITAL

The first visit following discharge from the hospital is critical in the long-term management of patients with a pregnancy loss. It is essential that these patients be brought back early for outpatient counseling, preferably during the first week after discharge. At this time, the physician may clarify issues and help the patient to express any anger that otherwise would increase as the patient begins to evaluate her experience once she is out of the hospital. The counselor must be able to accept a patient's anger, difficult as this sometimes may be. It is helpful to establish that the counselor is not there to defend the medical profession to a patient.

Follow-up Visit Very Early in the Postpartum Period

It is not redundant—and is often helpful—to bring a patient back to the office only days after her hospital discharge. Many issues do not surface before a patient returns home, and these can easily provide material for a meaningful and intense first counseling session. A patient scheduled for an outpatient follow-up visit very likely will feel the need for such an appointment as she begins to piece together what has happened.

Direct Discussion toward Immediate Issues

During the initial visit, it is appropriate to direct questions or suggestions toward events that have occurred during the first days following the pregnancy loss. Common feelings for patients

> The woman may experience intense emptiness at the thought of going home.
>
> Couples return to a house that will not be their baby's home.
>
> Many women have already set up the baby's room. Will they dismantle the crib and pack up blankets and diapers or just close the door to the room, to deal with it later?
>
> The woman has no appetite.
>
> The woman has no energy and has a diminished ability to perform a complicated task.
>
> The woman is unable to sleep; she has nightmares.
>
> The woman is preoccupied with thoughts and daydreams about her baby.
>
> There is a sense of utter despair or loneliness.
>
> There may be feelings of fear at anything or anyone.
>
> The woman may feel guilty that something she did or thought may have contributed to the pregnancy loss.

Figure 10.1. Woman's feelings about herself or her baby

with a pregnancy loss in the first week after discharge from the hospital are described in Figure 10.1. Recognizing that these conflicts can occur may help the physician focus his or her questions during initial outpatient visits. A tendency for inexperienced care providers is to overcounsel during this first visit. To do this is to overlook the needs of the patient at this stage in her recovery.

FEELINGS GENERATED BY ENCOUNTERS WITH OTHERS

Loneliness and Isolation from Family and Friends

1. "My family and friends avoid me." Relatives and friends represent the most important long-term support system for the couple. Unfortunately, few people are at ease discussing the death of a baby, regardless of family relationship. More commonly, family or friends are solicitous and attentive for the first day or couple of days after the woman returns home, only to become preoccupied once again with their own activities and commitments shortly thereafter. Worse, some family members or friends avoid the couple altogether. The misconceptions that motivate this avoidance behavior are simply that family members and friends may not know what to say and consequently are afraid that they will say the wrong things. They worry that if they say something "wrong" and the woman cries they will have caused her to be sad. They fail to recognize that the woman

Did the people in the hospital treat you well?

How did it feel to go home?

What was the hardest part for you once you returned home?

What do you think caused your pregnancy loss?

With whom do you talk about the death of your baby when you are at home?

How do your friends act? How are your co-workers responding?

What is the response of family members?

[If the father has gone back to work] How did his co-workers react?

How are the baby's siblings reacting? How did you tell them about what happened?

Do you have any questions for me?

Figure 10.2.   Questions pertinent to initial outpatient counseling visit.

often cries because someone, finally, has said, "Tell me how you feel." When family or friends stay away, the woman is apt to interpret this action as reflecting an uncaring and indifferent attitude.

2. "I run into friends or acquaintances who are unaware of my pregnancy loss." This often occurs in public places. Many women recount meeting members of their natural childbirth classes while out in public. In these circumstances, the woman is unsure whether to be honest and state what happened or to ignore the other person in order to avoid an unpleasant encounter, to either protect herself or "spare" the other. The questions listed in Figure 10.2 have proved helpful in encouraging the patient to discuss her problems during the first few days after discharge from the hospital.

SUBSEQUENT ISSUES AND CONFLICTS

Counseling Couples about Differences in Responses of Men and Women

Pregnancy loss affects every aspect of a couple's existence together. To properly counsel a couple who has experienced such a crisis, the obstetrician must be aware of these consequences and direct counseling to address these issues.

There are differences in the responses of men and women to a pregnancy loss. The response of each person is unique and is influenced heavily by past experiences, personality, and type of pregnancy loss. It is an understatement that a woman feels absolute responsibility for the fetus developing within her uterus. It is equally true that most women take full responsibility

**Fathers' Typical
Reactions to
Miscarriage**

for the consequences when a pregnancy loss occurs. Her partner may exhibit compassion, understanding, and a sense of personal loss when a fetus or neonate dies. However, he cannot realize the total sense of responsibility that the woman must endure as a result of the outcome.

The couple experiencing a miscarriage must deal with an additional problem. The woman has felt breast tenderness, nausea, and fatigue in the early part of her pregnancy. Before a fetus may be seen by ultrasonography, these physical symptoms are projected by the woman into the future child. Her hopes and dreams for this baby are the "pregnancy loss," when vaginal bleeding leads to discharge of tissue and then to a D & C. But what experience does the man have to enable him to bond with the baby? He may display considerable excitement when first learning of a positive pregnancy test. The man may begin to perceive loss when adverse events develop. But, he has no first-hand physical experience of the pregnancy before it is lost during the first trimester. He must accept the emptiness and physical pain described to him as real, although he is unable to share it.

Not physically affected by a miscarriage and most probably not as involved emotionally as is the woman with the loss of the baby so early in the pregnancy, many men quickly return to work and their usual leisure activities. Often, a man begins to question why his partner's grieving process is taking so long. A woman caught between her own reaction and that of her partner may question with anger how he could return to business as usual. The obstetrician, recognizing the destructive dynamics that are operating, may discuss with the confused couple how common this is and attempt to help each to understand the other's attitudes and reactions. Merely acknowledging that each interprets the event from a different perspective contributes greatly in opening communication between the man and woman.

Even when a stillbirth or neonatal death occurs, the response of men and women may be different. In the earliest days or weeks after the event, both parents may experience shock and disbelief in a similar manner. It is not uncommon for both to describe a lack of appetite, energy, and interest in daily activities. Each finds it a burden to carry out routine functions at home or work.

Within a few weeks, however, the reaction and mood swings for the couple become dyssynchronous. The man, by focusing on work or physical activity, may find a reprieve, however brief, from the heaviness of his baby's death. At other times, the woman may conscientiously refuse to think about the event. Unfortunately, if the couple does not communicate well during this period, these moments of one partner's resting

Obstetrician's Efforts May Help Couple Communicate with One Another

from the burden of the pregnancy loss may foster anger and resentment.

Soon conversations between the 2 people about their pregnancy loss stop. Although the couple may talk about other subjects, they avoid that which is most on their minds. In time, each is left alone and lonely to deal with emotions and pain incurred by their baby's death. The obstetrician must attempt to maintain a connection between the 2 individuals during this period of impaired communication if each is to understand the position and loneliness of the other.

Most men carry an additional burden after a pregnancy loss. Men are generally very poor at expressing their emotions. It is therefore not unusual when their male co-workers treat them as if nothing had happened. Only rarely will another man offer such words as, "I'm sorry; want to talk about it?" A man who says this usually has experienced a similar occurrence himself and, having known the terrible feelings of pain and loneliness, appreciates another man's needs under these circumstances. Unfortunately, many men are left alone, not understanding why their "friends" could be so uncaring.

Figures 10.3 and 10.4 offer questions that help the outpatient counselor assess parents' progress as they grieve for their baby. By discussing these issues in a thoughtful manner, the physician can provide patients recovering from a pregnancy loss with a series of suggestions for coping with events of the next days or weeks and can alert them to behavioral conflicts as they begin the slow process of healing.

Repeat any of the questions from the first visit that seem appropriate.

Provide more information about what may have caused the pregnancy loss. Search for any misconceptions, such as that sex, activity, or stress caused the loss.

Inquire more about feelings of anger and frustration. With whom does the patient feel she can talk?

How are the couple together and as individuals working through their grief? Are there problems with their sex life? What do they talk about from day to day?

Discuss support groups. Provide information as to their value for the couple.

Discuss subsequent pregnancies (when, risks, and so on).

Tell the patient that she will be called when final autopsy results are available.

Always finish each session with a statement of encouragement such as: "This has been very difficult for you, but I think you are responding in an appropriate and healthy way to the death of your baby."

Ask, "Do you have any questions for me?"

Figure 10.3. Guidelines for subsequent counseling sessions.

How is your appetite?

Are you sleeping as well as you normally do?

Are you having any nightmares? If so, can you describe them to me?

Are you having any family or sexual problems?

Figure 10.4.   Basic questions (which may be asked at any or all visits).

"HOW DO I TELL MY STILLBORN BABY OF MY LOVE?"

Writing a Letter to the Baby

For many couples, the single most unresolvable feeling is knowing that their baby died without knowing of their love, hopes, or dreams. The letter shown in Figure 10.5 was written by a man whose son was stillborn, and it illustrates this point.

Couples may be able to resolve their unfulfilled feelings when they are encouraged to write a letter to their son or daughter, to tell the baby of their feelings. The author often "begins" the letter for them during a counseling session by writing:

Dear [*name of baby*],
I am writing this letter to tell you of the hopes and dreams that I had for you and us but that I was never able to talk to you about. . . .

Writing such a letter sometime during the 2 weeks after delivery seems to capture parents' most intense feelings for their baby. When they write the letter, their tears will flow, but the results almost universally are very positive. The letter serves at least 2 purposes: (1) It crystalizes many of the unfocused thoughts that,

Dear Son,
    When I kissed you and left last night, I realized there were many things that I hadn't said to you. I forgot to tell you how proud mom and I were when we first found out she was pregnant with you. Grandma and Grandpa said you would be a boy; I thought so, too. I'll never get to buy you that baseball glove I saw at the store the other day. We'll never take those camping trips when your Grandpa and I would have taught you to fish. We won't ever have time to replace the old engine on my motorcycle. I was going to repaint the bike when you were old enough to drive it.
    During your mom's pregnancy, I made a lot of plans for you and me. I guess all dads do that. I'll just have to keep these dreams in my heart until we meet again.
    Mom and I will love you forever.

Dad
(June 1983)

Figure 10.5.   Father's letter to his stillborn son.

if left alone, weigh people down with an aching heaviness; and (2) it provides a permanent record of the love and hopes invested in the child who will never be. For most couples, months and years will fade the intensity of their feelings. With time, they may not even be able to cry for their baby. At that point, they might wonder whether it ever was all so important. The letter documents that their love was real and that the intensity of their feelings when the baby died paralleled the sensation of loss people feel at the death of any loved one.

Keeping a Written Record to Capture Feelings

Some couples prefer to keep a journal of daily events and their thoughts in addition to or in place of writing a letter to their baby. They can add to the journal, recording dreams, as time passes. The author has never known a patient to throw away a letter or journal written after a pregnancy loss. The importance of writing while the feelings are most intense was illustrated by one patient, a writer, who misplaced a lengthy manuscript she had composed detailing events of her baby's death. Several months later, she attempted to recreate the work, only to find that her feelings were no longer as intense and that the style was less vivid. Fortunately, she later found her original manuscript.

WHICH PATIENTS RETURN FOR OUTPATIENT COUNSELING?

In the first 18 months after the Perinatal Support Service (PSS) was established at the University of Cincinnati, 185 patients experiencing a pregnancy loss were referred for outpatient counseling. (The reader is referred to Chapter 16 for a detailed description of the program and methods of patient care.) In Table 10.1, this group of 185 patients is subdivided by

TABLE 10.1
Sample of PSS Patients According to Type of Pregnancy Loss

	PERCENTAGE OF TOTAL SAMPLE	PATIENTS LOST TO FOLLOW-UP	PATIENTS RETURNED FOR PSS OUTPATIENT COUNSELING	PERCENTAGE RETURNED ACCORDING TO TYPE OF LOSS
Stillbirth				
<13 weeks	31%	34	24	41%
13–20 weeks	22	23	18	44
21–28 weeks	11	12	8	40
29–44 weeks	14	11	14	56
Neonatal death	22	23	18	44%
Total	100%	103	82	Avg. = 45%

Who Returns for Outpatient Counseling?

type of loss. In this population of patients, about 55% refused to return for any outpatient counseling and were designated "lost to follow-up."

In an effort to characterize better those patients lost to follow-up, the author evaluated the demographic nature of this group and compared the results with those patients who did return for outpatient counseling. Eighty-two patients, upon discharge from the hospital, returned for outpatient counseling. After the initial office visit, each was offered the opportunity to return for continued counseling on a weekly basis. Many patients felt that 1 visit was sufficient; for others, repeated outpatient visits were required to adequately cover the issues. Table 10.2 compares type of pregnancy loss with the number of outpatient PSS visits. Most patients with a miscarriage felt satisfied at the end of 1 visit that genetic, medical, and psychologic issues had been addressed and therefore that no additional visits were needed. Patients experiencing a stillbirth or neonatal death at a more advanced gestation were less predictable, with 39% requiring 2 or more outpatient visits. These data suggest that, for many couples, the longer the pregnancy the more intense the grief reaction.

Next, the outpatient population was evaluated by age, race, marital status, number of prenatal visits prior to detection of the pregnancy loss (see Table 10.3), and whether they had experienced a prior pregnancy loss. These results do not support the myths that age, prior pregnancy losses, or other parameters commonly heard (see Figure 10.6) would make a patient more or less inclined to pursue outpatient assistance. Patients with no prenatal care were less apt to return for outpatient counseling than those without a prior pregnancy loss; but this was the only significant difference between those 2 groups in response to the offer of follow-up counseling. If those patients with first trimester losses (no prenatal care as a rule) are eliminated from

TABLE 10.2
Type of Pregnancy Loss Compared with Number of PSS Outpatient Visits

NO. OF PSS VISITS	<13 WEEKS	13–20 WEEKS	21–28 WEEKS	29–44 WEEKS	NEONATAL
1	20	13	2	7	8
2	4	4	2	1	6
3		1	3	1	3
>3			1	5	1

Total counseled as outpatients 82

> Young patients don't care when they lose a baby.
>
> It is worse if it's your first baby.
>
> Race makes a difference.
>
> Pregnancy loss means less to unmarried patients.
>
> Patients with prior pregnancy losses are more apt to seek help after this pregnancy loss.
>
> Patients with no prior pregnancy are less interested in help.

Figure 10.6. Myths about pregnancy loss.

TABLE 10.3
Demographics of PSS Patient Sample

	PATIENTS SEEN IN PSS FOR OUTPATIENT COUNSELING	PATIENTS LOST TO OUTPATIENT FOLLOW-UP	SIGNIFICANCE
Young patients (≤20 years)	38	30	N.S.
Older patients (>20 years)	65	52	N.S.
Race: Caucasian	44	34	N.S.
Black	58	47	N.S.
Marital status: Married	29	31	N.S.
Single	67	47	N.S.
Patients with prenatal care	56	56	N.S.
Patients without prenatal care	47	26	$p < .025$
Prior pregnancy loss	47	32	N.S.
No prior pregnancy loss	56	50	N.S.

N.S. = Statistically not significant.

analysis, even this distinction fails to differentiate those who do and those who do not return for outpatient counseling. Most surprising was the observation that patients who had experienced a prior pregnancy loss were not more likely to utilize outpatient counseling services.

LONG-TERM PSYCHOLOGIC ASSESSMENT

Important questions that must be considered during counseling of patients with a pregnancy loss are, "Is the response of this couple appropriate? Are these normal reactions from healthy patients experiencing a terrible event, or are they abnormal reactions that could lead to psychosis or suicide?" These questions are very important to patient care, and they heavily

**Questionnaire Used
to Evaluate Grief
Response**

influence the attitude of obstetrically oriented care providers. If these patients are normal, then their care in the postpartum period should be provided by obstetric care providers. If these patients are psychologically abnormal, then their care becomes the domain of the psychologist or psychiatrist.

Since December 1983, the PSS has administered a questionnaire to patients returning for follow-up. The Hopkins Symptom Checklist SCL-90 is used to evaluate all patients seen in the Outpatient Perinatal Support Service (1). The questionnaire consists of emotional responses to 90 questions, each scored from 0 (least) to 4 (most). The questionnaire takes about 15 minutes to complete, and it contains questions related to a range of human emotions. This device provides valuable information regarding 9 major areas of psychologic disturbance. The major categories emphasized in the questionnaire are given in Figure 10.7. (The reader is referred to Derogatis et al. (2) for a more extensive description of the evaluation and general application of the SCL-90 questionnaire.)

The author believes that no other group at this time has applied this questionnaire to patients experiencing a pregnancy loss. Conclusions resulting from the initial 10-month experience must therefore be viewed tentatively. No patients have objected to completing the questionnaire. Many, in fact, comment favorably after they have completed the 90 questions, asking, "How did I do?" Women and men are genuinely interested in answering the questions, and they appear to be sincere in their responses.

Answers to certain questions from the questionnaire are examined specifically. One such area pertains to questions concerned with "thoughts of ending your life" or "thoughts of death or dying." Patients indicating "quite a bit" or "extremely"

Somatization: Perceptions of bodily dysfunction.

Obsessive-Compulsive: Thoughts, impulses, and actions that are unremitting and of an unwanted nature.

Interpersonal sensitivity: Feelings of personal inadequacy.

Depression: Withdrawal, loss of interest or motivation, dysphoric mood, and affect.

Anxiety: Restlessness, tension, and panic attacks.

Hostility: Anger and hostile behavior expressed in thoughts, feelings, and/or actions.

Phobic anxiety: Fears of a phobic nature toward objects, crowds, and places.

Paranoid ideation: Hostility, suspiciousness, and delusions.

Psychoticism: Schizophrenic-like behavior, such as auditory hallucinations and external thought control.

Figure 10.7.   Major categories of psychologic disturbance (2).

to these types of questions are further questioned regarding any method or plan. Otherwise, the questionnaire of 90 questions scored into 9 categories offers insight into the patients response at several levels:

Advantages of Applying the Questionnaire

The questionnaire covers far more areas than could be addressed in a single counseling session.

The questionnaire indicates areas of abnormal psychologic adjustment that can be addressed in subsequent counseling sessions.

The questionnaire enables one to make counseling sessions more efficient. Questions marked by 3 or 4 ("quite a bit" or "extremely," respectively) are emphasized in the discussions; low-scored questions are usually not discussed unless the patient brings them up.

The questionnaire can be administered repeatedly, even at several visits extending over many months; thus it can indicate trends of recovery.

The questionnaire provides a rapid means of profiling a wide range of patients' emotional changes in response to the death of a baby. Composite results from the first 30 patients examined in this manner are shown in Figure 10.8. These results are compared with those of 700 normal patients screened in

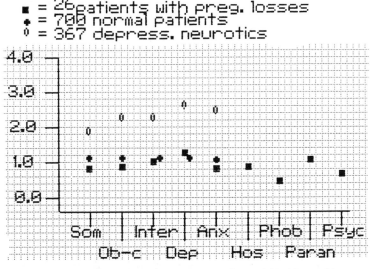

Figure 10.8. UC PSS pregnancy loss patients SCL-90 results compared with nonpregnant healthy and depressive neurotic patients. Note that assessment for Hostility (Hos), Phobia (Phob), Paranoic Ideation (Paran), and Psychotism (Psyc) were not carried out in the study of nonpregnant patients.

Oakland, California, and 367 patients who were known to be depressive neurotics (3). These results, although preliminary, suggest that these pregnancy loss patients are healthy individuals experiencing a terrible event in an appropriate manner. That this response to pregnancy loss is appropriate reaffirms the assertion that obstetric care providers should continue to serve patients' needs during the normal grieving period that follows a pregnancy loss. As a rule, these are not people who need the expertise—or expense—of a psychologist or psychiatrist. They are couples who need an interested and considerate obstetrically oriented listener and counselor. The author's experience strongly suggests that the obstetric care provider need not be afraid of these patients. Properly followed, they will not exhibit psychotic behavior that could be undetected by the uninformed care provider. The following discussion exemplifies the nature of the reaction to various types of pregnancy losses as indicated by the SCL-90.

Case Presentations

Figure 10.9 illustrates the questionnaire results from a 19-year-old who, during her second pregnancy, was determined to be carrying a live anencephalic baby at 28 weeks gestation. This patient had experienced a cesarean delivery with her first baby. After she learned about her baby's condition, the woman expressed a single desire for the management of her pregnancy, to carry the baby long enough so that, when she finally delivered, she and her baby could have a moment together before the baby died. The author obtained SCL-90 questionnaires at 32 weeks (squares) and 36 weeks gestation (circles), and then at 3 weeks

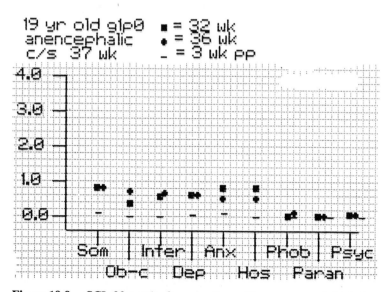

Figure 10.9. SCL-90 results from mother with an anencephalic baby.

postpartum (dashes). As the pregnancy progressed, the woman received intensive counseling and she began to accept the fate of her baby. At her request, the cesarean section was performed under epidural anesthesia. A cap was placed over the baby girl's skull defect, and the baby was wrapped and given to her parents immediately. She survived for about 5 minutes. While the woman's surgery proceeded, a glorious event occured as these 3 human lives expressed intense love for that brief time. And then the baby died. The follow-up questionnaire at 3 weeks begins to chart the progressive recovery that the woman experienced as postpartum counseling continued.

Identifying Patients with Abnormal Grief Response

What happens when the patient exhibits an abnormal response to the death of her baby? Can this type of questionnaire identify these patients? The author believes that it can. Figure 10.10 illustrates the results of a patient who experienced a neonatal death at 30 weeks. This case was presented in medical conference as follows: "This young woman at 30 weeks gestation was admitted with a placental abruption. She was taken to the delivery room and a cesarean section was performed, but the baby died." In conference, this case presentation generated a short medical discussion involving the management of placental abruption and the coagulation problems that can develop.

In her initial counseling visit at the Outpatient Perinatal Support Service, this patient said,

> You know, it was awful. I called the life squad because I had such a pain at home that I couldn't even get over to

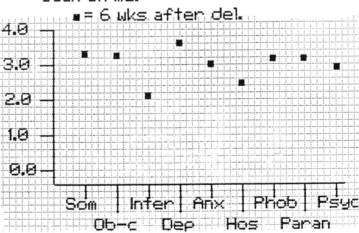

Figure 10.10.   SCL-90 results from patient whose pregnancy loss was complicated by a lack of support.

a neighbor's. The life squad delayed in coming to get me, then missed their turn coming to the hospital and had to take a couple of extra turns. I finally got up to labor and delivery. The resident came up and pulled the wrong chart. He said, "Well, you are not 30 weeks, you are only 15 weeks. Why haven't you been going to your clinic appointments? . . ." Meanwhile, the pain was getting worse. I was put in a room with a monitor and they went off to do another cesarean section. Then somebody walked in and said, "This patient is abrupting." I was rushed in for the section . . . and then my baby died.

The family history of this patient is as follows: She is a 31-year-old single parent, 1 of 9 children. Her 8 siblings live with their families on the same street; she is the only family member who lives several blocks away. Nobody comes to visit her. When she was in the hospital, no one came up to see her. It is no wonder that this patient would say, "They all just turned their backs on me." This example reminds us that all medical care has 2 sides, the side perceived by the patient and the side perceived by the medical system, which usually works well but which, every now and then, fails to meet a patient's needs.

CONCLUSION

What are the conclusions to be drawn from this type of data? Postpartum counseling for patients with pregnancy loss is truly an obstetric responsibility. Early postpartum counseling in the first week is essential. We can set aside the myths that we have created about these patients. We can educate our patients and we can let them educate us. We can reduce the numbers of malpractice lawsuits that emerge out of this group. Most lawsuits are the result of anger and ignorance stemming from the fact that no one takes the time to explain to these patients what has occurred. Consequently, they go home, their anger builds, and ultimately they go out to seek help elsewhere.

Obstetrician as Educator, Resource Person, and Concerned Counselor

The obstetrician as outpatient counselor, then, serves a pivotal role in the recovery of couples with a pregnancy loss. As an educator, he or she provides medical facts that clarify the events and decisions prior to the baby's death. As a resource person, the obstetrician can help the couple to understand that their reactions are appropriate and consistent with those of other couples under similar circumstances. Finally, the obstetrician's most important role is to maintain an ongoing dialogue between the man and woman during a time when loneliness and despair widen the distance between them.

REFERENCES

1. Derogatis LR, Lipman RS, Covi L: SCL-90: An Outpatient Rating Scale-Preliminary Report. *Psychopharmacology Bulletin* 9:13–17, 1973.
2. Derogatis LR: SCL-90R. Version Manual I. Baltimore, Johns Hopkins, 1977.
3. Derogatis LR, Lipman RS, Rickels K, Uhlenhuth EH, Covi L: The Hopkins Symptom Checklist (HSCL): A self-report symptom inventory. *Beh Sci* 19:1–15, 1974.

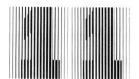

Office or Clinic Nurse's Role

SARA BERLEPSCH, R.N.

As a patient's advocate, the office or clinic nurse becomes protector, educator, and facilitator for parents as they encounter conflicts surrounding postpartum examinations, return office visits after a pregnancy loss, and possibly a subsequent pregnancy experience. The nurse's responsibilities after a pregnancy loss are influenced strongly by the type of clinic setting in which a patient is seen. In this chapter, responsibilities of the nurse in the private office and in the obstetric/gynecologic clinic will be discussed specifically.

SIMILARITIES AND DIFFERENCES IN THE PRIVATE OFFICE AND THE HOSPITAL-BASED CLINIC

Private Office: Opportunity for Relationships to Develop

How the office nurse deals with a family who has experienced a pregnancy loss can be affected by the type of setting in which a patient is seen. Nurses see families in 2 types of outpatient environments, the private office and the clinic setting.

In the private office, the patient often sees the same physician at each visit. She may have been a patient of the practice for some time and thus may be known by staff prior to her pregnancy. A sense of trust may already have been established. It is easier for the nurse to offer support to patients whom she already knows. The office setting is conducive to intimacy and personal attention.

Clinic Setting: Risk of Fragmented Care

In a clinic setting, the patient usually sees several different physicians during her pregnancy, which makes it difficult for a true physician-patient relationship to develop. She may receive her gynecologic care in an entirely different facility and therefore will be relatively unfamiliar with routines and staff in the obstetric clinic. Many clinic nurses make extraordinary efforts to develop a trusting and supportive relationship with patients even when the physical environment makes such intimacy difficult. Nevertheless, in a busy clinic where one-to-one relationships are difficult to establish, nurse and patient may be frustrated in their efforts to interact on more than a superficial level when a pregnancy loss occurs.

EXPLANATION

Nurse May Amplify and Reinforce Explanation

As a general rule, it is valuable for the office or clinic nurse to be present when parents are given information about their pregnancy loss. This exchange, however, usually occurs while the woman is in the hospital. If the nurse cannot be present, then she should discuss with the physician what was explained to the parents so that she is aware of the extent of information given them. After patients have finished talking with the physician, they may be unclear about what was said and may need someone to clarify and reinforce facts for them. News of a pregnancy loss is shocking and often it needs to be repeated. It is not that the nurse is better able to provide information or answer questions than a physician, but many patients view physicians with awe and find them inaccessible and intimidating. Hearing bewildering information from an authority figure may make such shocking news more difficult for some patients to comprehend, even though they have received a clear and thorough explanation.

WHERE PATIENTS ARE SEEN

Private Office

Family's Need for Privacy

Couples required to wait in a general patient waiting area may be engaged willingly or otherwise in casual conversation by other waiting patients. Thus, they may face troubling questions about the reason for their visit. For some, the uncomfortable experience of seeing newborn babies and hearing other patients talk about their pregnancies may be unsettling. Some insulation from this form of interaction with other patients should be offered by the nurse, and it usually is interpreted by parents as a sign of sensitivity. The patient and her partner may be escorted to a quiet room where they can wait to be seen. The nurse should let them know that staff is nearby and willing to talk with them while they wait, if they would prefer. The nurse should never give the impression that the staff is deserting the family because the issue of pregnancy loss makes them uncomfortable.

The physician and nurse should be careful to restrict all conversation regarding the family's pregnancy loss to the privacy of the office or examination room. Most patients do not appreciate having strangers hear details of their baby's death. In a private setting, the family may be more likely to ask personal questions, receive information, and express their emotions. A general patient waiting area is an unacceptable place for the doctor or nurse to talk with the family. Many patients not only cry when they are seen in follow-up for a pregnancy loss but may also exhibit anger. They should receive the courtesy of being able to express in private the emotions they feel at this time.

The Clinic

Hospital Clinic—Trauma of Returning to Location Where the Baby Died

When a patient has to visit an outpatient clinic in the hospital where her pregnancy loss occurred, the return visit can be a traumatic experience. Most patients prefer to return to a gynecologic clinic to avoid encountering pregnant women or women with babies. The staff should be aware of the stress that such a return visit places on bereaved parents. It is difficult enough for parents to return for care. They must be protected from the unfortunate chance that some uninformed well-wisher will say, "Oh, you had your baby! Is it a girl or boy?" As a simple method of avoiding embarrassment between staff and patients, the mother's chart should be marked by putting a colored label on the front of the chart or by highlighting their name in the appointment book so that the clinic staff will know that this family had a pregnancy loss.

Anger

During pregnancy, clinic patients may see many different medical personnel (for example, residents, staff physicians, medical students, nurses, aides, sonogram technicians, nutritionists, social workers, and financial counselors). This can make it more difficult for a family experiencing a pregnancy loss to talk about their grief. Because they have encountered so many different medical personnel during the course of the pregnancy, they may not have had an opportunity to develop a close relationship with any one person. Parental reactions to pregnancy loss under these circumstances can range from refusing to engage in conversation to directing widespread anger at the nurse, physician, or hospital. Such expression of anger by parents must not be taken personally. The family may feel guilt or anger that they cannot verbalize appropriately. Under conditions inherent in the clinic setting, they may not feel comfortable expressing their feelings to medical personnel they do not know personally. In this setting, the nurse may act as an important resource and liaison.

HELPING THE PREGNANCY LOSS PATIENT

Postpartum Discomforts

Nurse Can Tell Patients What to Expect Postpartum

During hospitalization for a pregnancy loss, patients should be advised about normal postpartum physical changes, which may serve to aggravate feelings of grief. Unfortunately, although postpartum instructions are a routine component of obstetric care when a healthy baby delivers, such advice may be overlooked (or consciously ignored) by care providers following the death of a fetus or newborn, as if the patient who has no baby were not going to experience normal postpartum events because she had a pregnancy loss. Omission of such information in the care of pregnancy loss patients also may be the result of early hospital discharge. It is advisable, then, for the office or clinic nurse to be aware of the dynamics by which she may become primary counselor regarding postpartum processes and recovery, which impact on a patient's grief reaction. As more patients are encouraged to return for counseling in the first week postpartum following a pregnancy loss (see Chapter 10, "Obstetrician As Outpatient Counselor"), their need to receive this type of information from their physician, midwife, and/or office or clinic nurse becomes an integral part of their continued obstetric care.

If at all possible, the nurse who sees pregnancy loss patients before and after delivery should describe typical postpartum physical processes that they will encounter. There may be perineal discomfort from an episiotomy or from lacerations. There will be postpartum vaginal bleeding. Women are often bewildered to hear that they will begin to produce breastmilk. It is hard for them to understand that the body still responds to the baby's need for nourishment although there is no baby to nurse. It can be a heartbreaking experience to a grieving woman to wake up and find her breasts engorged. These physical changes are a constant reminder to the woman that her baby has died. To be aware in advance that such things will occur will better prepare a woman to accept their occurrence.

Preparation for Followup

Flag the Chart; Seek Reports for the Physician

Before the patient returns for her postpartum examination, two important preparations should be instituted by the nurse. She should be certain that the chart has been flagged in some way to alert staff that this patient has experienced a pregnancy loss. Second, any information about the cause of the baby's death should be available for the physician to present to parents. This includes preliminary or final autopsy reports, surgical pathology reports, and genetic studies. If a written report is not yet available, a verbal report should be sought.

Physical Examination

Explaining Why an Examination Is Necessary

Even those who are aware of the emotional support needed to help parents grieve may not understand that follow-up procedures, which the patient must undergo, may be unusually uncomfortable or even distasteful. Reactions to pelvic exams following a pregnancy loss range from viewing it as a necessary evil to finding it extremely painful and embarrassing. A woman will say, "Why did he have to do a pelvic? It's bad enough to lose my baby." The nurse might explain ahead of time that it is necessary for the physician to check the size of the uterus, to ascertain the position of the baby and measure dilation of the cervix (if the baby is not yet delivered), or to evaluate the degree of vaginal bleeding. The patient should be told that information gained from these procedures enables the physician to evaluate her physical status more accurately. It may be helpful to reassure the patient that, although a pelvic exam at this time is unpleasant, the physician will be as brief and as gentle as possible. Gestures that can ease the discomfort of a physical examination are described in Figure 11.1.

OFFICE VISITS AS A MEANS OF EVALUATING THE GRIEF PROCESS

The office nurse has an important role in the overall gynecologic care of women who have experienced pregnancy loss. In this capacity, she may be the first medical professional to recognize that a patient is experiencing pathologic grief. Pathologic grief arises when the normal process of bereavement is suppressed or blocked. The circumstances under which this condition is most likely to occur are listed in Figure 11.2. Lindemann (1) has described symptoms of pathologic grief that may apply to a parent in response to a pregnancy loss. Indications that a person may be experiencing pathologic grief are given in Figure 11.3.

Office Nurse May Identify Pathologic Grief

The office nurse, seeing a patient months (or even years) after a pregnancy loss may believe that time alone is sufficient to distance a couple from the pain of their experience. Unfor-

Allow the patient to remain dressed during the initial discussion with the physician. If an examination is needed, give the patient time to change and drape herself appropriately. Do not hurry her.

Raise the back of the examination table to a 45-degree angle. No woman appreciates being positioned flat on her back for an examination.

Cover the metal stirrups with cloth or padding; metal foot rests are extremely uncomfortable for the patient with bare feet or wearing stockings.

Warm the vaginal speculum with hot water or a heating pad. Using a cold speculum is unnecessary and inconsiderate.

After the examination, allow the patient time to dress before the physician discusses results of the examination or issues related to the pregnancy loss.

When the visit has concluded, the patient may need a few moments alone to regain her composure before she leaves the office. Most patients who are upset or who have been crying in the office or examination room do not wish to exit into a waiting area filled with other patients before they have regained control over their emotions. Hurrying a patient at this point in the visit may be interpreted as an uncaring attitude on the part of office personnel.

Figure 11.1.   Easing discomforts during the physical examination.

Cause	Effect
She did not see or hold her baby after delivery. She has no mementos (pictures, identification wristlets) to remind her of her baby. The woman is being encouraged (or coerced) to forget about her baby and move on.	The woman is unable to accept that her baby is dead.
Lack of follow-up by medical personnel. No chance to talk with the physician about the medical course leading to her baby's death.	The woman feels that she has no medical support.
Overprotected by family and friends. Discouraged from grieving.	The woman feels that her personal need for support has not been met by family or friends.

Figure 11.2.   Ways in which normal bereavement may be suppressed or blocked after pregnancy loss.

tunately, this assumption is specious. In a survey of 56 women carried out 1–2 years after a neonatal death, Culbert (2) observed morbid grief reactions in one-third of the group. In a similar type of study, Rowe et al. (3) observed abnormal adjustment in 23% of patients queried. Of note in this latter series, 5 of 9 women who became pregnant within 5 months of the loss or who delivered a single surviving twin experienced morbid grief reactions (see Chapter 1, "Pregnancy Loss and the Grief Proc-

Remains busy so as to avoid confronting the reality of the loss.

Refuses to acknowledge the emotional impact of the loss.

Has psychosomatic complaints.

Experiences onset of valid medical conditions such as ulcerative colitis, rheumatoid arthritis, or asthma, whose cause in fact may be traced to the pregnancy loss.

Undergoes changes in relationships with friends or relatives leading to social isolation.

Harbors hostility against specific medical care providers.

Suffers a permanent loss of social involvement.

Displays a flat or unemotional affect.

Agitated depression.

Figure 11.3. Indications of pathologic grief (1).

ess," and Chapter 15, "Impact of Pregnancy Loss on Subsequent Pregnancy"). In a larger series, Lockwood and Lewis (4) observed that patients becoming pregnant within 6 months after a stillbirth delivery appeared most at risk for prolonged and unresolved grief.

Routine check-ups, therefore, may be an important time during which to evaluate a woman's emotional status following her pregnancy loss. The nurse may encourage her in a nonintrusive manner to talk about how she is doing. Is she comfortable around pregnant women? How is she dealing with insensitive, yet supposedly well-meaning, remarks? Does she have days during which she does not feel the intensity of the grief? Does she feel guilty that her pain has eased? The nurse has a unique opportunity during these office visits to ask simple questions that can uncover unresolved guilt, anger, or depression. If such problems are detected, these observations should be conveyed to the physician, who may then wish to schedule additional office visits to counsel the couple or refer them for outside professional consultation.

TELEPHONE CALLS FOR ADDITIONAL SUPPORT AFTER DISCHARGE

Further Opportunity to Assess Patient's Recovery

The office or clinic nurse is often a source of support to parents in the prenatal period. She provides and reinforces information, listens when parents need to talk, and acts as liaison between them and the physician. Many patients will turn to such a nurse for the same sort of support during the postpartum period following a pregnancy loss. A patient may call about a physical complaint ("It has been a week and I am still bleeding. How long does it last?"), when in reality all she really wants is someone with whom to talk. Her family may not be very helpful. Her husband may not understand why she still has crying spells. She may have difficulty coping with her other children's daily needs. She and her husband may be unable to talk together. Friends may avoid them. If a nurse receives such a telephone call, she should try to provide time to allow the woman to talk. Knowing that her nurse is willing to create time in a busy schedule to talk with her may provide the patient an essential link with the medical community during periods when family or friends are unable to provide this form of support.

During these telephone calls, the office or clinic nurse should assess the woman's statements to detect evidence of emotional instability or risk to life. Statements by patients that may serve as warning signs that the patient or her family are not reacting appropriately to pregnancy loss are listed in Figure 11.4. Occasionally, during a telephone conversation, a patient may describe behavior or activity (to the nurse) that seems unusual. This type of information should be relayed immediately to the physician, as it may indicate the patient's intense

Statement	Pathologic Response
I have no one to talk to about my feelings.	Isolation
I am so depressed.	Depression
I stay inside all day.	Isolation
I can't trust anyone.	Paranoia
I am losing control of my thoughts.	Psychotism
I should be punished for what has happened.	Guilt
I am not close to anybody.	Isolation
At times I am so anxious I can hardly breathe.	Anxiety
I am afraid I am going to hurt myself.	Self deprecation
I am afraid I will hurt one of my kids.	Hostility
My husband (boyfriend) and I can't talk about the baby's death.	Denial
My baby didn't die—he [she] is still in the nursery.	Denial
I don't feel sad about my baby's death.	Denial
Life isn't worth anything anymore.	Depression
I've had thoughts of ending my life.	Depression

Figure 11.4.   Statements that may indicate pathologic grief response.

struggle to adjust to her pregnancy loss. Examples of conflicted behavior encountered at the Perinatal Support Service at the University of Cincinnati during the past 3 years are described in Figure 11.5.

ENCOURAGING GOOD MEDICAL CARE AND PRECONCEPTION PLANNING

At some point, a couple may begin thinking about the possibility of another pregnancy. The office or clinic nurse may recognize that this issue is important based on questions or statements she hears from the patient. Because pregnancy loss may result from poorly controlled medical conditions such as hypertension, diabetes, or malnutrition, the nurse can help the patient to develop a plan for addressing any such problems preconceptually. The nurse may recommend to the patient a weight loss program or nutritional counseling. Medication should be reviewed by a physician. Certain medications may need to be changed to prevent possible fetal malformations from teratogenic drugs. Any questions about the pregnancy loss that have not been clarified should be clarified *before* the next pregnancy is undertaken. The more involved parents are in planning for their next pregnancy, the easier it is for them to cope with fears of another pregnancy loss. Couples need to know that they are doing everything possible to prevent another loss from occurring. (For a complete description of issues of concern during a subsequent pregnancy, the reader is referred to Chapter 15.)

A woman who continued to visit her baby's grave every day several months after her stillbirth.

A woman who lost her job 2 months after a miscarriage because of poor attendance that began after her pregnancy loss.

A woman who screamed out during the funeral service for her stillborn baby that the hospital had killed her baby.

A woman whose newborn baby had died who visited the emergency room on multiple occasions for various minor complaints.

A woman who called repeatedly for sleeping medication.

A woman who informed the nurse she never went out of her house after her baby died.

Figure 11.5. Pathologic responses of women after pregnancy loss.

SETTING THE STANDARD OF CARE

The importance of the nurse in a busy office or clinic is often overshadowed by the impressive array of technical procedures, ultrasound techniques, and laboratory tests that dominate current obstetric care. Nonetheless, day-to-day activities on which quality patient care is based are often dictated by the attentiveness and commitment to patient care exhibited by the office or clinic nurse. When events develop that result in a pregnancy loss, this commitment by office or clinic nurses to their patients is heightened further. Some, however, may not readily recognize their true value in the care of these unfortunate patients.

The nurse can set the standard of care for these patients by understanding the dynamics of patient flow in a clinic or office, by listening to subtle and not-so-subtle pleas for help from distressed parents, and by providing an empathic relationship to these patients. In this role, the nurse becomes an important complement to the caring physician when both of them make an effort to be involved in the slow and often painful recovery of the couple with a pregnancy loss.

REFERENCES

1. Lindemann E: Symptomatology and management of acute grief. *Am J Psychiatry* 101:141–148, 1944.
2. Culbert J: Mental reaction of women to perinatal death. In Morris N (ed): *Psychosomatic Medicine, Obstetrics and Gynecology.* 3rd International Congress. New York, S Karger, 1972, pp 326–329.
3. Rowe J, Clyman R, Green C, Mikkelsen C, Haight J, Ataide L: Followup of families who experience a perinatal death. *Pediatrics* 62:166–170, 1978.
4. Lockwood S and Lewis IC: Management of grief after a stillbirth. *Med J Aust* 2:308–311, 1980.

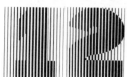

Genetics and Pregnancy Loss: Value of Counseling between Pregnancies

PETER ST. JOHN DIGNAN, M.D.

The geneticist has only recently become an integral member of the medical team caring for a couple with a pregnancy loss. Like the pathologist (see Chapter 13, "Value of the Perinatal Autopsy"), the role of the geneticist is to gather facts in order to explain past occurrences and to interpret future risk. These facts, in turn, are obtained from taking a careful family history (pedigree) and from inquiring about a previous miscarriage or stillbirth, or by studying the genetic makeup of the parents themselves. Many questions exist in the minds of patients and care providers, however, as to procedural issues, types of tests, and the correlation of prior pregnancy losses and future risk. In this chapter, the author addresses the following questions:

1. What is the correlation between genetic makeup of the parents and pregnancy outcome?
2. Which chromosomal abnormalities of the embryo are most often associated with a pregnancy loss?
3. Do environmental factors influence pregnancy outcome?
4. Are there genetic differences between early and late gestational losses?
5. What are the proper methods to collect tissue samples for cytogenetic analysis from a pregnancy loss?
6. How does the geneticist serve as a counselor?

Incidence of Spontaneous Abortion

It generally is accepted that 15% of clinically recognized pregnancies spontaneously abort (1). However, when conceptions are followed from implantation (about the tenth postconception day), this figure increases to at least 45% (2). Thus, most spontaneous abortions go unnoticed. Estimates of the rate of all spontaneous fetal losses have been as high as 78% (3), but the exact frequency in the population is unknown and would be difficult to determine.

"Natural Screening Process"

Many spontaneous abortions have been observed to be abnormal. In 1956, Hertig et al. (4) reported that 13 of 34 human embryos examined less than 17 days postfertilization were grossly abnormal and would have aborted early in gestation. In another study, gross pathologic changes or localized anomalies were found in 81% of zygotes lost earlier than the fourth month of gestation (5). It has been estimated that 95% of abnormal pregnancies spontaneously abort (6). Therefore, it appears that embryo and fetal losses are not rare events in humans and that these losses are often a means of selective termination of abnormal products of conception. The mechanism that produces this "natural screening process," which eliminates abnormal embryos and fetuses, has been termed by Warkany (7) "terathanasia." How it works is unknown and can only be conjectured. Knowledge of the frequency of these losses and the high incidence of associated abnormalities can be of some comfort to couples who have suffered a pregnancy loss in helping them to understand that they are not alone and that seldom are they at fault.

RECURRENCE RISKS FOR FETAL LOSSES

The recurrence risks for couples who have a history of a spontaneous fetal loss depend on the woman's prior reproductive history, her age, and other factors. However, empirical data from Warburton and Fraser (8), who studied couples with at least 1 liveborn child, indicate that the chance for a recurrent abortion is 24% after 1 fetal loss, 26% after 2 consecutive losses, and 32% after 3 consecutive losses. Poland et al. (9) found that the recurrence risk for another fetal loss is about 46% for a couple who have no live children and who have had at least 1 fetal loss. These are empirical risks combined from cases that probably abort for many different reasons.

CHROMOSOME ANOMALIES AND FETAL LOSS

The most common factor associated with fetal loss is that of chromosome anomalies. Anomalies are distributed evenly between the sexes. Fifty percent of early spontaneous abortions have chromosomal errors (10). Therefore, chromosome errors occur 100 times more frequently in abortuses than in term infants. If only first trimester losses are considered, the percentage of chromosome anomalies is even higher.

Trisomy

Trisomies as a group account for half the total chromosome anomalies, with trisomy 16 being the most frequent. Most trisomies are the result of meiotic nondisjunction during gametogenesis. Nondisjunction is the failure of chromosomes to move to opposite poles during the anaphase of cell division. More rarely there is mitotic nondisjunction in the zygote or early embryo. The phenotypes in many of the trisomic abortuses, if they have recognizable structures, often are different from those seen in their liveborn counterparts. However, many trisomies are so disruptive to embryonic and fetal development that recognizable fetal parts are rarely seen. This applies particularly to trisomies involving the larger chromosomes such as trisomy 16, which is usually associated with an empty sac or an extremely stunted embryo. Studies have demonstrated that, when the first abortion examined has normal chromosomes, 81% of subsequent abortions also have normal chromosomes. However, when the first abortion is trisomic, about 70% of subsequent abortions also are trisomic but the specific chromosome involved is not always the same (11). These data suggest that nondisjunction is not always a random event and that some couples have a higher-than-average risk of having trisomic conceptions. A gene that causes nondisjunction has been identified in *Drosophila*. Although such a gene may exist in humans, its presence has not been proven. Amniocentesis or chorionic villous sampling should therefore be considered for all women who have had a trisomic abortus. Couples who have had a trisomic abortus are frequently of advanced parental age. The relationship to advanced age has not been observed with polyploidy, monosomy, or translocation abortuses (10).

Monosomy

Monosomy X is the most common single chromosome anomaly in human abortuses. It is reported to occur in 20 to 25% of chromosomally abnormal pregnancy losses. Epidemiologic studies suggest that 99% of conceptuses with this anomaly are aborted. The phenotype can range from an empty sac to an apparently normal fetus, or the more recognizable fetus with nuchal hygromata and lymphangiomata (10).

Polyploidy

Polyploidy, where there is a complete extra set or sets of chromosomes, occurs in another 20 to 25% of chromosomally abnormal fetal losses. The majority are triploids with 69 chromosomes. This condition usually arises from fertilization by 2 sperm (dispermy) or from failure of 1 of the maturational divisions of either the ova or the sperm so that a diploid gamete is produced. Two-thirds of triploids have XXY sex chromosome complement; most of the rest are XXX. XYY constitution is seen in less than 3% of all triploid fetuses. The reports of phenotypes vary from intact empty sacs, amorphous embryos, or apparently normal fetuses, to those with multiple malformations of the brain, neural tube, face, and limbs. Placental changes are common with hydatidiform degeneration in early abortuses and partial hydatidiform moles in later fetal losses. There appears to be no correlation between the degree of placental lesions and the severity of fetal malformations. This suggests that triploid fetal losses are determined by the degree of placental pathology rather than the severity of the fetal malformations (12).

Structural Chromosome Anomalies

Although structural chromosome anomalies (translocations, deletions, duplications, and rearrangements) are relatively rare and account for about 5% of chromosomal abnormal aborted fetuses, they are an important cause of repeated early abortions in humans (10). Most are translocations that occur when a fragment of 1 chromosome becomes attached to the broken end of another. If there is a mutual exchange of fragments, without a loss of genetic material, this is a balanced reciprocal translocation. Such individuals will be phenotypically normal, but they can have reproductive problems depending on the type of meiotic segregation that the involved chromosomes undergo. The zygote can be normal, a balanced translocation carrier like the parent, trisomic for part of a chromosome, or monosomic for part of a chromosome. The last 2 alternatives often are associated with an abortion of the fetus. In about 4% of couples with repeated early spontaneous abortions, 1 parent, often the woman, will have a reciprocal translocation. When, in addition to the patient's history of spontaneous abortions, a fetus is found to have a major malformation, 14% of the parents have a balanced translocation. A second type of translocation that occurs in spontaneously aborted fetuses is a Robertsonian translocation. This results when acrocentric chromosomes (chromosomes with the centromere very near to 1 end) break near the centromere, resulting in a translocated chromosome with 2 long arms. The inactive short arms are usually lost during cell division. Robertsonian or centromeric translocations account for half of the unbalanced translocations found in spontaneous abortions. Half of these are "de novo" rearrangements. Parents who are translocation carriers have been reported by a number of authors to have conceived trisomic fetuses where the extra chromosome was unrelated to the translocated chromosomes (13).

EXPOSURE TO ENVIRONMENTAL AGENTS

Teratogens

Exposure to environmental agents present at the time of conception or during gestation is of constant concern to parents.

High-level ionizing radiation, carbon monoxide, and aminopterin have been reported to cause fetal losses when the pregnant woman has had significant exposure. Other substances such as alcohol, tobacco, diethylstibestrol (DES), certain anticancer drugs, and hypoglycemia-producing agents have all been implicated, but the evidence that they cause abortions is tenuous. Several reports have shown an epidemiologic relationship between coumadin taken by the woman and increased reproductive losses (14). In the clinical situation, it is rare to find an environmental exposure that poses a significant risk to the mother; but this should not lull the clinician into a false sense of security. There is more than ever a responsibility for the care provider to obtain thorough medical and environmental histories. Obstetricians and geneticists should inquire into not only prescribed drugs, but also self-administered over-the-counter medicines, work and hobby exposures, and possibly the nutritional practices of couples with a history of fetal loss. Where there is a positive history, standard references and reviews should be consulted (15, 16, 17) before couples are counseled. Commonsense can encourage couples to avoid any excesses or insults prior to conception and beyond if they are contemplating another pregnancy.

LATE FETAL LOSSES

Chromosome Anomalies among Stillbirths

Fetal losses after 20 weeks gestation are classified as stillbirths. In spite of various degrees of maceration, all stillborn fetuses require complete necropsies that include whole body roentgenographs and clinical photographs. Handling of tissues for cytogenetic analysis is presented in Table 12.1. (For a discussion of the pathologic evaluation of the products of conception, the reader is referred to Chapter 13, "Value of the Perinatal Autopsy.")

Approximately 5% of stillbirths have chromosome anomalies. It is not rare for them to have apparently normal phenotypes. The most common chromosome errors are trisomies, which make up 60% of all chromosome anomalies. Trisomy 18 is found in about half of all trisomic stillborn fetuses. Parents should be forewarned that tissues of stillborn fetuses often fail to grow in culture.

COUNSELING AND FETAL LOSS

Who Should Receive Genetic Counseling and When?

Until recently, couples who had suffered a fetal loss rarely were given a comprehensive explanation of the event. Ideally, every fetal loss should be evaluated and the parents provided

TABLE 12.1
Handling of Tissues for Cytogenetic Analysis

	MATERIAL REQUIRED	COLLECTION	STORAGE	PRECAUTIONS	EXPECTED SUCCESSFUL GROWTH
Abortus	Fetus, sac, or umbilical cord tissue	Collect tissue under sterile conditions and place in Eagle's MEM or equivalent tissue culture medium. If there is no medium available, place the tissue in a sterile air-tight container and cover the tissue with sterile gauze moistened with sterile saline or water.	Tissue should be processed as soon as possible. If storage is necessary, place the container in a refrigerator at 4°C. The tissue may be processed up to 24 hours after collection if it is stored in medium.	Maternal placenta or decidua is useless. Material from suction curettage is useless as it is not sterile and it is impossible to identify fetal tissue. Never place tissue into formalin or saline. Never freeze tissue.	Approximately 60%.* About 50% of successful cultures are expected to show an abnormal result.
Stillbirth	Fetus or umbilical cord tissue	Skin can be cultured from a large fetus or stillborn by wiping an area of the abdominal wall three times with alcohol. Remove 2 cm of full thickness skin with sterile scissors or scalpel blade. Place into tissue culture medium.	Tissue should be processed as soon as possible. If storage is necessary, place in a refrigerator at 4°C until processed. The growth failure rate will increase with storage.	Never place tissue into formalin or saline. Never freeze tissue.	Approximately 5%.* About 5% of successful cultures would show abnormal results.
Parents' blood for lymphocyte chromosome analysis	Whole blood	Collect 5–10 ml in a syringe with 0.5 ml of sodium heparin.	Should be processed as soon as possible but will grow in culture up to 48 hours at room temperature.	Usual precautions in performing a venipuncture. No preservatives should be used.	Approximately 100%.* If done for 3 or more spontaneous abortions about 6% of cultures would have an abnormal result.

* Percentages may vary in different laboratories.

with an understanding of the possible cause, recurrence risks, and possible prevention of the disorder. However, to cover all fetal losses would place an overwhelming burden on healthcare systems. Consequently, there is debate about who should be evaluated and to what extent. Many authorities agree that couples who have had 3 consecutive early fetal losses should be evaluated and counseled comprehensively. Some would also encourage full evaluation of couples with 2 consecutive losses, while couples with their first loss would be supported and reassured that fetal losses are common, usually are sporadic, and often involve a natural selection process (1).

The objective of counseling should be to provide useful information to couples so that they can make informed decisions regarding future pregnancy. The emphasis should be on educating the couple, not on influencing their decisions. In many instances, after all possible information has been gathered and considered, no cause for the pregnancy loss will be found. However, if the process is done well, parents will be relieved of many of their concerns.

Conducting a Genetic Consultation

A family history is taken and a pedigree is constructed. The reproductive history is fully explored. Whenever possible, records are checked. A morphologic examination of the products of conception should be done, including a cytogenetic evaluation. Complete clinical photographs are always helpful. When the products of conception are not available, then chromosome evaluation of the parents is considered. If there are 2 or more unexplained consecutive early spontaneous abortions, or if a fetus had a major malformation, the parents' chromosomes are analyzed. Other investigations into the causes of early spontaneous fetal losses routinely are done by obstetricians; these are reviewed in detail by Simpson (1). Areas of concern are blood cell and HLA incompatibilities, uterine malformations or tumors, maternal chronic diseases including endocrine conditions, and maternal infections.

PRENATAL DIAGNOSIS

Indications for Prenatal Diagnosis

Genetic counseling for couples who have had multiple pregnancy losses should include discussion about not only the possibility of additional fetal loss, but also the possibility of bearing a liveborn abnormal baby. It is clear from this review that both risks may be increased, given a history of spontaneous abortion. The following situations warrant consideration of prenatal diagnosis: women who are 35 years of age or older; women who have had either a liveborn baby or a pregnancy loss who was trisomic; and confirmation of a balanced translocation in 1 parent. A difficult decision is posed by the case of chromosomally normal parents who have had repeated fetal losses when the chromosomes of these fetuses are unknown. It is possible that any of their losses could have been a trisomic fetus. If this were the case, these parents could be at an increased risk for having another trisomic conceptus, but the magnitude of this risk is unknown. Additionally, women who have fetal losses with neural tube defects should be offered prenatal diagnosis in subsequent pregnancies.

When the ultrasonographer detects a fetal anomaly, late second or third trimester amniocentesis may be indicated to detect a possible chromosome anomaly. Presence of an omphalocele, for example, increases the possibility that the fetus may have a trisomy 18 chromosomal defect. For investigation under these circumstances, amniotic fluid should be cultured in Chang's medium for the best possible growth success rate.

CONCLUSIONS

Genetic counseling of couples with fetal loss can be of both practical and psychologic benefit. The information is often provisional. But if attention is given to collection and evaluation of the data, counseling can be provided to couples so they can understand and interpret their risks for future pregnancies. The interest and thoroughness of the genetic counselor who has empathy and tact can be of benefit in easing parents' adjustment to their tragedy.

REFERENCES

1. Simpson J: Repeated suboptimal pregnancy outcome birth defects. *Original Article Series*, vol XVII, no 1, pp 113–142, 1981.
2. Miller JF, Williamson E, Glue J, Gordon YB, Grudzinskas JG, Sykes A: Fetal loss after implantation. *Lancet* II:554–556, 1980.
3. Roberts C and Lowe C: Where have all the conceptions gone? *Lancet* I:498–499, 1975.
4. Hertig AT, Rock J, Adams E: A description of 34 human ova within the first 17 days of development. *Am J Anat* 98, 435–493, 1956.
5. Stratford B: Abnormalities of early human development. *Am J Obstet Gynecol* 107:1223–1232, 1970.
6. Haas J and Schottenfeld D: Risks to the offspring from parental occupational exposures. *J Occup Med* 21:607–613, 1979.
7. Warkany J: Terathansia. *Teratology* 17:187–192, 1978.
8. Warburton D and Fraser F: Spontaneous abortion risks in man. *Hum Genet* 16:1–25, 1964.
9. Poland B, Miller J, Jones D, Trimble B: Reproductive counseling in patients who have had a spontaneous abortion. *Am J Obstet Gynecol* 127:685–691, 1977.

10. Carr D: Cytogenetics of human reproductive wastage. In Kalter H (ed): *Issues and Reviews in Teratology 1*, New York, Plenum Press, 1983, pp 33–72.

11. Lippman-Hand A: Genetic counseling and human reproductive loss. In Porter I and Hook E (eds): *Human Embryonic and Fetal Death*. New York, Academic Press, 1980, pp 299–314.

12. Ornoy A, Kohn A, BenZur A, Weinstein D, Cohen M: Triploidy in human abortion. *Teratology* 18:315–320, 1978.

13. Wolstenholme J, Faed M, Robertson J, Lamott M: Chromosome abnormality in couples with histories of multiple abortions: the outcome of pregnancies subsequent to ascertainment and study of familial translocation carriers. *Hum Genet* 63:45–47, 1983.

14. Hall J, Pauli R, Wilson K: Maternal and fetal sequelae of anticoagulation during pregnancy. *Am J Med* 68:122–140, 1980.

15. Schardein J: *Chemically Induced Birth Defects*. New York, Marcel Dekker, Inc., 1985.

16. Shepard T: *Catalog of Teratogenic Agents*. Baltimore, Johns Hopkins University Press, 1980.

17. Warkany J: *Congenital Malformations, Notes and Comments*. Chicago, Year Book Medical Publishers, Inc., 1971.

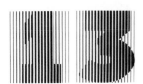

Value of the Perinatal Autopsy

JAMES R. WOODS, Jr., M.D.
ROBERT BENDON, M.D.

The autopsy is an essential component of patient care following a pregnancy loss. For the patient, the autopsy may answer the fundamental question, "Why did my baby die?" The obstetrician may correlate prenatal management decisions with autopsy results. The academic community benefits from a better understanding of processes leading to death.

Refusal of Autopsy May Result from Professionals' Insensitivity

It is a formidable loss to the medical community when an autopsy is not performed after the death of a fetus or newborn. Failure to obtain parents' permission to conduct an autopsy may be attributed to an insensitive approach by the physician or others. There are individual parents who will refuse to permit an autopsy for their infant, no matter how well the benefits are articulated. In general, though, parents can make the appropriate decision concerning an autopsy when a full, considerate explanation of the procedure and its value is presented. Without an autopsy, parents are left with many questions and few answers. As time goes by, they come to feel the full brunt of this omission. Without an autopsy, the obstetrician is forced to evaluate prenatal care for answers and may be as frustrated as the parents at the inability to construct a cause-and-effect relationship between the course of the pregnancy and its outcome. Finally, the medical community asks, "What will we do differently next time to prevent this occurrence?" but realizes that without autopsy results this may be an unanswerable question.

The importance of the autopsy is generally acknowledged among obstetricians and pediatricians. However, many simple questions about the autopsy exist that are not often addressed in medical school or during residency training. In this chapter, the perinatal autopsy will be analyzed to answer the following questions:

1. What are medical objectives of the autopsy report?
2. What findings from the autopsy will be most helpful to parents and to the woman's care providers?
3. What is an appropriate protocol for carrying out an autopsy?
4. What special tests may be requested in selected cases to broaden findings at autopsy?
5. What is the proper method of obtaining tissue for analysis?
6. What are the pitfalls in collecting or transferring specimens of tissues that may limit analysis?
7. What factors limit the amount of information that can be obtained from an autopsy?
8. How do autopsy findings correlate with "cause of death"?

PURPOSE OF THE AUTOPSY

Explanation of Death; Evaluation of Recurrence Risks

The purpose of the perinatal autopsy is to determine the pathogenic process that has led to death. A clear explanation may help parents and care providers accept the baby's death as a reality. For example, specific information may dispel a mother's unfounded feeling of guilt that she or her partner caused their baby's death. An important purpose of the autopsy is to evaluate potential risks of recurrence in the patient's subsequent pregnancies. The discovery, at autopsy, of underlying infection or maternal disease (for example, diabetes mellitus or systemic lupus erythematosis) may be critical to medical care of the patient between pregnancies or during her next pregnancy. Freeman et al. (1), from a collaborative study within 19 institutions, evaluated subsequent pregnancy outcomes of 308 patients who had experienced a prior stillbirth. Those patients with no medical or recurring obstetric condition encountered the same incidence of intrauterine growth retardation, abnormal fetal heart rate patterns in labor, and perinatal deaths as did the general population. In contrast, patients with a prior history of hypertension or stillbirth complicated by intrauterine growth retardation exhibited a statistically higher incidence of abnormal antepartum tests for fetal wellbeing or of premature labor with the next pregnancy than did their control group. With proper prenatal care, none of the 308 patients experienced a repeat stillbirth.

Autopsy as a Tool for Advancement of Scientific Understanding

A secondary goal of the perinatal autopsy is to further scientific understanding of fetal loss. Accurate diagnosis of congenital anomalies or specific infections provides important epidemiologic information. The correlation of pathologic findings with detailed clinical findings ultimately may explain mechanisms for such common problems as premature labor, premature rupture of membranes, chorioamnionitis, or placental abruption. Perinatal implications of more uncommon disease entities such as systemic lupus erythematosis or maternal herpes simplex may also be advanced. Finally, the autopsy should be used to verify prenatal diagnoses determined on the basis of such techniques as ultrasound or amniocentesis.

Unfortunately, autopsy results may be inconclusive as to cause of death. Some limits are inherent in the autopsy, as when autolysis (cellular breakdown) occurs as a normal postmortem process. In the case of an intrauterine death, for example, the fetal body is inaccessible for some period following death, and this unavoidable delay can influence the effectiveness of tests that are to be conducted. In other cases, an autopsy may be inconclusive because our knowledge of physiologic mechanisms of fetal death is still incomplete.

Approach to Conducting the Autopsy

There are many aspects of autopsy examination that may be applied toward a better understanding of the cause of fetal death. Components of the perinatal autopsy examination are listed in Figure 13.1. A realistic approach to the perinatal autopsy is to treat each case as an individual diagnostic problem. The clinical history is reviewed before the autopsy is begun. Gestational age is of marked significance. After a careful external examination, appropriate procedures should be planned, such as histologic evaluation of the fetus or placenta, x-rays of the fetus, karyotyping, bacterial or viral cultures, or other special studies. The autopsy should be modified, based on the findings, as dissection proceeds. Throughout this process, pathologist and obstetrician should work together to determine the optimum information that may be obtained from the autopsy.

THE FETUS

Physical Inspection

Maceration poses a major problem in analysis of a stillborn fetus at autopsy, but it never should be used as justification (or rationalization) for not performing an autopsy or for not seeking autopsy permission. Autolysis is rapid in the intrauterine environment, even without bacterial decay, and it complicates interpretation of many postmortem findings. This is because of

Procedure	Diagnostic Purpose of the Procedure
1. *Physical inspection* of the fetus or newborn and placenta with photographs of entire body/placenta; examination of each internal organ	Presence or absence of maceration Gross fetal anomalies Placental or umbilical cord anomalies Trauma Placental hemorrhage/infarction
2. *Whole body x-rays*	Lethal bone dysplasias/skeletal abnormalities Gas formation in the fetus
3. *Histology* Fetus Placenta	Gestational age Acute versus chronic stress Viral/bacterial infections Chorioamnionitis Duration of meconium exposure Hemorrhage/infarctions
4. *Microbiologic cultures* Fetal lung, aerobic/anerobic cultures Placental (subamniotic) cultures Viral cultures	Fetal infection
5. *Genetic evaluation* (Fetal skin, cardiac blood sample, or placenta)	Karyotype of fetus or newborn (See Chapter 12.)
6. *Other* Kleihauer-Betke analysis Maternal TORCH titers	Fetal/maternal hemorrhage Fetal viral infections

Figure 13.1. Components of the autopsy evaluation.

unknown effects of fluid shifts between tissue compartments and because of leaking of substances such as hemosiderin out of the cells. The most apparent change is slippage of skin, which varies in extent from requiring pressure to elicit it to the spontaneous shedding of all epidermis during delivery and handling.

Maceration Should Not Preclude an Autopsy

Rayburn et al. (2) suggest that absence of, minimal, or significant maceration may allow one to assess the time elapsed since death as less than 8 hours, 8 to 24 hours, or greater than 24 hours prior to delivery, respectively. Others (3) have correlated the degree of autolysis with cases of known postmortem intervals in order to provide a general estimate of time of death. The authors' experience and that of others (4) suggest that the degree of maceration is not very useful for determining exact time of death, because of its rapid course at core body temperature. Moreover, the effects of meconium staining, gestational age, oligohydramnios, and fetal hydrops may influence the appearance of maceration.

Gross organ malformations usually can be determined by careful dissection even of the very soft tissue, but important brain malformations may be obscured by liquification. External lesions such as a cystic hygroma or neural tube defect can be seen readily, even with advanced maceration. Hydrops is reliably maintained in many severely autolyzed specimens. However, flattening resulting from postmortem compression can mimic anatomic deformities from oligohydramnios. In a recent case in which a prenatal ultrasound demonstrated posterior nuchal edema, the macerated fetus showed only redundancy of the skin.

Photographic Documentation

Photographic documentation as part of the external physical examination is important in differentiating dysmorphic from edema/maceration-induced bodily changes (4). Such photographs offer a reliable reference while the autopsy is carried out.

Whole Body X-Rays

Selective Use of X-Rays in Perinatal Autopsies

Whole body x-rays of the fetus are important for identifying fetal bone dysplasias or skeletal abnormalities. There is some controversy, however, as to whether all fetuses should be x-rayed or only those having obvious external abnormalities. Cremin and Draper (5) reported their prospective assessment of 60 stillbirths and 40 infants dying as neonates. In all cases, routine radiographs were obtained prior to surgical autopsy. These x-rays included an anterior-posterior film with legs abducted and knees in contact with the cassette and a lateral film with one arm and one leg in contact with the cassette. This study did not detect any skeletal abnormalities or bone dysplasias that were not obvious during external examination. In this series, positive findings on x-ray included anencephaly, spina bifida, hydrocephaly, talipes equino varus, phocomelia, and congenital syphilis. The investigators concluded that x-rays are not recommended routinely for all babies but should be performed if fetal abnormalities are noted on physical examination. In a more recent report, Winter and Sandin (6) x-rayed 488 consecutive infants dying as stillbirths or neonates. Appropriate x-ray diagnoses were made for 7 dwarfs in this series. Moreover, x-ray results were essential in the diagnosis of 1 of 282 babies with no external abnormalities and 1 of 99 babies with external abnormalities. The authors in this study concluded that if radiographs were performed on all stillbirths and babies dying in the newborn period 16% would exhibit some x-ray findings. Had these authors x-rayed only those babies with obvious physical findings or dwarfism, only 22% of babies in this series would have been radiographed, but 146 of 191 radiographic abnormalities would have been detected. Based on the findings from these series, selective use of x-rays for evaluation of stillbirths and dead newborns is indicated.

Cremin and Draper (5) also noted that gas commonly was documented by x-ray in the pharynx and on 2 occasions in the stomachs of stillbirths. No x-rays demonstrated the presence of intravascular gas. In a recent report (7), gas was documented in the cardiac chamber, great vessels, and liver cavity of a stillbirth septic with Escherichia coli. Because intravascular gas can form within 1 hour of death (8), the rare occurrence of this phenomenon does not appear to justify the routine use of x-rays to seek this diagnosis alone.

Organ Weights

Effect of Autolysis on Organ Weights

In his monograph, *Perinatal Pathology*, Wigglesworth (3) suggests that, at minimum, the brain, heart, lungs, spleen, liver, thymus, kidneys and adrenals should be weighed at autopsy. The reader is referred to this monograph for a listing of average newborn organ weights according to gestational age. Unfortunately, the significance of fetal organ weights following prolonged in-utero death remains controversial. Autolysis results first in softening and then in liquifaction of tissues so that organ weights in macerated fetuses will eventually decrease. Care should therefore be taken in interpreting the low weight of an organ in the event of advanced autolysis. Despite the limitations that maceration and organ liquification pose, their presence should not prevent the pathologist from performing these measurements.

Histologic Evaluation

Importance of Obstetrician's Clinical Data

Regardless of tissue autolysis, histologic evaluation of fetal organs can be diagnostically useful. As in all autopsies, tissue samples from the fetus or neonate should be taken as needed to address specific questions. In addition, the authors routinely obtain a standard number of representative sections from specific organs: (1) the thymus, to evaluate involution; (2) the lung, to examine for aspirated materials and viral inclusion bodies and to assess gestational age; (3) the kidney, for viral inclusion bodies and determination of gestational age; and (4) the liver, for evidence of hemosiderin (the stored form of intracellular iron) and viral inclusion bodies. The obstetrician can help the pathologist in this diagnostic process by verifying as well as possible the stated gestational age, time of fetal death, prenatal ultrasound findings, and other clinical information relevant to the perinatal outcome.

Bacterial Cultures

Culturing the Fetal Lung

Bacterial cultures from the stillbirth or dead newborn may provide important indications of undiagnosed infection. The value of positive results, however, depends on whether infection existed prior to delivery or was the result of contamination during the delivery process. The authors routinely culture the fetal lung, because it is continuous with the amniotic fluid in utero yet is protected from contamination during delivery. The finding of aspirated neutrophils in the fetal lung is evidence of infection occurring prior to death.

Results of several recent studies raise questions as to whether fetal infection should be considered during the autopsy evaluation of a stillbirth or dead newborn, in the absence of premature rupture of the amniotic membranes (9–12). As part of the collaborative Perinatal Project of the National Institute of Neurological and Communicative Disorders and Stroke, Naeye and Peters (9) identified 107 stillbirths and 223 newborns dying shortly after birth, all of whom had congenital pneumonia. In every case, fetal membranes were intact prior to onset of labor, and placental evaluation demonstrated acute inflammation of extraplacental membranes, acute umbilical phlebitis, and inflammation of the chorionic plate. Positive cultures were obtained from 76% of lung samples and 49% of blood samples. More recently, Ross et al. (11) in a prospective study of 22 stillbirths were able to identify lung isolate (group B beta-hemolytic streptococcus) in only 1 case. Royston and Geoghegan (12) reviewed the histology of 145 macerated stillbirths. In their series, only 2 stillbirths demonstrated frank congenital pneumonia in the presence of intact amniotic membranes. The collective results of these studies suggest that the true risks of congenital infection with intact fetal membranes remain to be established.

Genetic Evaluation

Obtaining Specimens from Placenta Immediately upon Delivery

If the fetus has multiple congenital anomalies, even if minor, genetic evaluation is indicated since phenotypic diagnosis may be in error. A sample of fetal skin may be taken for chromosomal analysis (karyotyping). To obtain a sample of skin for analysis, the authors routinely clean the area with an alcohol swab and aseptically place an ellipse of skin into a refrigerated bottle of transport media. Unfortunately, cells from the skin of a stillbirth may not grow if intrauterine death occurred days or weeks before delivery. An alternative approach is to obtain cells from viable placental villi. This method should be selected immediately after delivery, before the placenta is placed in formalin (see Chapter 12, "Genetics and Pregnancy Loss: Value of Counseling Between Pregnancies").

FETAL CONDITIONS REQUIRING SPECIAL CONSIDERATION

Acute versus Chronic Stress

A critical question in many perinatal autopsies is whether the fetus was healthy until an acute fatal insult occurred or if he or she died because of a chronic stress process. This question may be evaluated even when the fetus is severely macerated. The clinical obstetric history or visual inspection of the placenta or umbilical cord may identify placental abruption, a true knot in the cord, or an episode of maternal trauma as the acute cause of fetal death. In the absence of any evidence of these events, meconium-stained amniotic fluid or fetal squame cells, vernix, or meconium in the fetal lung, resulting from fetal gasping, may suggest an acute event as the cause of death (4).

Signs of Chronic Intrauterine Stress

The chronically stressed and malnourished fetus exhibits very little subcutaneous fat. Another clue to prolonged stress is involution of the thymus. Thymic involution is considered a subacute steroid-induced stress response. This determination is based on visual inspection of the area occupied by the thymus and on its size contrasted with that expected for gestational age. In some cases, histologic evidence of reparative gliosis in the brain or follicular formation in the spleen suggests chronic intrauterine stress.

Nonimmune Hydrops

Common Etiologies

Nonimmune hydrops is a clinical syndrome occurring approximately once in 3000 pregnancies wherein the fetus develops some variation of subcutaneous edema or massive hydrops. Once Rh isoimmunization is ruled out, this complex condition becomes a major challenge to the obstetrician, pediatrician, and pathologist. In 1984, Holzgreve et al. (13) reported the outcome in a collected series of 50 pregnancies characterized by fetal ascites and generalized edema. In every case, the fetus was alive at the time diagnosis was made. Overall perinatal mortality in this group was 82%. The most common etiologies were cardiac anomalies (22%), chromosomal disorders (14%), congenital anomalies (12%), alpha thalasemia (10%), and twin-twin transfusion (8%). Of note, in only 16% of the babies was no definitive cause for nonimmune hydrops established. These results and the authors' own experience indicate that autopsy evaluation should include the procedures shown in Figure 13.2.

Fetal Trauma

Importance of Distinguishing Antepartum and Intrapartum Injury

Birth trauma is responsible for 1 to 2% of all perinatal deaths (14). In most cases, a clinical history of a difficult delivery or one requiring significant fetal manipulation for delivery should alert the pathologist to the possibility of birth injury. During autopsy, careful inspection should be carried out to document intraabdominal or intracranial hemorrhage. The Falx cerebri and tentorium should be inspected for tears. Additionally, the cervical and thoracic vertebrae should be examined grossly and, if needed, by x-ray. When interpreting the findings, the pathologist must recognize that fetal injury may occur in

Procedure	Evaluate For
Fetal	
Gross autopsy	Cardiac anomalies
	Sequestrated lobe of lung
	Pulmonary hypoplasia
Stains of cardiac conduction pathways	Cardiac arrhythmia
Complete blood count and indices	Hematologic disorders (alpha thalasemia)
Blood typing, antibody studies, and Direct Coombs Test	Rare blood type incompatibilities
Viral cultures/maternal TORCH titers	Fetal infection
Genetic karyotyping	Turner's Syndrome
	Down's Syndrome
Metabolic tests	Gaucher, Tay Sachs, other metabolic disorders
Maternal	
Maternal Glucose 6-phosphate dehydrogenase, Pyruvate Kinase carrier state	Fetal RBC enzyme deficiency
Maternal Kleihauer-Betke analysis	Fetal-to-maternal transfusion

Figure 13.2.   Procedures included with perinatal autopsy evaluation for nonimmune hydrops.

utero prior to labor or delivery. Sims et al. (15) carried out analyses of 433 consecutive stillbirths, 25 of whom exhibited periventricular-intraventricular hemorrhage or gliosis. All 5 stillborn fetuses who exhibited gliosis had died prior to labor. From these results, the authors cautioned that one must distinguish prelabor events from intrapartum events, because both types can be associated with permanent brain injury.

THE UMBILICAL CORD

Specific Cord Lesions

Perinatal death is often attributed to umbilical cord accidents (16, 17). However, the pathologist may have difficulty correlating clinical events with pathologic changes—or the lack thereof—within the substance of the umbilical cord. Cord prolapse may be a cause of fetal death; however, in the absence of specific cord lesions, only an unequivocal clinical history would enable the pathologist to establish this as the cause of death. In cases where fetal or neonatal death is preceded by fetal heart rate decelerations from umbilical cord compression, inflammation of the umbilical cord may be the only finding. Distinctly abnormal umbilical-placental lesions that may be noted on gross inspection include marginal insertion of the umbilical cord at the placental edge (battledore placenta), velamentous insertion of the cord, and true knots in the cord itself. Uncommon lesions include umbilical vein thrombosis, ulceration, and tumor or hematoma within the cord. Ghosh et al. (17) recently reported 12 cases in which cord complications were believed to be the cause of fetal or neonatal death. Six cases involved cord stricture and torsion, 2 had true knots, and single cases involved a short cord, an umbilical vein thrombosis, an aneurysm, and a perivascular hemorrhage at the fetal end of the cord. The authors cite observations by Brown (18) that relatively new knots in the cord may be differentiated from old knots by the absence of marked grooving at the site of the knot. Moreover, old knots tend to lose Wharton's jelly, which is not seen with new knots. Twisting of the umbilical cord, particularly at the point where it enters the fetal abdomen, is a common finding if intrauterine death occurs prior to the onset of labor. Torsion of the cord at the fetal abdomen occurring after death may be distinguished from torsion preceding and possibly causing death on separation of the fetus from the placenta. Postmortem twisting will not remain twisted (17). Other findings suggestive of torsion prior to death include thrombosis and edema opposite venous obstruction as evidence of hemodynamic alterations.

The length of the umbilical cord should always be measured, and the clinical diagnosis of nuchal cord (cord around the fetal neck) or cord prolapse must be communicated by obstetrician to pathologist.

THE PLACENTA

The perinatal autopsy is not complete without a thorough visual and histologic inspection of the placenta (19). When an autopsy request is refused by parents, evaluation of the placenta alone may provide answers as to cause of death. Unfortunately, the placenta frequently is discarded as an unimportant byproduct of pregnancy, even after delivery of a stillbirth or premature newborn. Careful gross and histologic assessment of the placenta often provides valuable information as to cause of death. Unlike the fetus, the placenta does not undergo autolysis or maceration following intrauterine fetal death. It therefore offers a valuable resource for detection of intrauterine infection, chronic intrauterine fetal stress, and maternal vascular disease.

Typical Assessment of the Placenta

Assessment of the placenta may be done in a number of ways. Although each institution's methods vary somewhat, typical assessment follows that proposed by Benirschke and Driscoll (20) to include:

Visual assessment of the placenta and umbilical cord;

Serial slicing of the placenta;

Examination of areas of frank hemorrhage or infarct;

Microscopic evaluation of abnormal areas, placental margins, and membranes.

In a series of 360 spontaneous abortions or stillbirths, Ornay et al. (21) observed a high degree of hydatid degeneration (44%) in first-trimester (less than 12 weeks gestation) losses, especially in association with a blighted ovum. Between 13 and 18 weeks, the incidence of hydatid degeneration markedly decreased (2.9%), but inflammatory lesions occurred in 38.6% of the cases. For stillbirths over 25 weeks, vascular lesions predominated (37.5%), although inflammation was frequently observed (25%).

Despite the apparent value of microscopic evaluation of the placenta, Mueller et al. (22) suggested that, when resources were limited, karyotyping and histopathology could be used selectively. This proposal, although perhaps economically sound, evoked protests from other investigators who strongly advocate inclusion of histopathology as an essential component of the perinatal autopsy (23, 24). More recent studies have provided additional support for microscopic evaluation of the placenta (11, 25). Based on his experience with 38 normally formed stillbirths and 53 normally formed babies dying within 24 hours of delivery, Naeye (23) found a 53% incidence of chorioamnionitis, defined as acute inflammation extending through the fetal membranes. In 2 other series of stillbirths or neonatal deaths, chorioamnionitis was documented in 56% (24) and 20% of placentas (26). In a review of 89 placentas following delivery of a stillbirth, Rayburn et al. (2) found that placental examination supported the clinical history and fetal autopsy in 77% of cases, was not consistent with the clinical impression in 11%, and was the only definitive finding in 11%. From this experience, the authors express a strong argument for histological evaluation of the placenta during all perinatal autopsies.

INFECTION

Chorioamnionitis

A common problem in the perinatal autopsy is evaluating the clinical significance of chorioamnionitis (27–30). Pathologically, this condition is diagnosed by the presence of neutrophils in fetal membranes. Bacteria are presumed to migrate from the vagina through the cervical barrier into the chorionic-decidual layer where most of the inflammatory cells are seen (10). The plausibility of this route of infection is supported by the strong correlation between presence of inflammatory changes in the fetal membranes and length of time that fetal membranes have been ruptured prior to delivery. In Naeye et al.'s series, 15 of 48 cases of chorioamnionitis were preceded by premature rupture of the membranes (10).

Most commonly, neutrophils are densest at the chorionamnion junction. The finding of neutrophils only in the subchorionic fibrin of the intervillous space is considered evidence of early chorioamnionitis. Although neutrophils are presumed to come from maternal blood, the pattern of neutrophil infiltration has not been shown to be important (10). Frequently, histologic changes consistent with chorioamnionitis may appear in the absence of clinical infection. Nevertheless, subclinical chorioamnionitis is associated with neonatal morbidity, prematurity, and premature rupture of the membranes (10, 4, 25).

Common Organisms Found on Culture

The mechanism by which chorioamnionitis causes fetal or neonatal death is complex and poorly understood. In some cases, a pathogen recognized for its virulence such as group B beta-hemolytic streptococcus may be cultured. Recent studies, however, have suggested that the most common organism associated with chorioamnionitis is Ureaplasma urealyticum (29). In 1 series of 33 perinatal deaths, U. urealyticum was cultured in 78.8% of cases, compared with 32.3% of control patients

(25). In this group of patients, pathogenic stains of bacteria or viruses were recovered from 27.3 and 20% of cases, respectively. Chlamydia was not found to be a contributing pathogen. Ross et al. (11) obtained vaginal cultures from 154 women experiencing preterm labor or intrauterine fetal deaths. Among those patients with intrauterine fetal deaths, mycoplasma species (57%), U. urealyticum (32%), and listeria monocytogenes (16%) were the most common organisms recovered.

Viral Infections

Viral infections in the perinatal period must also be considered during histologic evaluation of the placenta for evidence of intrauterine infection. Intrauterine infections by syphilis, toxoplasmosis, rubella, cytomegalovirus, and herpes are often associated with a plasma cell infiltration of placental villi. This histologic finding is positive evidence of a reaction to a foreign antigen within the villi. However, fatal in-utero infections may occur without any visible placental reaction. Likewise, placental involvement may occur without fetal infection. Notably, cytomegalovirus (CMV) placentitis without fetal infection has been observed (31). More recently, CMV infection was associated with an infected hydropic stillbirth and an uninfected second twin (32). Viral cultures and special stains (gram stain for bacteria, silver stain for fungus) should be undertaken during the postmortem examination whenever there are clinical suspicions and/or lesions suggestive of sepsis. When applicable, these results should be correlated with maternal antibody titers (33).

Inflammation Unrelated to Infection

Certain histologic changes may occur in the placenta that are unrelated to the outcome of the pregnancy. Acute inflammation in the uterine decidual layer is a common finding in spontaneous abortion, in premature labor, and even in some term labors. Thus, inflammation of the decidua does not necessarily imply infection, but rather it may be a part of normal tissue reaction during labor.

Certain substances in amniotic fluid may induce a reaction in the amniotic membranes. Miller et al. (34) exposed placentas *in vitro* to varying concentrations and durations of meconium. Surface staining was noted within 1 hour of exposure and was proportional to length of exposure and concentration of meconium. In contrast, pigment penetration and uptake by macrophages were primarily dependent on length of exposure alone. Eight of 11 placentas exhibited meconium pigmentation in macrophages after 1 hour. The presence of meconium pigmentation in macrophages within the chorion took somewhat longer, but pigmentation was noted in all placentas by 3 hours. Umbilical cord staining was observed at 1 hour with 5% meconium and at 15 minutes with 10% meconium.

HEMORRHAGE

Fetal-to-Maternal Hemorrhage

Fetal or maternal hemorrhage can be associated with fetal death. Lesions that cause serious fetal hemorrhage include ruptured vasa previa, torn placenta previa, and amniocentesis with penetration of a large fetal vessel. An often overlooked cause of fetal hemorrhage is fetal-to-maternal bleeding (35,36). This condition can be documented by performing a Kleihauer-Betke analysis on maternal blood to determine the presence and amount of fetal red blood cells. In a series of 29 stillbirths who died without an obvious cause, 4 fetuses (13.8%) experienced blood losses of 147 to 240 ml into the maternal circulation, amounts estimated at 30 to 66% of the fetal-placental blood volume (35). In a later report, 3 cases involving fetal-to-maternal transfusions of 270, 355, and 460 cc fetal blood were documented (36). The author of this study commented that the Kleihauer-Betke analysis is most accurate when maternal blood is obtained before delivery, because during the delivery process all patients experience some degree of fetal-to-maternal transfusion.

The presence of thrombi of fetal blood in the intervillous spaces of the placenta is a common finding and is usually considered innocuous. The laminated appearance of these thrombi suggest that they result from sluggish flow of fetal blood into the maternal intervillous space.

Findings Associated with Placental Abruption

Retroplacental hemorrhages of varying sizes are the morphologic findings associated with placental abruption. In some cases, they may have occurred in early pregnancy, as shown by an old placental infarction overlying a pale hematoma devoid of hemoglobin. In more acute cases, such hemorrhages may compress the overlying placenta, causing acute infarction. The latter may be recognized only by villous congestion. At times, there is almost no pathologic evidence of placental abruption except for hemorrhagic disruption of the adherent decidua basalis. In all hematomas, the initial site of hemorrhage is within the basal decidua.

Not infrequently, clinically significant placental abruptions are associated with smaller, older hemorrhages or infarcts in the membranes or hemosiderin-laden macrophages present in the base of the placenta. Retroplacental hematomas are relatively frequent findings in nonmacerated second trimester stillbirths. Whether these hematomas reflect conditions leading to abruption or are a primary cause is unknown. Even when it does not cause fetal death, this type of bleeding may compromise the fetus by pooling blood in nonperfused, infarcted villi and by reducing functional placental volume acutely. Thus, even small or old retroplacental hematomas should be noted and correlated with the clinical history.

Breus Mole

Another type of hemorrhage not infrequently associated with fetal death is massive subchorionic hemorrhage (Breus Mole). This type of hemorrhage, in the authors' experience, appears to involve maternal blood and is usually associated with hemorrhage at the placental margin. In some cases of large retroplacental hemorrhages, however, slices of the placenta have demonstrated tracking of blood to form subchorionic hemorrhage. Thus, Breus Mole may be a variant of placental abruption. This form of hemorrhage is different from subamniotic hemorrhage found at delivery, which results from damage to a fetal umbilical cord stem vessel. The latter type of acute hemorrhage presumably results from traction on the umbilical cord at the time that the placenta is extracted. Postmortem investigation for fetal death from pregnancy-related hemorrhage requires clear communication between pathologist and obstetrician.

IMPROVING CLINICIAN-PATHOLOGIST COMMUNICATION

The obstetrician (and neonatologist) can improve the quality of the perinatal autopsy by providing the pathologist with complete clinical information. The autopsy is a professional consultation. The better the communication between pathologist and clinician, the more fruitful the autopsy is likely to be.

The Perinatal Autopsy as a Professional Consultation

Adequate communication, however, requires more of the pathologist and the obstetrician or pediatrician than an exchange of the clinical history and the autopsy findings. The pathologist must actively demonstrate to the clinician what the autopsy can and cannot explain. Likewise, the clinician for his or her part should not accept autopsy reports that are superficial or that fail to address important questions. Unanswered questions or dissatisfaction with the autopsy report should be discussed constructively with the pathologist. From such discussions, improvements and new ideas regarding approaches to the autopsy and use of its findings inevitably will be generated. In cases with unusual maternal disease or fetal complications, the pathologist should be consulted prior to autopsy. He or she may need to prepare tissue rapidly for electron microscopy, biochemical study, cell culture, or frozen immunohistology. This kind of preparation should also extend to study of the placenta. The obstetrician is responsible for seeing that tissues reach the pathologist in appropriate condition. Viral or cytogenetic studies cannot be carried out on formalin-fixed tissue, but all too often spontaneously aborted fetuses with obvious malformations or skin lesions are simply placed in formalin and treated as routine pathologic specimens. If the pathologist cannot be contacted immediately, the specimen should be refrigerated in moist gauze.

CONCLUSIONS

The autopsy often clarifies the cause of a perinatal death. Use of the information obtained by autopsy varies from genetic counseling to epidemiologic monitoring, from confirming new diagnostic modalities to suggesting new models of pathophysiology and new treatment strategies. In some cases, autopsy information will be difficult for the obstetrician or pediatrician to act on (for example, CMV infection). At other times, the information will be disconcerting to the patient, as when it raises such questions as, "Where does chorioamnionitis come from?" "Could I have an abruption again?" or "Why don't you know the cause of my baby's malformation?" Unfortunately, such questions point to real gaps in our knowledge. The autopsy will exclude with certainty many possibilities, even if it cannot answer all questions. At the very least, the autopsy should cause the obstetrician, neonatologist, pathologist, and even the patient to ponder with enhanced effectiveness the unanswered questions in the case.

REFERENCES

1. Freeman RF, Dorchester W, Anderson G, Garite TJ: The significance of a previous stillbirth. *Am J Obstet Gynecol* 151:7–13, 1985.
2. Rayburn W, Sanders C, Barr M, Jr, Rygiel R: The stillborn fetus. Placental histologic evaluation in determining a cause. *Obstet Gynecol* 65:637–640, 1985.
3. Wigglesworth JS: Performance of the perinatal autopsy. In Wigglesworth JS (ed): *Perinatal Pathology*, Philadelphia, WB Saunders Co, 1984, p 29.
4. Manchester OK and Shikes RH: The perinatal autopsy: Special considerations. *Clin Obstet Gynecol* 23:1125–1134, 1980.
5. Cremin BJ and Draper R: The value of radiography in perinatal deaths. *Pediatr Radiol* 11:143–146, 1981.
6. Winter RM and Sandin BM: The radiology of stillbirths and neonatal deaths. *Br J Obstet Gynaecol* 91:762–765, 1984.
7. Jasnosy KM, MacPherson TA, Mazer T: Escherichia coli gas production in a fetus. *Am J Obstet Gynecol* 150:1001, 1984.
8. Quisling RG, Poznanski AK, Roloff DW: Post-mortem gas accumulation in premature infants. *Pediatr Radiol* 113:155, 1974.

9. Naeye RL and Peters EC: Amniotic fluid infections with intact membranes leading to perinatal death. *Pediatrics* 61:171–177, 1978.

10. Naeye RL, Maisels MJ, Lorenz RP, Botti JJ: The clinical significance of placental villous edema. *Pediatrics* 71:588–594, 1983.

11. Ross SM, Windsor IM, Robins-Brown RM, Ballard RC, Adhika M, Fenn DB: Microbiological studies during the perinatal period. *S Af Med J* 66:598–603, 1984.

12. Royston D and Geoghegan F: Amniotic fluid infection with intact membranes in relation to stillbirths. *Obstet Gynecol* 65:745–746, 1985.

13. Holzgreve W, Curry CJR, Golbus MS, Callen PW, Filly RA, Smith JC: Investigation of nonimmune hydrops fetalis. *Am J Obstet Gynecol* 150:805–812, 1984.

14. Gresham EL: Birth trauma. *Pediat Clin North Am* 22:317–328, 1975.

15. Sims ME, Turkel SB, Halterman G, Paul RH: Brain injury and intrauterine death. *Am J Obstet Gynecol* 151:721–723, 1985.

16. Corkill TF: The infant's vulnerable life-line. *Aust NZ J Obstet Gynaecol* 1:154, 1961.

17. Ghosh A, Woo JSK, MacHenry C, Wan CW, O'Hoy KM, Ma HK: Fetal loss from umbilical cord abnormalities—a difficult case for prevention. *Eur J Obstet Gynecol Reprod Biol* 18:183–198, 1984.

18. Brown FJ: On the abnormalities of the umbilical cord which may cause antepartum death. *Br J Obstet Gynaecol* 32:17–20, 1925.

19. Fox H: The pathology of the placenta. In Fox H, Langley FA (eds): *Postgraduate Obstetrical and Gynecological Pathology*, Oxford, Pergamon Press, 1973, pp 409- 439.

20. Benirschke K and Driscoll SG: *The Pathology of the Human Placenta.* New York, Springer-Verlag, 1967.

21. Ornay A, Salamon-Arnon J, Ben-Zur Z, Kohn G: Placental findings in spontaneous abortions and stillbirths. *Teratology* 24:243–252, 1981.

22. Mueller RF, Sybert VP, Johnson J, Brown AZ, Chen W-J: Evaluation of a protocol for post-mortem examination of stillbirths. *New Eng J Med* 309:518–522, 1983.

23. Naeye RL: The investigation of perinatal deaths. *New Eng J Med* 309:611–612, 1983.

24. Jones NL and Esterly JR: Perinatal autopsies. *New Eng J Med* 310:393–394, 1984.

25. Quinn PA, Butany J, Chipman M, Taylor J, Hannah W: A prospective study of microbial infection in stillbirths and early neonatal death. *Am J Obstet Gynecol* 151:238–249, 1985.

26. Turkel SB: Perinatal autopsies. *New Eng J Med* 310:394, 1984.

27. Naeye RL and Ross SM: Amniotic fluid infection syndrome. *Clin Obstet Gynecol* 9:593–607, 1982.

28. Fox H and Langley FA: Leukocyte infiltration of the placenta and umbilical cord. *Obstet Gynecol* 37:451–458, 1971.

29. Kundsin RB, Driscoll SG, Monson RR, Yeh C, Biano SA, Cochran WD: Association of ureaplasma urealyticum in the placenta with perinatal morbidity and mortality. *N Engl J Med* 310:941–945, 1984.

30. Hameed C, Tejani N, Verma U, Archbald F: Silent chorioamnionitis as a cause of preterm labor refractory to tocolytic therapy. *Am J Obstet Gynecol* 149:726, 1984.

31. Hayes K and Gibas H: Placental cytomegalovirus infection without foetal involvement following primary infection in pregnancy. *J Peds* 79:401–405, 1971.

32. Morton R and Mitchell I: Neonatal cytomegalic inclusion disease in a set of twins, one member of whom was a hydropic stillbirth, the other completely uninfected. *Br J Obstet Gynaecol* 90:276–279, 1983.

33. Sever JL: TORCH tests and what they mean. *Am J Obstet Gynecol* 152:495–498, 1985.
34. Miller PW, Coen RW, Benirschke K: Dating the time interval from meconium passage to birth. *Obstet Gynecol* 66:459–462, 1985.
35. Laube DW and Schanberger CW: Fetomaternal bleeding as a cause of unexplained fetal death. *Obstet Gynecol* 60:649–651, 1982.
36. Fay RA: Feto-maternal hemorrhage as a cause of fetal morbidity and mortality. *Br J Obstet Gynaecol* 90:443–446, 1983.

CHAPTER

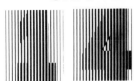

Peer Support Group Network

CAROLE BONNO

In recent years, peer support groups for parents grieving a pregnancy loss have gained credibility. Parents have asserted that they have a need for such self-help groups, and the community has learned to respond. A peer support group is a unique way for parents to help themselves and others through their intense period of grief. The group is a place where people feeling pain, anger, and confusion because of a baby's death can turn to others who have suffered the same tragedy. Strong bonds form among members of the group. These bonds remain even when parents cease to need the support group, as their mourning gradually subsides. Parents whose baby dies before or shortly after birth grieve intensely for their lost baby, a fact that has not been widely acknowledged in our society. Support groups for parents undergoing this crisis are growing in number, acting both to focus attention on this problem and to relieve the terrible loneliness and suffering of mothers and fathers who endure such a loss.

This chapter is designed to clarify the role, identity, and structure of peer support groups. Additionally, recruitment of and delegation of responsibilities to group volunteers, the telephone as a method of outreach, and the logistics of running a monthly peer support group meeting will be discussed.

PARENTAL EXPECTATIONS OF A SUPPORT GROUP

The desire to be understood and to have feelings accepted by others becomes critical during the period of grief. A parent who comes to a pregnancy loss support group needs and can expect the following:

1. A support group puts parents in touch with others who understand what they are going through. Because parents may not know anyone else who has suffered a devastating pregnancy loss, feelings of isolation and loneliness are overwhelming. Sharing their experience with others who have had a similar loss helps parents understand that they are not alone. They discover that their feelings are not unique and that they are responding appropriately to their loss.

2. A support group helps to stimulate communication between couples. Although a couple is grieving for their baby, it is unlikely that both parents can grieve at the same pace. For example, the woman might wish that her partner would be less protective and would discuss his feelings with her. Support group encounters provide a neutral setting in which a couple may open up to each other, either during a meeting or afterward.

3. Grieving parents need to talk about their baby and their entire experience. The support group provides parents with many new sympathetic listeners who are interested in their story. This is important because parents usually arrive at their first meeting at a point when their friends and family may have already returned to their own activities and thus are less patient with the parents' need to talk about their experience. The support group may be the only place where parents can talk about their baby or just say the baby's name out loud. Also, hearing about how other couples work through daily activities as they grieve gives parents insights about themselves as well as a gauge to check their own recovery.

4. A support group reassures parents that their grief is appropriate and valid. Grief can produce bizarre behavior that can be very frightening. Parents learn from each other how grieving for a pregnancy loss will affect their lives for a long time and how others have responded to these feelings.

5. Support groups provide information through lectures, books, reprints of pertinent articles, and poetry. Discussions during meetings are of value, too, because individuals dare to bring up issues that no one else will, and this allows parents to share their feelings about taboo topics.

SUPPORT GROUPS TO MEET PARENTS' NEEDS

The group most often will start out very small, but with a clear set of objectives. Two people or 2 couples to lead the group are sufficient to begin. Ideally, the people founding the group should share a philosophy and also complement each other's skills. Some important skills include the ability to lead a group meeting, a background in social work, and good telephone counseling techniques. The cofounders have to create a strong and united entity. Because they must work together intensively, compatibility is crucial. It is realistic to expect that 6–9 months of preparation will be needed before the first parents' meeting can be held. Because of the range of decisions that must be made regarding the operation of the group, plans may move slowly.

Types of Support Groups

There are, generally speaking, 3 types of support groups: educational, professionally facilitated, and peer. A group may be identified as one of these types in particular, or it may combine aspects from each to form a hybrid type, adapted to a community's needs and resources.

Educational Support Group

The educational support group might operate as a series of meetings extending over 4–6 weeks. A sample format of topics to be covered might include those listed in Figure 14.1. Topics can be presented by core members of the group or by professionals who are knowledgeable in each area. Since the process of grieving lasts longer than a 4- to 6-week program, a regular monthly support group meeting, another meeting to be held 1 month later, or one-to-one counseling may be offered in conjunction with the 6 sessions as a follow-up.

Professionally Facilitated Group

The second type of support group is the professionally facilitated group. This group may include the participation of a

Week 1: Explore the basis and goals of the group, then have parents introduce themselves as desired and describe their losses.

Week 2: Explain the stages of grief and how they manifest themselves in people's lives.

Week 3: Suggest ways of dealing with others (for example, spouse, children, family, friends, and co-workers).

Week 4: Discuss how people feel about themselves and how the loss affects their marriages.

Week 5: Summarize the elements of healing.

Figure 14.1. Sample format for educational support group.

social worker, nurse, chaplain, psychologist, or doctor. Usually, a hospital-directed support group has these professionals as staff members and can call on them for advice. Along with professionals, it is helpful to have trained parents aid in facilitating the group. Some people contend that support groups cannot be run by professionals who have not themselves experienced a miscarriage, stillbirth, or neonatal death. However, the professional person who wants to work with the support group usually has a vital interest in parents' recovery from their loss because they have seen them during their crisis or have had contact with similar patients in the past.

Parents sometimes feel constrained in the presence of a professional, particularly one in a healthcare-related field such as nursing or social work. Often, parents feel angry about treatment they received when they lost their baby. The professional associated with the support group may not have been involved directly with parents who attend meetings. Yet, that care provider's presence may inhibit parents from expressing strong, painful feelings that need to be vocalized. Leaders of a professionally facilitated support group must be aware of this possibility. They may find that they need to exert extra effort in setting parents at ease. This objective can be accomplished, giving parents the opportunity to share both positive and negative feelings.

Peer Support Group

The third type is the peer support group, which is run by parents who have experienced a pregnancy loss, have worked through their grief, and want to help others. The balance of this chapter explores the peer support group.

GETTING STARTED

People interested in establishing a pregnancy loss peer support group usually have experienced the loss of a baby. They understand the need for such a support group in their community. They have the most important asset for this work—good will—but they also need specific skills. If there are any bereavement support groups in the area, the founders should attend some of their meetings and seek advice from their leaders. Other support groups, no matter what their focus is, can serve as examples of differently structured programs. By attending such meetings, the founders of a new support group can pick up pointers on facilitating a group and choosing a format. They also can ask for advice and recommendations from professionals. Obstetricians, social workers, mental health agencies, or anyone else involved in care of bereaved patients can provide first-hand information on helping parents as they grieve over a pregnancy loss.

Gathering Information for the Group

A further way to prepare for the support group is to read. Helpful professionals can suggest journals and periodicals that teach one how to respond effectively to the bereaved. Many excellent books are available in libraries that describe the normal grieving process, give actual accounts of parents' experiences, point out problems most parents will encounter, and list addresses of local and national support groups (See "Suggested Resources" at the end of this chapter). These support groups are willing to send educational material on request. The people working in these groups are a special network of individuals who will encourage new leaders and help them to get started.

To Affiliate with a National Group or Remain Independent

Another issue to be decided is whether the new group should join with a national support group or should remain independent. There are advantages to joining an already existing support system. The training program usually is well organized and conducted by professionals who are available for consultation as needed. The name of the group, pamphlets, and a format are standardized. For individuals forming a group in a community where none yet exist, association with a national group can add to the new group's credibility. It is necessary, however, to take into consideration that national groups might charge an annual fee, have a set format that cannot be changed, or impose certain restrictions or expectations on the new chapter that may not accommodate the objectives of the new group's leaders.

An alternative approach is to develop as an independent group. The program can be tailored to the particular needs of the community, within the limits of the group's resources. There can be enormous satisfaction when an independent group has been established successfully. Although the main objective is to aid bereaved parents by telephone or at meetings, there is a natural "ripple" effect in the medical community. Once established, the support group is able to speak for parents so that changes are made in the way parents are treated by medical personnel when their baby dies.

As the founders create plans for the support group, they have to decide what services their group will provide. It is wise to start small and add services as the group grows. For example, a volunteer training program is an immediate need, whereas issuing a newsletter can be postponed until later. Some services that might be offered over the course of time are suggested in Figure 14.2. Some of the options listed are ambitious and will require experience, skill, and personnel. It is best to choose an

Parent meetings

Volunteer training program

Resource library

Telephone counselors

Individual visits to home or hospital

Pamphlet for distribution (to hospitals, religious congregations, and/or group obstetric practices)

In-hospital seminars by group members

Newsletter

Sharing information with interested professionals and with other bereavement groups

Community education and workshops

Figure 14.2. Services that may be offered by a support group.

initial program that is reasonable and more limited in scope and then to add other features as the group's skills, personnel, and confidence increase.

Location

An important feature to determine is where group meetings will take place. Until the group is well established, it might be preferable or necessary to meet in the homes of core members. After a few meetings, bereaved parents may, on a rotating basis, offer their homes as a meeting place. A home offers a comfortable setting for parents, and in the beginning this location might put everyone more at ease. Many successful support groups meet in homes and have been doing so for as long as 10 years. However, in a home there are distractions to consider, such as ringing telephones or unavoidable interruptions by other family members. Furthermore, after a while, membership may outgrow the home setting.

A good possible meeting place is in a church or synagogue, which usually has good facilities to meet the need for privacy. A community organization or a local business might also have meeting rooms available. Colleges and schools are other possibilities to consider. Even a local hospital is a possibility, but the group's affiliation or lack of affiliation with the hospital might need to be articulated. As the group becomes recognized, helpful professionals may be able to suggest other appropriate meeting places. Every facility has advantages and drawbacks. It is important to select a site that is centrally located with ample parking spaces available.

Atmosphere

More important than location is atmosphere. The reason that people attend a meeting is that they have experienced a pregnancy loss. Parents are there to talk about their baby. They are not as interested in physical surroundings as they are in the atmosphere of care and concern provided them.

Pamphlet

Two other points to consider are pamphlets and referrals. A pamphlet is the means of informing the general public about the peer support group. Primarily, though, it acts as an invitation to bereaved parents to make contact. The pamphlet should be simple, well written, and clear. It is useful to look at other bereavement pamphlets for ideas. A pamphlet can be typewritten with limited information, or it can be more extensive in scope. If the group has financial resources or contacts who may offer design, typesetting, and printing services free or at a reduced price, the design and production of the pamphlet can be more elaborate. The following information should be included in the pamphlet:

Name of the support group;

Group's philosophy;

Services provided;

Method of contacting the support group.

If telephone numbers are included, be sure to add the area code, an extension number if necessary, and the phone contact person's name. A second person's name and number can be added to the pamphlet for parents' convenience. A permanent mailing address for correspondence is also helpful, either one member's home address or a post office box number. The pamphlet may also include a logo, the location and time of meetings, or a brief history of the group. The color of the pamphlet is another choice to consider. It is considerate to avoid pink or blue, since these colors are widely associated as baby colors and might add to parents' discomfort.

Referrals

The pamphlet will be important as the group seeks referrals. There are several good places to begin for referrals. Obstetricians and pediatricians—starting with the members' own doctors—should be informed of the group's services. Head nurses on the maternity floors and newborn nurseries of local hospitals are also important contacts. It is inappropriate for the support group to request a list of bereaved parents' names from doctors or the hospitals because such information cannot be made public. Usually the hospital staff is willing to inform patients of the support group's existence while they are hospitalized and give them a pamphlet before their discharge. It is then up to the parents themselves to make contact with the group. Sometimes a doctor, friend, or member of the clergy will get permission from newly bereaved parents to have someone from the support group call them directly.

Other referral sources to consider are childbirth educators, LaLeche League, community clergy, funeral directors, and women's service organizations. The group can be listed in the telephone book, as well as with citywide hotlines and mental health agencies. Announcements that a meeting is scheduled, noting that there is no admission charge or fee of any kind (which is usually the case), may be printed for free in the community events listings of a citywide newspaper. Smaller community newspapers may be prompted to write a story about the support group because they are always seeking features about local residents and their interests.

FINDING VOLUNTEERS

The first class of volunteer counselors recruited to help the peer support group probably will not have been involved with any support group before. As the group expands over time, the next class of volunteers will have had the experience of coming to the support group initially as bereaved parents. With training, these individuals can make the transition more smoothly from parent to volunteer. The overall motivation for becoming a volunteer, however, is the same for the first and all subsequent training classes—to help bereaved parents. However, if the idea that parents grieve after suffering a pregnancy loss is new in the community, the initial group of volunteers may have experienced feelings and problems that are not an issue for subsequent volunteers. The first volunteers may be angry because they did not receive any support from others, because their doctors and other care providers did not acknowledge the significance of the loss, because their hospital experience caused them unnecessary emotional pain, or because no choices were offered to them and they now wish that things could have been done differently. The support group offers volunteers a means of resolving these feelings. Gradually, they can see that, because of their efforts, subsequent bereaved parents will be treated more compassionately.

Screening Volunteers

Those who interview prospective volunteers usually can judge whether a new volunteer will be an effective counselor. Often, a "gut feeling" about a volunteer is valid. If the person fills conversations with judgmental remarks such as, "Parents shouldn't feel like that," "Parents have to put the loss behind them and go on," or "All you have to do to feel better is . . . ," then it is probable that this candidate would not be a good volunteer for the group. The group needs volunteers who are compassionate, nonjudgmental, and good listeners. Volunteers should know the group's history—how it was formed and its

Infertility problems

Adopting children

A pregnancy loss while unmarried

A difficult pregnancy that required bedrest and/or hospitalization

Loss of twins (or loss of 1 twin)

Loss of a baby during a second marriage

Figure 14.3. Some experiences that may affect individual responses to pregnancy loss.

philosophy, achievements, and future goals. The "mix" is important, too. It is advisable to look for people who have had a variety of experiences connected with their losses. Volunteers may have had, among them, a wide range of experiences (such as the examples given in Figure 14.3), all of which impinge on responses to a pregnancy loss itself. A group composed of volunteers whose losses occurred under many different circumstances thus may be able to "match" a volunteer with, for example, a newly bereaved mother whose premature newborn was the only child of a second marriage. Each kind of experience adds dimension to volunteers' ability to be understanding and makes the group more effective overall. It is helpful, moreover, to have husband-and-wife teams participate in group leadership.

VOLUNTEER COUNSELOR'S ROLE

When it comes to training volunteer counselors, there are 2 completely different schools of thought as to the issue of training. One group believes that volunteers need training in marriage, family, and child counseling, psychology, and social work; the other group believes that all that is needed is to put grieving people together in a room and let them talk. Perhaps both approaches can be justified, but the author will concentrate on a modified approach to training that comprises both views.

Defining the Role   The volunteer counselor needs to understand his or her role in the support group and to know what is expected in the way of duties and responsibilities. So that prospective volunteers may see how the group works, they should be included at a staff meeting. This gesture gives them both a realistic view of the group's workings and an opportunity to decide if they can be comfortable working with the group before they have made a real commitment. Another way to help them decide is to let them be hostesses at (monthly) parents' meetings. This screening process also benefits group leaders because only the sincerely committed will continue on with formal training.

Volunteers also have to understand the scope of their authority. Even though they may carry the title of counselor, they must remember that they do not and should not take the place of professional counselors. If a bereaved parent or couple requires more help than the group is capable of providing, volunteers need to discuss this with him or her and possibly will be able to refer the person to an appropriate professional.

Confidentiality

Confidentiality is another issue that volunteers must recognize. Because of the situation, parents often confide in group members about angry feelings they have toward a physician or the hospital. The support group and its representatives should be perceived uniformly as a receptive, sympathetic, and confidential ear. Parents should feel reassured that group leaders will not criticize their experience or gossip about them.

Another important resource to utilize in training volunteers is the literature. Books and articles on treating grieving parents, written by professionals for their colleagues, are valuable. Also, videotapes about bereavement counseling can be rented from some national support groups (see "Suggested Resources"). These tapes can be brought in periodically and shown to a large group or to several small groups over a few days. Opening a group discussion after the viewing reinforces important points to be drawn from the film and furthers the education and experience of all volunteers, old and new.

ABILITY TO LISTEN

Learning to Feel Comfortable with Silence

Listening skills for individual counseling and for leading a group discussion are vitally important. This is probably the area in which volunteers feel most insecure, and it is the skill that is most difficult to teach. There are books and national support group articles concerned with listening skills that are of great benefit as training tools (see "Suggested Resources"). Volunteers must become comfortable with silence, able to resist the urge to jump in and "save" the conversation. Learning to use "I think" or "I feel" statements is helpful because stating generalizations about grief can intimidate newly bereaved parents. These parents do not attend a group meeting or call on the telephone to hear a speech. They must be encouraged to talk and to express painful feelings.

Volunteers should learn to share their experiences, both helpful and negative, with group members. This invites parents to reveal their feelings, knowing that the volunteer will be nonjudgmental. As feelings surface, parents may laugh or cry.

Tissues should be available at all meetings. When tears or poignant moments occur, volunteers should be encouraged to do what they feel is natural and comforting—to clasp a hand or place an arm around the parent's shoulder.

Learning the Process of Grief

New volunteers need to know the stages of grief in detail, how each stage manifests itself, and what parents say when they are in each stage. Volunteers should be alerted to identify unresolved grief. It is important to recognize a parent who "gets stuck" in a phase of grieving, who may need professional counseling. (The reader is referred to Chapter 1, "Pregnancy Loss and the Grief Process," for this information.)

Role Playing

Skills in facilitating a group meeting can be learned by role playing. However, the artificial situation can make first-time participants self-conscious. An effective alternative is to have volunteers observe the dynamics of group meetings. If the group divides into smaller groups at meetings, a new volunteer can be paired with a more experienced one. This pairing gives the new volunteer a chance to gain confidence in running a meeting while benefiting from watching a role model—the experienced volunteer.

Attending Seminars

Seminars and conferences on loss, grief, and bereavement counseling are important for all volunteers to attend. Although the material sometimes may not be new to any volunteer, hearing it again always helps as reinforcement. Such meetings are a good source to get ideas for new goals and to generate enthusiasm among volunteers. They often put group leaders in touch with others in the community who share the group's concerns. Meetings also provide an opportunity for group volunteers to form and broaden a network of local people and to share information.

Making Referrals to Other Organizations

Volunteers should be given a list of local mental health services and hotlines for referrals in the event of an emergency. "Suicide" is a word bereaved parents may use at times. It is vital that volunteers learn to respond to any such reference in a calm manner. They need to be able to determine how serious the person's threat is and what measures, if any, should be taken. Note that volunteers should be reminded that they are not to give medical advice even for those who coincidentally might have medical knowledge.

Resolving Personal Responses

It is well to advise new volunteers that, as they review their own pregnancy losses during their training period, old and often unsettling feelings may arise that they thought were resolved. On the other hand, as they continue on into expanded roles in the support group, they may find themselves even better able to adjust to their personal experiences with pregnancy loss because of their involvement in the program. This adjustment comes from new insights they gain, which they might express by saying, "My baby's death had a purpose. I am more compassionate now toward people, and I am able to help others who have had a loss."

WORKING WITH PARENTS ON THE TELEPHONE

Special Demands on the Telephone Contact Volunteer

Not every volunteer can or should make the commitment to serve as a telephone contact for the support group. This is a special role that requires a dependable, dedicated individual who understands as fully as possible the responsibilities of the job. Those whose names are on the support group's pamphlet should be available most of the time at the phone numbers listed. Because calls can come at any time of the day or evening, these contacts need to be prepared to respond whenever the telephone rings. This role demands flexibility and tact, and it requires a commitment from a few special people. Other members of the contact's family should be willing to answer the telephone courteously at all times. The bereaved parent (most often the woman) usually calls when she is feeling very sad and is in need of immediate help. The main job of the telephone contact is to be a sympathetic and patient listener.

Obtaining Information from the Caller

The initial phone call may take from 30 to 45 minutes. Unless the group's telephone contact is going to continue talking with this parent on a long-range basis, she acts merely to put on a "bandaid," not engaging to assume the role of the caller's volunteer counselor. The contact should listen to this caller and then later try to match her up with a volunteer whose loss and attitudes seem compatible. Inevitably, there will be times when the contact cannot talk when someone calls for the first time. Whenever this happens, the contact should explain that his or her time is limited at the moment and then arrange to call back at a specified time that is convenient for both. The contact needs to be sure that he or she has the caller's name and phone number. The caller may be reluctant to telephone again for fear that she will be calling back at another inconvenient time.

If a woman is crying when she calls, the contact should be sympathetic but not overindulgent. It is helpful to provide information about the support group, their library, or telephone counseling, in order to give the caller a moment to compose herself. In the initial telephone conversation, it is better not to talk too much about meetings. This decision benefits both parties. The caller may want time to consider whether to make an "obligation" to attend a meeting; the contact might need to assess, to the best of his or her abilities, how this caller will fit in at a meeting. Such screening must be very courteous and, if possible, completely undetected by the caller. If the experienced contact feels that a caller has a psychologic problem that would disrupt meetings, it is better that she be dealt with on a one-to-one basis or even that she be referred for professional help. This type of problem occurs very rarely, but it is of value to note because group leaders have an obligation to protect other parents and themselves at meetings.

The initial conversation requires commonsense and good listening skills on the part of the contact person. He or she should develop a technique to elicit information in an unforced manner and to assess the caller's needs, while at the same time he or she is helping the caller feel more comfortable in talking about her loss with a stranger. The contact should ask open-ended questions and accept whatever information the caller is prepared to offer at that point. It is better to say, "May I ask what kind of a loss have you had?" rather than rattling off, "Did you have a miscarriage, stillbirth, or neonatal death?" A series of such questions can be intimidating, as if the contact had a clipboard and were filling in a questionnaire with the caller's answers. It is not important to know the caller's obstetrician's name or her religion. On the other hand, there is information that the contact should note as the caller provides it during the course of the conversation, such as when she mentions her husband's name, the baby's name, her children's names, and when the pregnancy loss occurred. The contact should note these facts so that they can be integrated into later conversations.

Bereaved parents are very vulnerable when they make their first telephone call. The conversation should not sound like an exam. Likewise, it is best for the contact not to overwhelm the caller with her own story. However, it is appropriate, and usually quite helpful, to share similar experiences. This type of exchange makes the parent feel understood.

Identifying the Caller's Particular Needs

The first conversation may be a means to identify problems. For instance, if the woman has young children, the contact can discuss how difficult it is to grieve when one also has to care for a toddler who demands constant attention. Or the contact can talk about relating to a confused child who does not understand why his mother is crying or where the baby is. There may be communication problems between the 2 parents that can be discussed. Sometimes if the contact talks about his or her loss, or simply says, "It's okay to grieve for your baby," that is what the caller needs to hear.

To conclude the conversation, the contact should be certain that he or she has the caller's phone number and complete name correctly. The contact should be listening during the conversation to determine what services the support group can provide this caller. He or she may then discuss how further contact with the support group should be made. Sometimes, the caller states that she prefers to initiate any future contact and does not want to be phoned. More often, the caller is relieved to have taken the first step, and she welcomes the offer to have subsequent calls made to her. If the caller wants to talk to someone who experienced a similar pregnancy loss, she should be told that such a volunteer will call her soon. It should not be left to the parent to make this subsequent call. It takes enough courage for her to make the first call to the group's contact; it is unlikely she will make a second call to a stranger.

The group's contact should give all pertinent information about the caller to the designated volunteer. If there seem to be any problem areas, the volunteer should know about them. This type of exchange makes it possible for the volunteer to mention her own feelings on any such topic in a natural way, rather than having to confront the woman with privileged information. When the volunteer speaks with the woman, she should encourage her to telephone at any time and then ask for permission to call again. If the group's next meeting is several weeks away, the volunteer counselor could ask if the woman would like to receive some articles that discuss issues related to her type of pregnancy loss. All phone calls initiated by the woman should be interpreted as an indication of need. The woman might be reluctant to call the volunteer counselor for help even when she is feeling sad. She may call on the pretext of asking the time or date of the next meeting when she really has a need to talk.

Group leaders must try to cultivate a strong, reliable telephone network. Between meetings, the telephone can be a lifeline for grieving parents. This is especially the case when a loss first occurs, because it is a time when parents are feeling confused and isolated and are afraid that their feelings are abnormal. The telephone network makes possible a vital bond between parent and volunteer. The phone conversations that take place in the first weeks allow the volunteer to show his or her sincere concern for the parent, and the parent begins to feel comfortable and able to trust the volunteer with his or her real feelings. The communication that is established through the use of volunteer telephone counseling has a profound effect on parents' ability to experience the normal grieving process.

Not all telephone calls will be from parents whose baby died. Relatives, friends, and even a grieving parent's co-workers may contact the group for advice. They may want to ask what they can do for the bereaved family. Such calls indicate a desire to help grieving parents, and this source of support should be nurtured as much as possible.

When appropriate, it is recommended that the volunteer telephone counselor refer to parents as mothers and fathers, rather than as wives and husbands. Some parents who become involved with the group will not be married. If the baby was a couple's first child, moreover, probably no one but support group members will refer to them as parents, and bereaved parents generally want and appreciate this recognition.

MAINTAINING A HIGH-QUALITY LEVEL OF SERVICES

Once the core group of volunteers is working well together, it is important to maintain that level of quality. It is, however, normal to have staff turnover. There is a natural time when each volunteer will reduce his or her duties and then retire from the group. Some people move out of town and some go on to work in bereavement teams with a church, while others' family priorities change, especially after subsequent babies arrive. Occasionally, after a volunteer has had a successful pregnancy, she finds that she has reached a new level of resolution, and she moves away from her involvement with other newly bereaved parents. This is a natural and healthy pattern.

Preventing Burnout   Group leaders should take care that people do not need to leave the group because of burnout. Due to many demands on emotions and personal time, burnout is particularly common in the case of volunteer work such as a support group. Figures 14.4 and 14.5 show stated reasons for and symptoms of burnout. It is important to recognize the causes and symptoms of burnout and to make an effort to forestall it. All of these symptoms produce feelings of guilt that add to the dilemma.

Group leaders must offer sincere public praise, reinforcement, and appreciation for volunteers' efforts. Grieving people can take but they cannot give. It is important for volunteers to come to terms with the fact that parents usually are unable to express their appreciation for the group's work. Volunteers must

---

I do not know my limitations and try to do too much.

I want to give advice and become upset when it is not taken.

I want recognition for all the work I have done.

I do not feel I have adequate skills or training for my job.

Others place unrealistic expectations on me.

My work is taken for granted by other staff members.

My views or suggestions are not being considered. The group is run by a clique and there is no room for me.

Figure 14.4.   Stated reasons for burnout.

I put off calling parents I know I should be calling.

I miss important meetings.

I am irritable with parents' grieving and their problems.

I do not really listen to parents when they speak.

I wish I were somewhere else instead of at a parents' meeting.

I get used to hearing about the loss of a baby.

Figure 14.5. Symptoms of burnout.

provide each other mutual support. For instance, a volunteer might work very hard on a presentation for a parents' meeting. Parents listen attentively but are quiet during the discussion and do not give feedback to the speaker. Volunteers should remember to thank the speaker later for his or her presentation and for not only being well prepared but for sharing personal experiences with the group as well. After the meeting, parents usually tell their own volunteer counselor how the talk touched them, that it was the first time anyone said what they have been feeling, and that they have thought about the talk often. These comments should be passed on to the speaker. It will reassure him or her that the talk was well received and was helpful. This will also give the speaker confidence to talk on other occasions.

Using Each Volunteer's Special Talents

All volunteers need to be invited to voice their thoughts concerning group matters. Brainstorming yields many new ideas, encourages discussion, and lets everyone know that this input is important, needed, and valued. Each volunteer has some special gift that should be identified. Someone with good business skills is the ideal person to manage correspondence. Another might excel at reviewing new books and articles for the group's library. Someone else with a flair for getting publicity may undertake to make the group known in the community. It is the responsibility of group leaders to look for the talents that each volunteer possesses and to allow them to put their skills to use.

Group leaders themselves are vulnerable to burnout, especially if they are unable to delegate responsibility. Practically speaking, delegating responsibility is a necessity. If a leader cannot assign tasks and rely on volunteers to do things as she herself would do them, then she will be the first one to experience burnout. Sharing responsibilities helps the entire staff, so that no one person carries most of the burden.

Looking for each volunteer's skills and then delegating responsibilities that are compatible with those skills gives shy members the encouragement they need to take on more duties. They should always be aware of the group leaders' support and guidance privately and publicly. If a group leader needs to correct a volunteer, this action should be made in a constructive manner in private. A leader may have tireless energy to give the support group. She may have to learn to appreciate the amount of time that volunteers *do* offer and not to ask for more. Volunteers must feel free to refuse to work with a new caller without having to provide an explanation when a leader asks them to take a call from a newly bereaved parent. For example, some volunteers may decline to take responsibility for a new caller because they do not feel comfortable speaking to unmarried parents or to someone who has had an elective abortion. Volunteers' attitudes and beliefs should be respected as much as are any of the grieving parents' circumstances and feelings.

Finally, group leaders must take time to appreciate the joy that comes in seeing staff members develop into capable leaders. Capable successors eventually will be needed as the group develops over time. There should be a natural evolution in the leadership of the support group.

MEETINGS WITH PARENTS

One of the most rewarding times for support-group volunteers can be at parents' meetings. Meetings are a time when group members can acquaint themselves with parents whom they have met through phone calls. Regular meetings also offer an opportunity for volunteers to see how parents are resolving their grief as time passes. The meeting room should be an emotionally comfortable place where parents do not even have to speak to know that they are being understood. In this room, parents are made to feel normal. Everyone in the room has lost a baby. However, as soon as they leave the meeting, they go back out into a world where their situation is far from universal. In the outside world, it seems that everybody has healthy babies except them.

Informing New Parents What to Expect at Meetings

As volunteers describe meetings to new parents, they should tell them what to expect. If new parents have not been prepared, they might be surprised or offended to hear people make light-hearted comments before or during the meeting. Parents usually worry about what would happen if they cry. Some of them feel very shy about appearing for the first time at a meeting. Quite often, parents confess that they have driven around the block several times before entering the building where the meeting is being held. Anything that volunteers can do to ease parents' apprehensions before a meeting will be helpful. When a volunteer who is expecting a newly bereaved parent will not be able to attend the meeting, she should ask another volunteer to greet and sit with the new member.

Most groups hold their meetings once a month in the evening. An alternative is to have bimonthly meetings—one meeting at night and one during the day—which are even better suited for helping parents get through their first difficult months of grief. Bimonthly meetings make the group more accessible and are particularly recommended if the group does not have enough telephone volunteers available to attend to the needs of all newly bereaved parents between meetings. The number of parents who attend a given meeting does not reflect on the meeting's effectiveness. At the beginning, attendance at meetings is very small. This should not be viewed as failure and group leaders should not feel discouraged. It is easier to lead a small group and then work up to larger attendance as the group's confidence and number of volunteers increase.

Parents who do come, even if few in number, are in need of assistance. Usually, parents who have experienced a stillbirth or neonatal death come to meetings as a couple for several months. The father then may stop attending meetings, and the mother continues to come alone for another 4 or 5 months. In the author's experience, parents who have experienced a miscarriage rarely come together as a couple unless the person who referred them to the group has motivated them by emphasizing the benefit for each parent. Women usually come alone for 3 or 4 months and then return for more support as their due date approaches. Many women, regardless of the type of loss, return when they are pregnant again, and they seek support intermittently until the subsequent baby is born.

EXAMPLE OF A TYPICAL MEETING

Hostesses should arrive early to prepare the meeting room before parents arrive. The library must be set up, refreshments arranged, and chairs moved to form a circle. As parents arrive, they should be greeted by a hostess or, preferably, by the volunteer counselor to whom they have been assigned. They should be welcomed as friends. A hostess can see that parents get a nametag and fill out the sign-in sheet, if the group has one. Nametags should be worn by all volunteers. If time permits, parents should be shown the library. A volunteer can offer suggestions and direct parents' attention to article reprints or books dealing specifically with their type of pregnancy loss. But, no one should hover over parents. Couples usually find that they wish to talk to each other as well as with their volunteer counselor at this point. Women who have come alone often introduce themselves to each other and begin to talk as they look over the literature available.

Group members may indicate that it is time to begin the meeting by moving toward the circle of chairs and sitting down. Others will follow. Sitting with new parents gives them added reassurance and comfort. Often, parents come at the last minute or are late, so a volunteer should be seated near the door to greet them. This arrangement downplays parents' embarrassment and lessens the disruption. Try to start on time. The group leader for the evening should begin by doing the following:

Introduce her or himself;

Welcome everyone;

Mention the location of restrooms;

Inform parents when and where the next meeting will be held;

State the topic of the next meeting and the speaker's name.

The group leader should explain the group's ground rules (for example, that no one is obliged to speak). If there are any announcements to make or other business matters to be addressed, they should be mentioned at this time.

Either the speaker or someone else can introduce the topic and the speaker for the evening's meeting. If one of the group's volunteers is speaking, the talk might be expected to last from 10–15 minutes. If a panel discussion is presented, the time will be longer. If a talk is given by an invited speaker, he or she usually will want more time, and time for questions and answers should be included.

Dividing into Smaller Groups

If the evening's program is short and a large number of people are present, the entire group might divide into smaller groups of 8 to 10 to facilitate discussion. A useful way to divide the group is by type of pregnancy loss. If possible, a volunteer who has experienced a particular type of loss should act as that group's leader. As need arises, there may also be another group for those who are pregnant, with pregnant volunteers or volunteers who have had successful pregnancies subsequent to their own pregnancy loss as leaders. These women will be focusing on the future, but still need support because the last pregnancy ended unsuccessfully—otherwise, they would not attend meetings.

If those in attendance do split into smaller groups, each group will break up at different times. There should be time left for the entire group to socialize following the structured part of the meeting. Refreshments can be offered at this point or they can be available throughout the meeting so that parents and counselors may take them as desired. Refreshments should be simple and easy for parents to carry and eat. There will be a natural drifting away after people have socialized for some short period. The volunteers can collect the group's things and straighten up the room while some parents still remain talking with each other or with volunteers.

ORGANIZATIONAL GUIDELINES

Organization is essential to keep things running smoothly. But it is not advisable to become so organized and regimented that the group's functioning becomes sterile. Flexibility is a key ingredient because the group exists for parents and parents' needs change. The need for a constitution might not be obvious until the volunteer staff has increased to a point where it no longer is possible to function without one. Then, a constitution can be an effective mechanism by which the support group can state its purpose and the roles of the staff.

Funding

Although funds may not be a concern at first, some income is necessary. Group expenses are incurred for printing of pamphlets, purchasing books, funding volunteers' fees for seminars, and providing refreshments. In order to cover these expenses, members may want to seek donations. It may be helpful to achieve tax-exempt status because it stimulates donations from corporations. Group members need to consider organizing a fundraiser. Smaller donations come occasionally from grateful parents who have benefited from the group's work. Another small source of income can come from asking volunteers and parents attending the meetings for a dollar or two to go toward the expenses of photocopying articles and buying books.

Staff meetings, apart from the monthly or bimonthly parents' meetings, are extremely important. They provide all volunteers an opportunity to give their input about the program and the format that should be used at parents' meetings. When staff members are unable to attend a meeting, it is useful to send a copy of the unapproved minutes to them soon after the meeting so that everyone is equally informed. Other than addressing business topics that affect the support group (see Figure 14.6), members can broaden the group's activities by offering educational services to meet the needs of the community. Volunteers can go out as speakers, and printed materials may be provided by the group to hospitals or churches. Some of these services can earn Continuing Education Units for professionals who are involved with the group or who attend these in-service meetings.

Going directly into hospitals can effect changes in the way parents are cared for before, during, and after the loss of a baby.

1. Review and evaluate the effectiveness of the last parents' meeting.
2. Plan the next parents' meeting. It is appropriate to plan several months ahead, especially if guest speakers are needed. Some groups have a rotating schedule of set topics, while others like to mix new topics with ones used before.
3. Set or reevaluate goals for the support group. Members should seek to deepen the group's referral lists. This would include making the group known to the entire community as well as to specific people who provide care for bereaved parents.
4. Duties should be assigned by the staff. There is a natural tendency to allow more experienced volunteers to take on the visible roles, such as speaking at parents' meetings. Newer staff members should be encouraged to speak up and ask for these assignments. When a group leader judges that a newcomer would be the appropriate choice for a job, she might ask that person directly for help. This shows confidence in the staff, encourages everyone to participate more, lightens the load for everyone, and gives each volunteer the feeling that she or he is valued and needed.
5. Professionals should be invited to speak to volunteers on subjects related to the group, to review national support group movies, or to discuss new books or articles that have been added to the library.

Figure 14.6. Sample of business that might be covered at a staff meeting.

Many policy changes have occurred because of support-group volunteers who have visited hospitals to educate staff about what is helpful, what options are available, and what a positive difference their care can make.

CONCLUSION

The well-established support group is able in many ways to help parents who have experienced a pregnancy loss. The group's support and comfort can help them directly by offering meetings, telephone contact, information, and other resources. Healthcare providers can benefit greatly from the educational influence that support-group members can offer, which indirectly helps parents more than they often realize. As more support groups reach hospitals and professionals who encounter patients with pregnancy losses, the services offered families will be improved and refined. The work to be accomplished by the support group is limited only by the imagination of its dedicated volunteers.

SUGGESTED RESOURCES

Reading for Support-Group Leaders

Berezin N: *After a Loss in Pregnancy—Help for Families Affected by a Miscar-*

riage, a Stillbirth, or the Loss of a Newborn. New York, Simon & Schuster, 1982.

Borg S and Lasker J: *When Pregnancy Fails—Families Coping with Miscarriage, Stillbirth, and Infant Death.* Boston, Beacon Press, 1981.

Church MJ, Chazin H, Ewald F: *When a Baby Dies.* Oak Brook, IL, The Compassionate Friends, Inc., 1981.

Fischhoff J and Brohl NO: *Before and After My Child Died—A Collection of Parents' Experiences.* Detroit, Emmons-Fairfield Publishing Co., 1981.

Friedman R and Gradstein B: *Surviving Pregnancy Loss.* Boston, Little, Brown & Company, 1982.

Ilse S and Burns LH: *Miscarriage—A Shattered Dream.* Long Lake, MN, Wintergreen Press, 1985.

Johnson J, Johnson M, Cunningham J, Ewing S, Hatcher D, Dannen C: *Newborn Death.* Omaha, Centering Corporation, 1982.

Kübler-Ross E: *Death: The Final Stage of Growth.* Englewood Cliffs, NJ, Prentice-Hall, Inc., 1975.

Kushner HS: *When Bad Things Happen to Good People.* New York, Avon Books, 1983.

Peppers LG and Knapp RJ: *Motherhood and Mourning—Perinatal Death.* Philadelphia, Praeger Publishers, 1980.

_____: *How To Go On Living after the Death of a Baby.* Atlanta, Peachtree Publishers Ltd., 1985.

Schiff HS: *The Bereaved Parent.* New York, Penguin Books, 1977.

Schweibert P and Kirk P: *When Hello Means Goodbye.* Portland, OR, University of Oregon Health Sciences Center, 1981.

Resources for Information (Audiovisual Programs, Workshops, and so on)

1. Centering Corporation
   Box 3367
   Omaha, NE 68103–0367
   (402) 553–1200
   Booklets, books, workshops, videotapes (for example, "To Touch Today").

2. Pregnancy and Infant Loss Center
   1415 E. Wayzata Boulevard, Suite 22
   Wayzata, MN 55391

3. The Compassionate Friends
   National Headquarters
   P.O. Box 1347
   Oak Brook, IL 60521
   (312) 323–5010

Training Materials for Volunteer Counselors

Cordell AS and Apolito R: Family support in infant death. *JOGNN* 281–285, July/Aug 1981.

Crout TK: Caring for the mother of a stillborn baby. *Nursing 80* 70–73, April 1980.

Davidson CS and Goldenberg R: Report on counseling elicited by symposiums on fetal death. *Contemp Obstet Gynecol* 13:13–23, Mar, 1979.

Horowitz NH: Adolescent mourning reactions to infant and fetal loss. *Social Casework* 551–559, Nov 1978.

Jiménez SLM: Grief counseling: when doctors are too distant and relatives too distraught, educators can help grieving parents. *Childbirth Educator* 42–47, Fall 1978.

Kennell JH, Slyter H, Klaus M: The mourning response of parents to the death of a newborn infant. *New Eng J Med* 283:334–349, 1970.

Knapp RJ and Peppers LG: Doctor-patient relationships in fetal/infant death encounters. *J Med Educ* 54:776–780, 1979.

Kowalski K and Osborn MR: Helping mothers of stillborn infants to grieve. *Matern Child Nurs J* 29–32, Jan/Feb 1977.

Kushner L: Infant death and the childbirth educator. *Matern Child Nurs J* (4):231–233, 1979.

Lewis E: Mourning by the family after a stillbirth or neonatal death. *Arch Dis Child* 54:303–306, 1979.

_____: The management of stillbirth: Coping with an unreality. *Lancet* 2 619–620, 1976.

Quirk TR, O'Donohue N, Middleton J: The perinatal bereavement crisis. *J Nurse-Midwife* 24(5):13–21, 1979.

Sahu S: Coping with perinatal death. *J Reprod Med* 26(3):129–132, 1981.

Stringham JG, Riley JH, Ross A: Silent birth: mourning a stillborn baby. *Social Work* 322–327, July 1982.

Wilson AL and Soule DJ: The role of a self-help group in working with parents of a stillborn baby. *Death Educ* 5:175–186, 1981.

Wooten B: Death of an infant. *Matern Child Nurs J* 6:257–260, 1981.

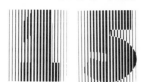

Impact of Pregnancy Loss on Subsequent Pregnancy

JANET KIRKSEY, R.N.

The issues surrounding pregnancy loss are manifold. One area that must be addressed separately is that of subsequent pregnancies and the particular needs of expectant parents who previously experienced a pregnancy loss. This chapter presents many of the issues that parents attempting a subsequent pregnancy confront.

ATTEMPTING A NEW PREGNANCY

The decision to become pregnant again following a pregnancy loss is an extremely difficult one. Most couples want to have another baby. In fact, they might be talking about another pregnancy and asking questions about it even while the woman is still hospitalized following her pregnancy loss. One or both of them may be very impatient to start another pregnancy. However, there also is a strong fear that makes the couple ambivalent toward trying again. Fears of another failure and another death make the decision agonizing. Even when both parents are eager to try again, the conflict remains. One day, the woman may be determined to become pregnant as soon as possible, and the next day, she may be terrified at the thought of going through another pregnancy. When couples do decide to try again, they often find the wait unbearable. It is a relief when they finally have confirmed the new pregnancy. Then, there is no turning back.

On the average, physicians recommend that, following a pregnancy loss, another pregnancy not be attempted for 2 to 4

When?

menstrual cycles. However, it is difficult to find sound medical information that substantiates this recommendation. Very often, couples feel that this suggestion is offered on an arbitrary basis. Perhaps some medical "reasons" for postponing the attempt to conceive again should be explained to the couple. When no information is provided, the dilemma the couple faces is additionally burdensome in a period of their lives that already is very stressful. Parents want to try to have another baby; but their doctor has advised them to wait, without telling them why they should wait for a given amount of time. If the couple proceeds to attempt a new pregnancy anyway, their fears and guilt, if this new pregnancy fails too, may be aggravated.

It is very helpful, then, for the physician to discuss the rationale for postponing conception with the patient. Waiting at least 2 to 4 months generally allows a sufficient interval for return of normal menstruation. The emotional impact of grief is more unpredictable and varies from person to person. It should be mentioned to patients that a pregnancy conceived 3 months after a pregnancy loss means that the expected date of confinement for the current pregnancy will be close to the first anniversary of the previous loss. The anniversary date can be a very anxious and difficult time for people.

For the woman who miscarries, an emotional readiness may appear after 2 to 3 periods. This may also coincide with a physical readiness. Conception immediately after the loss may carry a higher risk for recurrent miscarriage, due to an inadequate luteal phase (1). The first menstrual period usually starts between 30 and 35 days after an early pregnancy loss (1–4). For pregnancy losses later in gestation, the first period is less predictable and may occur anywhere from 4 to 8 weeks postpartum.

Couples should be advised to use contraception when they resume intercourse (usually after the postpartum bleeding stops) because some women may ovulate prior to their first period. Foam and condoms or a diaphragm are recommended if the couple plans to try to conceive after only 2 or 3 periods. Oral contraceptives or an intrauterine device are not recommended methods of short-term contraception.

During the months that a couple is using contraception, it is also helpful if the woman establishes her ovulatory pattern. The most accurate means of doing this is to record her daily basal body temperature (BBT) in an effort to properly time conception. Some physicians feel that fertilization involving aged gametes increases the likelihood of spontaneous abortion (5, 6).

Attempting another pregnancy is often an anxious time for both partners. Life becomes centered on the woman's menstrual cycle and a vigil for the physical indications of pregnancy. If the ovulation chart dictates when intercourse must occur, the spontaneity of a couple's sexual relationship may be diminished or lost. Performance anxiety, impotence, or decreased libido may be a problem. The fear of not becoming pregnant is offset by the fear of becoming pregnant. If a menstrual period comes, it is both a disappointment and a relief.

ISSUES

Choices in Healthcare

Changing Physicians

For couples facing a new pregnancy after a pregnancy loss, a primary decision that they should make is whether or not to continue with the healthcare professionals whom the woman saw in her previous pregnancy. Although most couples do not complain about the medical care that the woman received previously, some do question if the woman received the best care available. The couple should review events leading up to the loss and think about the care provider's course of action. Patients may switch to a new obstetrician even if they are not overtly critical of the former one's care. They may be suspicious of care that the former physician provided. They are apt to have learned a great deal about pregnancy by this point, and they may "shop" for better medical care by calling the Academy of Medicine or other medical associations or by asking for advice about physicians from nurses, other care providers, and friends.

Unresolved Anger

There are 2 other reasons why parents may choose to see another physician. The first reason is that they do not want to repeat the same routine with the same medical team. Some parents state that they would feel uncomfortable seeing the same care providers and delivering at the same hospital because it would remind them of a painful episode in their lives. Caring physicians and their staff, therefore, should not be offended if a woman does switch to another medical group. It is one means of a couple's assimilating what has happened to them and moving on with another pregnancy. The second reason that women choose different healthcare providers is because of unresolved anger. Anger may be directed at the physician and/ or staff for insensitive treatment at the time of the baby's death and thereafter. Frequently, women complain that their physicians seemed uncomfortable during a follow-up visit and that they felt rushed. They feel that they are not given enough time during the office visit to talk about their experience, nor are they encouraged to ask questions about prenatal care or the baby's delivery (see Chapter 5). This cursory behavior, often stemming from the physician's personal insecurity in the face of a professional failure, is interpreted as insensitivity and is a common reason why women switch to another physician after a pregnancy loss. Parents need to feel that their physician understands how the loss impacted on their lives. Special effort should be made to ensure that the physician and the rest of the staff are aware of a patient's poor obstetric history. An uninformed nurse who sees, for example, the notation $G_2 P_1$ on a woman's chart might ask her the age of her first child. This is an awkward question for the woman, one which is asked frequently. In the obstetrician's office where the woman receives prenatal care during her subsequent pregnancy, the staff should attempt to be sensitive to the patient's needs.

PATIENT'S INTEGRATION OF HER PREVIOUS PREGNANCY EXPERIENCE

Patients Need Information

Women want to be told, sometimes several times, details about their birth experience. This is true when the outcome has been successful. It is more of a necessity when the outcome has been unsuccessful. Seeking information about the pregnancy loss helps women integrate this critical experience into their lives. Men who were present at the delivery frequently have to answer their partners' seemingly endless questions about the sequence of events during labor and delivery. Women must depend on these observations most heavily when they have received sedation that renders them incapable of remembering the experience clearly themselves. Even the most sympathetic man may lose his patience when his partner wants to know more than he himself can relate to her. Such questioning indicates the strong need the woman has to fix into her consciousness a traumatic event that was overwhelming when it occurred.

Internalization

The process of internalizing the previous pregnancy loss may or may not be completed before another pregnancy is under way. Indeed, it is likely that a subsequent pregnancy provides an appropriate means for a woman to examine her past pregnancy experience. The anxiety that she will never again be able to conceive—a fear common among women after a pregnancy loss—is now irrelevant. The new pregnancy serves as a positive goal and to some extent detaches the woman from her previous loss, so that she may begin to consider it with some objectivity. She now can focus her attention on the general issue of childbearing and its meaning in her life. Usually, she will spend time reading books about pregnancy, where she can find sections that discuss problems of concern. Looking forward to the delivery of this baby, she imagines how different this experience will be—a safe, vaginal delivery; the baby will be alive; she will hold her baby; and she will cry with joy and grief. Although the actual birth probably will be quite different from what she expects, those daydreams have a significant healing effect on the woman recovering emotionally from her previous loss.

Ambivalence toward the New Pregnancy

When a new pregnancy is confirmed, it is not always a happy occasion. Often, women fear that they have made the wrong decision or that they have become pregnant too soon. During this period, they need reassurance that the ambivalence they are experiencing is common, even for women who have not suffered a bad pregnancy outcome previously. These feelings will not impact physically on this pregnancy.

Protecting Herself   For many couples, the first trimester stirs up emotions and unresolved issues regarding the previous pregnancy. Many families say that the father and other family members see a future, while the mother sees her past. During this time, women also report a feeling of detachment, which they claim they prefer to feel toward the new baby. They want to shield themselves from getting hurt, should anything go wrong. As outsiders' and the woman's own attention to the new pregnancy increases, so does her sense of guilt. She has a feeling of betrayal to her previous baby. This occurs more intensely for those women who carried their babies closer to term or who experienced neonatal death. Families who have had therapeutic abortions for genetic reasons also report these feelings.

"HIGH-TECH" PREGNANCY: DOING EVERYTHING RIGHT THIS TIME

Prenatal Diagnosis   When the previous pregnancy has concluded disastrously, a couple's anxiety and fears, both founded and unfounded, might be greater than normal. Issues regarding perinatal diagnostic testing need to be discussed. Pertinent information and the rationales in support of or against a patient's having amniocentesis or sonograms performed need to be explored. Many parents during a subsequent pregnancy opt for more testing than is probably necessary. The tests eliminate some of their anxiety. Indeed, maternal anxiety is a valid factor to be considered in determining what testing will be done, even when the previous pregnancy would not have had a better outcome if a particular test had been carried out. Of course, the risks of the test may be greater than the benefit of the information to be ascertained by it (7). Pros and cons should be weighed by the couple and the physician in a thorough discussion of this issue. However, for many couples, the information provided by these tests gives great comfort. For others, placing themselves in a situation where they might have to make the decision whether or not to continue the pregnancy is too great a risk in itself.

Each couple contemplating amniocentesis needs to be assessed thoroughly. The anticipated psychologic benefit of amniocentesis should be weighed as a factor in the decision to perform this procedure much as are clinical ones such as maternal age or a family history of chromosomal anomaly. Sonograms help parents because they establish unequivocally that the new baby is really "there" and alive, dispelling denial of the new pregnancy. Having parents view their baby in utero promotes bonding, which is especially critical for those who have suffered a previous pregnancy loss.

If the previous pregnancy was twin or triplet, many mothers fantasize that the new pregnancy too will be a multiple gestation. Seeing a single fetus during a sonogram confirms, vividly, that this is not a continuation of the previous pregnancy. Parents realize intellectually that the new baby is not a replacement for the one lost. However, they may have expectations that a new baby will take away much of the pain they have been feeling. When the loss involves a multiple gestation, this issue is more difficult to resolve. A multiple gestation is a unique situation that may never again be duplicated by this couple. This represents a loss in itself.

Extreme Responses   In some cases, a woman who is pregnant again following a pregnancy loss may have a more extreme response to pregnancy and her own prenatal care. A woman with a strong need to deny the pregnancy may take very poor care of herself, smoking cigarettes, using drugs, and consuming excessive alcohol, or neglecting her diet and her vitamin supplements. This behavior may stem from the attitude that, "I did everything right last time, and look how little good it did." More commonly, a woman will be very concerned to do everything "perfectly." As a consequence, her obstetrician may receive many more phone calls from her and may need to answer more questions for her than for his or her other pregnant patients.

STRESSES DURING THE SUBSEQUENT PREGNANCY

Resolving Old Fears   Regardless of how many assurances are offered a pregnant woman during her subsequent pregnancy, most women report that they cannot start thinking about the baby until they pass the point where the previous loss occurred. If an intrapartum

**The Need for
Emotional Support**

death occurred, obviously the period of heightened anxiety extends through delivery.

During the late second and the third trimesters, as the pregnancy continues without complication, women report that they receive less and less support. This is probably because most people, nonprofessional and professional, view the new pregnancy as resolution to the grief period precipitated by the other baby's death. Seeking out someone who will listen attentively to their concerns becomes very important to women at this time. This is a period when the woman once again needs to talk about her previous birth experience. Doing so seems to help her to regard the previous and current pregnancies as distinct, nonintersecting events. This is more likely to be the case for the patient whose next pregnancy occurs soon after her loss. It can be a very frightening and confusing time if the woman is not helped by care providers to understand the dynamics by which each pregnancy impacts on the other.

The current pregnancy tends to diminish sympathy about and interest in her previous experience from the woman's family and friends. This issue, therefore, is one to which her healthcare providers need pay particular attention. During routine prenatal appointments in the second or third trimester, it is very important for her obstetrician or nurse to ask the woman if she has someone with whom to talk about her previous pregnancy outcome and her fears about this pregnancy. This will offer the woman an opportunity to talk about her anxious feelings at a time in her pregnancy when she may feel quite alone.

**Value of Support
Groups**

If the woman has no other outlet, the concerned professional may arrange for her to talk informally with a former patient who has undergone experiences similar to her own, or he or she may advise the woman about support groups that are available in the community. Peer support groups established for parents grieving for a pregnancy loss are frequently an excellent source of support for parents in a subsequent pregnancy. The care provider should advise the woman to call the contact person of such a group in order to learn what means of support are available in this particular set of circumstances. The group may hold special meetings for pregnant women and their partners, or they may welcome a pregnant woman at a general meeting. A volunteer for the support group can become a telephone contact for the woman going through this difficult phase of her pregnancy. (The reader is referred to Chapters 5, 10, 11, and 14 for further discussion of care that professionals and peer support groups may offer to this group of pregnant patients.)

ANGER

Late in pregnancy, new forms of anger may surface. Usually, this anger is directed at issues or events over which women have no control, such as the lack of innocence regarding potential outcomes of a given pregnancy. Once a woman has suffered a pregnancy loss, she may begin to hear of and read about other tragic outcomes that are possible. Her anxiety can become generalized—it is unlikely that the same tragedy will happen again, but there is always the possibility that something different will go wrong this next time. There also can be anger at the wearisome stress of pregnancy itself. It may seem unfair to a woman that she has to go through this process again and have only 1 baby when by this time she should have had 2.

Sense of Failure

Feelings of anger (and jealousy) may be directed at relatives', friends', and even at strangers' apparent ease in attaining successful pregnancies. This anger may mask failure as a woman, a sense of being incapable of fulfilling a basic biologic function. This fear of failure in a subsequent pregnancy is very real. For this woman, another failure would confirm her suspicion that she cannot achieve that which every other woman can achieve effortlessly.

Other Sources of Anger

A woman may feel angry that others around her do not appreciate their good fortune. She may even voice strong disapproval at the way relatives and friends treat their own children, thinking, "If she had been through what I have been through, she would never do that to her baby." If the woman actually does reprove other parents' behavior, this could strain important relationships, undermining the support network that she needs during her pregnancy. If she says nothing, she may feel increasing anger at others, which is detrimental not only to those relationships but also to her own state of mind.

Sources of Anxiety

Another source of anger concerns the nature of presumably well-intentioned comments that parents receive as the subsequent pregnancy progresses and nears its conclusion (see Figure 15.1). These statements often imply that it is wrong for the couple to cherish their dead baby's memory or even to mention the baby's name. Couples can be offended by phrases such as "your new baby," which they may interpret to mean that the "old" baby is of no value and can be replaced, much in the same way one purchases a new vacuum cleaner or a pair of eyeglasses. Couples who can share between themselves the frustration and pain that such remarks can cause may be sufficiently supportive of each other to fend off these remarks. If the man is inured to such comments and does not share his partner's sensitivity to them, then the woman needs to find some arena in which she can express her feelings. A peer support

> "You should be over your other baby's death."
>
> "You ought to forget about that other baby."
>
> "Now, you'll really have a baby [you didn't last time]."
>
> "This baby will make you forget all about the other one."
>
> "This baby will replace your other one."
>
> "You shouldn't ever tell your new baby about the other one."
>
> "This baby is *really* going to be special."

Figure 15.1. Examples of inappropriate remarks to parents during a subsequent pregnancy.

group network is an invaluable place for women to share experiences and perhaps to prepare themselves to respond to thoughtless, insensitive, or misguided remarks.

Even normal bodily changes consistent with a healthy pregnancy may fail to evoke joy. Casual remarks made by a care provider or friend such as, "You're gaining faster this time," or "You look smaller this time," can engender needless concern. Innocent statements may be interpreted by the expectant woman to mean that there is a grave problem. Her heightened sensitivity during this period needs to be recognized by care providers.

STRESS ON THE MARITAL RELATIONSHIP

Differing Responses of Men and Women

A baby's death can have an irrevocable effect on the parents' marriage. The death of a child is unnatural, violating the order of nature. No other type of death has equal impact on the married couple. When a spouse loses a parent or sibling or friend, he or she will grieve more intensely than his or her spouse, for whom the death is to some extent indirect. When a spouse dies, the survivor grieves alone. Only when their offspring dies does a couple experience analogous grief. Yet, it is impossible for each to grieve in exactly the same way. Because they are married and because they are grieving for their child, couples may expect to share their grief. Most couples soon realize, as they fail to synchronize their responses to the death, that no 2 people can grieve alike. This realization may run counter to their basic concepts of marital commitment. The frustration that results can lead to long-lasting resentment, anger, and discord (8).

An additional source of conflict between parents is that the woman's need to talk about her pregnancy loss and events surrounding the baby's death frequently is greater than her partner's. Men often want to put the previous experience behind them and look to the future sooner than women do. During these periods of conflict, support groups can offer an important resource for a woman to turn to, relieving some of the pressure that can build up for both partners.

Sexual Relationship

A subsequent pregnancy often dovetails with the grief process precipitated by the other baby's death. The new pregnancy and its continuation may place a great stress on a marital relationship. Bad marriages can get worse, and the best of marriages suffer some strain. Women admit that pregnancy consumes their thoughts, and often their attitude is very pessimistic. Men, on the other hand, typically continue their work and routines, and they expect a good outcome. A man's anxiety level is usually substantially lower than a woman's. When the focus of the woman's attention is on her pregnancy and not on the marital relationship, she may not feel comfortable having sexual relations. Sexual intercourse may have been linked unconsciously with the previous pregnancy's outcome. To engage in sexual intercourse in this pregnancy may create great fear for this baby. Unfortunately, the man may perceive this response by his partner as rejection or even as punishment. Unresolved misunderstandings about sexual activity during pregnancy can cause long-term anger and a permanent change in a couple's relationship.

BEING GOOD PARENTS TO OTHER CHILDREN IN THE FAMILY

Response of Siblings

If there are older children in the family, demands are placed on parents who, on the one hand, may still be grieving for their dead baby and, on the other hand, are endeavoring to cope with a subsequent pregnancy that inevitably is stressful. For many parents, it may seem that the burdens placed on them at this time are more than they can endure. Their marriage and their family have suffered an overwhelming blow with their baby's death. Surviving siblings are struggling with their own emotional pain and guilt concerning the lost brother or sister (see Chapter 1, "Pregnancy Loss and the Grief Process" and Chapter 8, "Social Worker: Hospital Advocate for the Immediate and Extended Family"). With the additional impact of a subsequent pregnancy, the strain on all family members may be enormous. At a time when parents' inner resources seem to be utterly depleted, parents find that they have to offer much more support and understanding to their surviving children. Perhaps recognizing the crisis that they are undergoing can help keep the family united and communicating with each other. With very young children, though, parents have the responsibility to sustain their children's sense of security and of being important in the family. Older children demand an increased level of interaction that can exact its own toll because they comprehend more and require more explanation and emotional comfort.

Involving Children in the New Pregnancy

Deciding how to discuss the subsequent pregnancy with surviving children is paramount. Based on their children's level of understanding, parents should explain as much as they feel comfortable with and as much as they determine their children need to know. For example, there is always a period of extreme anxiety while a couple with a history of a baby with a genetic abnormality awaits amniocentesis results regarding the subsequent pregnancy. They may choose not to discuss the current pregnancy or the possible decision to seek a therapeutic abortion with their other children. Individual needs in each family's case dictate the extent of involvement that parents will want their children to have in the subsequent pregnancy. If the outcome is expected to be successful, parents should make an effort to give their children a sense of optimistic anticipation about the forthcoming baby. A reasonable goal is for the family, parents and children alike, to recapture as much as possible any normal, joyful feelings that accompanied the previous pregnancy.

UNREALISTIC EXPECTATIONS

"Perfect" Parents

Expectations that parents place on themselves after a fetal or neonatal death are often unrealistic. This occurs because of the "bargaining" that takes place (9). It is common for a woman to think and even say, "If I get pregnant again, I'll never complain about anything, even morning sickness," or "If I can have this baby, I'll be the *best* parent in the world." Then, with the subsequent pregnancy and with the healthy baby's birth, parents find that they cannot always live up to the unrealistic "bargain" they have made, and they may feel guilty for "failing." Parents need to set more realistic goals for themselves. Because a baby dies and another one is born does not mean parents are marked for life and will be judged differently if they complain of the burdens or minor irritations regarding pregnancy or of the major changes brought about with the baby's arrival.

The death of one's baby is often a profound although deeply painful experience. Parents who have undergone this misfortune do not necessarily gain a special set of qualities that make them "better" parents than couples who have not experienced such a loss. But, it often happens that parents who have suffered the death of their baby approach any surviving and any subsequent children with enhanced appreciation, patience, and sensitivity. All of these traits can have a strengthening effect on the family's life together. Even if parents do come to feel that this is true, they almost always also protest that they did not have to lose a baby to learn that lesson.

ALLEVIATING STRESS VIA PROFESSIONAL INTERVENTIONS

Need for Continued Support

During the third trimester of a pregnancy following a previous loss, a meeting not related to routine prenatal care should be arranged between expectant parents and obstetrician. At this meeting, continuing management of the pregnancy should be defined. Parents may wish to describe hypothetical situations and events that are a source of anxiety, in order to explore the obstetrician's and their own attitudes and expectations regarding them. They might want to know how the hospital would manage various situations medically. Prematurity and postmaturity management are typical examples of issues that parents want to discuss at this time. The necessity of or desire for nonstress testing and other measures of fetal wellbeing are also appropriate subjects. For parents, this process marks a new level of resolution to the pregnancy loss, and it demonstrates an acceptance of the current pregnancy. But parents' reluctance to "bother the doctor" may mean that someone else has to initiate such a discussion.

An interview with the pediatrician is of equal value. Many families want their own pediatrician present at delivery of their baby. This is not always possible or necessary, particularly in a teaching hospital with pediatricians in attendance. An agreement regarding this issue needs to be reached before the advent of the baby's delivery. Questions of a hypothetical nature posed to the pediatrician may concern management of a baby of questionable viability. Attitudes about aggressively treating premature infants or infants with anomalies may be explored, with the mutual understanding that no decisions have been made if problems discussed do arise.

Both parties—the family and their physicians—must feel comfortable with each other's attitudes to ensure that the pregnant patient and her baby receive satisfactory medical care. Other resources to which parents may turn for additional information are the obstetric and the pediatric nurse and the support group, where couples who have gone on to have subsequent babies can provide information that may be helpful.

Sympathetic attitudes from relatives, friends, or members of the church community can be very beneficial to the couple but may not be consistently present. Relatives and friends may have little awareness of how stressful the subsequent pregnancy can be. The physician, nurse, social worker, or family's clergy might be the couple's only source of compassion and support during this difficult episode in the family's life.

ISSUES SURROUNDING THE BIRTH OF THE NEXT BABY

Bonding during Pregnancy and after Birth

Holding Back

Bonding during the subsequent pregnancy can be a difficult process for the woman. Her ambivalence toward the current pregnancy can affect a woman's bonding with her baby. Feelings stirred up by her previous pregnancy experience can make a woman want to shield herself from the possibility of feeling that much pain a second time. She may simply express this need, saying that she is holding back her love "in case something happens again." Despite these precautions, most women know intuitively that to lose another baby would be just as painful as it was the first time. Fathers and the couple's own parents, as well as other relatives and friends, feel this conflict also, although usually it is to a lesser extent.

Putting off the Nursery

One manifestation of this attitude is that of being "consciously unready." Many couples will delay purchasing clothes or a crib for the baby. Within their home, they may even have purposely not defined a room or part of a room for their baby "just in case. . . ." By ignoring material aspects of the anticipated birth, these couples attempt to shield themselves emotionally from the commitment to and fear of the loss of this baby. At some point in the subsequent pregnancy, nearly every woman says, "When I can hold this baby in my arms, then I'll worry about the nursery." No one who has had to dismantle the nursery following a baby's death is eager to set herself up again for that contingency. It is a very natural and common conflict for women pregnant again after a pregnancy loss to put off preparing the baby's nursery.

Belief that things might work out successfully this time overtakes women at different points in their subsequent pregnancies. For some, the desire to prepare the baby's room is strong in spite of the previous loss, although others may never have stored away the items in the dead baby's room; so the nursery is ready long before the due date and stands as a symbol of hope. Some women begin gingerly to "feather the nest" once they have safely passed the point at which the baby died in the previous pregnancy. And there are women who simply will not set up a nursery, refusing relatives' or friends' offers to throw a shower for them, until this new, healthy baby is safely delivered and even already at home. As a rule, women want very much to prepare the baby's nursery and they delay doing it only to protect themselves.

Delivery

Where?

The milieu of this subsequent delivery usually is an issue for consideration, especially for the woman. If her previous delivery occurred at home or in an alternative birth center, she may choose the more imposing environment of a sophisticated hospital. Conversely, if the previous delivery was "high tech," she may seek out surroundings that are more natural or home-like. Options available to her depend largely on the practices of the professionals to whom she turns for her prenatal care. The woman may find that she would have to switch to another healthcare group if she wants services not offered by her own care provider. Within the range of choices open to her, the woman's requests should be considered seriously, as long as she is healthy and there is no reason to doubt the health of the baby. Information to support or deny her wishes regarding the delivery should be presented forthrightly.

Joy and Grief at the Birth

Care providers notice sometimes after they deliver a much-desired, healthy baby that parents seem detached and remote from their baby for a time after delivery. There is a lag period before some couples can express joy at the birth of their baby. This occurs because parents cannot believe that they have obtained their goal, the birth of a healthy baby. Also, with this new life, realization of the magnitude of their previous loss becomes striking. In fact, some parents may grieve more for their other baby as they bond after birth with their subsequent one. This transition phase can cause great sadness. Many women fear that, once they have this new infant, no one will remember the dead baby. Eventually, they find that they do not have to forget the past in order to enjoy the present—and the future. The past becomes less painful as time goes on, and with the new baby new memories are generated.

For many couples, the birth of their healthy baby symbolizes attainment of a long-sought goal and opens a new chapter in their lives. For some, however, the previous pregnancy loss is an ongoing menace that the healthy newborn's existence fails to eradicate. The previous baby's death can lend a prophetic aura to the family's sense of anxiety over their new baby. During delivery, common obstetric events may support the couple's fear that this baby will not survive either. A cesarean section becomes a failed vaginal birth. An abnormal fetal heart rate pattern during labor, even if it is of no clinical significance, evidences impending death or compromises the baby's chances for a full and healthy life. When the newborn in the hospital's nursery exhibits an elevated serum bilirubin level or a low blood glucose level, the parents' unspoken conviction is that their greatest fear is going to be realized again.

Feelings of Continued Failure

In these responses, the common emotion is that of repeated personal failure that is not eliminated by the birth process alone. Particularly when there is a less than "perfect" birth experience, as with a midforceps delivery or an unanticipated cesarean section, delivery is not a healing experience such as parents may have imagined. It is hard to accept the reality that each pregnancy is a discrete event with its own circumstances and outcome. It is difficult for parents not to compare deliveries and contrast the events surrounding each. Care providers sensitive to these attitudes in the early postpartum period may say, "Some couples still worry, even after their healthy baby has been delivered, that something terrible will occur. Do you have any of these feelings yourself?" In the authors' experience, such fears recede in the early weeks after delivery as the couple bonds with their baby. For parents who have had a baby die, there may always remain an air of vulnerability that makes them more nervous, more protective, or more easily alarmed about their healthy children than they might otherwise be. Clearly, pregnancy loss is a continuum, the assimilation of which is unique for each couple and each set of circumstances.

Next Baby's Sex

No parent wishes for anything other than a healthy baby. There are, naturally, preferences at different times for a girl or for a boy. Almost universally, when the healthy newborn has arrived, even when one or both parents would acknowledge that they are somewhat disappointed with the baby's sex, everyone adjusts readily. Those who previously have suffered a loss, however, may learn that the sex of the next baby stirs up unresolved issues. Many parents hope that the subsequent baby will be of the other sex, so that they will not fuse the identities of the 2 babies. Others actually would prefer an infant of the same sex as the previous baby, particularly if they did want a baby of that sex very strongly during the last pregnancy. There does not seem to be a way of predicting this desire. It can, however, make parents, especially women, feel guilty when the baby is not of the hoped-for sex.

PREGNANCY LOSS AND THE COUPLE WITH INFERTILITY PROBLEMS

Loss of a "Premium" Pregnancy

In a sense, almost any pregnancy is "precious." Even when there has been great ambivalence at the beginning of pregnancy, families usually have made accommodations—both physically and psychologically—so that the baby is welcomed and loved by the time of delivery. In the case of the woman with infertility problems who has achieved conception, however, the adjective "precious" acquires enhanced poignancy.

Infertility

A couple who has undergone extensive medical intervention to become pregnant has exhibited seemingly unlimited dedication and desire for a child. Both partners have had to suppress embarrassment, anger, and dismay at having to attempt conception under the scrutiny of a group of medical experts. The couple's most intimate act together has been discussed, investigated, and proscribed. The woman may need to have her physician examine her postcoitally. The husband may be required repeatedly to produce semen specimens in the sterile atmosphere of a urologist's or gynecologist's office. Either partner may have undergone exploratory or corrective surgery. Terminology used to explain any problems uncovered can be demoralizing. For example, the couple may hear that the woman's vaginal mucus is "hostile" to her husband's sperm. The husband's semen analysis may classify him as "subfertile." The couple, uncomfortable about sharing what is happening with acquaintances or co-workers, may find the need to leave work for medical appointments stressful. Medications prescribed to correct problems or stimulate ovulation are expensive. Nothing about the conception of a baby under these circumstances is spontaneous or natural.

Often, the infertile couple attempting to conceive is older than most people having babies. They may have married at a relatively older age or delayed starting their family while the woman pursued her own professional career. The likelihood that there will be infertility problems increases with age (10). The couple may have used up even more time trying to conceive, both before and after they sought medical assistance. The time required to investigate the causes of a couple's infertility consumes additional months. Adoption sometimes ceases to be possible because of the trend toward lowering age limits for both parents at the time of application for adoption. This makes the quest for conception that much more crucial for the couple desiring a baby.

When pregnancy finally has been achieved, the woman still may not be able to enjoy the luxury of routine prenatal care. Tests may be conducted either because they are warranted or because her physicians are cautious in her case. Usually, there are more frequent prenatal check-ups—constant reminders that this is not a normal, simple pregnancy.

Pregnancy loss under these circumstances, then, can be devastating. As it is, people with infertility problems struggle with feelings of failure that are hard to overcome. The loss of a pregnancy after a conception is tragic, especially for the woman because it is her body that has failed. She has failed herself, her precious baby, her husband, and her care providers. What appears to be so easy for everyone else seems to be impossible for this couple and this woman. The couple's desire for a baby already has caused much sorrow and anxiety, and the achievement of conception gave them joy and hope. It is hard for the couple not to feel bitterly victimized by circumstances beyond their control when the pregnancy ends with a loss.

Deciding Whether or Not to Pursue Another Pregnancy

The issue of whether or not another pregnancy should be attempted is intensified. To do so means beginning all over again. The average, fertile couple trying to conceive after a pregnancy loss waits anxiously and impatiently for the woman's ovulation. The couple with infertility problems is under extreme stress waiting for ovulation, which may have to be stimulated. They wonder if it is worthwhile. After everything they have been through, they still do not have a baby. They question themselves and everything else, trying to figure out why this had to happen to them. To this couple, life is unfair.

The couple with infertility problems will not get pregnant again right away. Failed ovulation, irregular menstrual periods, and other medical issues may provide a physical obstacle to attaining pregnancy. Additionally, the couple has to regather the will to pursue such an objective. If they do make the decision to try again, the period of uncertainty while they wait can be more draining than anything up to that point. When another pregnancy is conceived at last, parents are again on the horizon of the life they have been yearning to lead. The 9 months to follow may be very expectant and very painful ones for them.

WILL THIS FAMILY ALWAYS BE INCOMPLETE?

Even with the birth of the subsequent baby and after discharge from the hospital, reminders persist that the family who has lost a baby is "different." The seemingly innocent question "And is this your first baby?" dredges up the past. It takes the parents some time and perhaps some experience to decide on an appropriate response to that question. Even years later, questions about the children in the family may make parents reminiscently sad. One woman mentioned having this feeling when she completed a form for a class reunion. The form asked her to list the number of living children and the number of children no longer living. She greatly appreciated the opportunity to "count" her stillborn son in her biography for the class reunion.

How any given family will adjust to a pregnancy loss depends on many factors. The responses vary from a family's putting the event completely behind themselves to their dwelling on the loss interminably. The normal course is between these 2 extremes. As time passes, families cease to talk about what happened and concentrate on the living children in the family. One question most couples consider is whether or not to commemorate the baby. There are several components to this issue:

Deciding how to memorialize the baby;

Telling younger children who never knew the baby;

Determining what place the baby's memory has in the family's history.

Memorializing the Baby

Families who want to memorialize their dead baby find many ways to do so. There are personal memorials, often a special piece of jewelry, a tree planted in memory of the baby, or a plaque or photograph displayed in the home. If the baby was buried, the grave becomes a memorial whose significance is eternal, even if family visits to the grave tend to decrease as time passes. Some families sponsor flowers in the baby's name at religious services, particularly on the anniversary of the baby's death, on holidays, or on some other date of special meaning to the family. Occasionally, parents will make donations to some cause that they associate with their loss, such as a research fund at the hospital where the baby was delivered or a support group where the parents received comfort while they grieved for their baby.

Melding Family Needs and Past Memories

What, if anything, to tell other children in the family about the dead brother or sister is a matter of personal choice. Most parents realize that they must be very careful in how they convey the story to their other children as they are growing up. Naturally, how children will perceive the event for themselves cannot be controlled; if they are old enough when the woman loses a baby, they will be aware on some level of the event and their parents' reaction to it. Parents have more control over how to let their children know what happened when the children are born after the loss or, at any rate, are much too young at the time to understand what has happened. Obviously, parents manage this with greater or lesser success for many reasons. If the dead baby is held up as an idealized angel, other children may struggle to be perfect, too, which can lead to emotional problems. On the other hand, it is possible for parents to communicate the love they felt for the dead baby and complement it with the love they feel toward their living children. Children who are aware of their sibling and and are sad that he or she is not alive, but who are not threatened by this knowledge will feel loved because of their parents' experience.

Ultimately, parents have the responsibility to fit the loss of their baby into their family's life. With acceptance of the event, parents find their own means of remembering and referring to their baby. There is no right or wrong way to accomplish this. There are no guarantees that a family's method of integrating this loss will last for the rest of their lives. A couple will find their own way to forget and remember, to let go and hold on, to feel sad and to love their baby forever after.

WHEN THERE IS NO SUBSEQUENT PREGNANCY

For several reasons, there may be no subsequent pregnancy for a woman or couple after a pregnancy loss (see Figure 15.2). For some couples this may be a matter of choice; for others, there may be no choice. The couple unable to have another baby may adopt and find a sense of contentment with the family they create in this way. Sometimes, not even adoption is possible, for reasons such as parents' ages, expense and time involved, or shortage of babies available for adoption. As a consequence,

---

The baby who died was unplanned; the couple does not strongly desire to have a larger family.

The mother is unwed and does not want to rear a child as a single parent.

The relationship ends; the married couple divorces in the time following the baby's death.

Infertility problems are overwhelming; the couple cannot have another baby, or the couple is unwilling to undertake the protracted quest for conception again.

The pregnancy loss was too painful for one or both parents; another pregnancy is too frightening to contemplate.

Genetic counseling has revealed chromosomal disorders that compromise or rule out the couple's chances of having a healthy baby.

Figure 15.2.   Reasons why there may not be a subsequent pregnancy after a loss.

a couple who very much wanted children may need to adjust to a life that is childless. Through the years, such couples may have to fend off thoughtless and unwittingly cruel comments about their being too selfish and self-centered to have had children. Whether or not they explain the circumstances to others is their own decision. How they adjust to this turn of events and find different sources of satisfaction and happiness is a personal endeavor that no outsider can or should attempt to influence.

CONCLUSIONS

The decision to become pregnant again represents the desire for a child that outweighs parents' fear of a new pregnancy after a failed one. Families need to know that, with time, the acute pangs of loss diminish. They need to hear that there is no calendar to dictate their schedule of grief. Physicians need to know this, too. Each pregnancy loss impacts differently on each couple. It is impractical and misleading to imply that a new pregnancy should not be attempted until a specified period for mourning has passed. Certain feelings and levels of resolution do not occur until a new pregnancy is conceived, progresses, and concludes successfully.

Caring for families undertaking subsequent pregnancies carries with it a burden. This special care also can provide some of the most rewarding experiences in one's professional life. These patients need strong, supportive physicians and other healthcare providers, not only to bring the new pregnancy to term with a good outcome, but also to help with the resolution of grief for the other baby who did not live. Such sympathetic care is only possible when healthcare providers have an understanding of how pregnancy loss affects a family. They need to appreciate the impact of pregnancy loss on subsequent pregnancy and to be prepared to address an individual family's special needs. Families have the responsibility to seek out care providers whose philosophy parallels their own and who are competent to provide the highest standard of medical care possible. Both parties need to recognize that there are no guarantees and that the attempt to bear a healthy baby represents a cooperative agreement between prospective parents and the medical community.

REFERENCES

1. Lahteenmaki P and Luukkainen T: Return of ovarian function after abortion. *Clin Endocrinol* (Oxf) 8:123–132, 1978.

2. Sullivan C: The return of reproductive capacity following spontaneous abortion. *Am J Obstet Gynecol* 63(3):671–673, 1952.
3. Boyd E and Holmstrom E: Ovulation following therapeutic abortion. *Am J Obstet Gynecol* 113(4):469–473, 1972.
4. Hallet R: Cyclic ovarian function following spontaneous abortions. *Am J Obstet Gynecol* 67(1):52–55, 1954.
5. Iffy L and Wingate M: Risks of rhythm method of birth control. *J Reprod Med* 5(3):11–15, 1970.
6. Guerrero R and Rojas OI: Spontaneous abortion and aging of human ova and spermatozoa. *New Engl J Med* 293:573, 1975.
7. Short EM: Genetic disorders. In Burrow GN and Ferris TF (eds): *Medical Complications during Pregnancy*. Philadelphia, WB Saunders Company, 1982, pp 109–144.
8. Peppers LG and Knapp RJ: Husbands and wives: incongruent grieving. In *Motherhood and Mourning—Perinatal Death*. New York, Praeger Publishers, 1980, pp 66–79.
9. Kubler-Ross E: Third stage: Bargaining (V). In *On Death and Dying*. New York, Macmillan Company, 1969, pp 82–84.
10. DeCherney AH and Berkowitz GS: Female fecundity and age [Editorial]. *New Engl J Med* 306(7):424–426, 1982.

Perinatal Support Service Formats

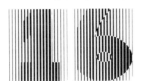

Perinatal Support Service at the University of Cincinnati

JAMES R. WOODS, Jr., M.D.
REVEREND BERT A. KLEIN

Discharging Pregnancy-Loss Patients into a Nonsystem Environment

The concept of a Perinatal Support Service (PSS) at the University of Cincinnati originated over a weekend in May 1983. That weekend, we (a hospital chaplain, Bert Klein, and a perinatologist, James Woods) were involved in caring for 2 quite different patients, both of whom had experienced intrauterine fetal deaths. One was a young professional, married to a professor at the university, whose baby had died at 30 weeks. We were inducing her into labor. Down the hall, a clinic patient was being induced under the same circumstances. The second woman was unattractive, overweight, alone, and on public assistance. During the course of both patients' labors and deliveries, we began to make some observations.

We contrasted the experiences of these 2 patients and how the staff cared for them. Certainly both patients received similar, good medical care. The attractive, professional couple, however, was surrounded by willing nurses, physicians, and other staff because they were interesting and easy to talk with. Nobody voluntarily sat at the bedside of the other patient just to talk and keep her company. The 2 women's hospital experiences thus were quite different. But their situations after discharge would not be so very different. When they were ready to leave the hospital, we became concerned about what would happen to them as they tried to pick up the pieces and carry on with their lives. Probably both would benefit from family and friends' expressions of sympathy at first. But, after a week or so, support for these women and their partners would dwindle. Who would spend the time with them that would help them in the long run to cope with this personal crisis?

DEVELOPING AN IN-HOSPITAL AND EXTENDED OUTPATIENT APPROACH TO CARE

Need for Level of Standard Care

It became clear to us, as we discussed these 2 patients, that if we did not establish a consistent approach to patients with pregnancy losses, we would be sending these women and others who would follow out into a world in which they very likely would remain confused and uninformed. They would be left to come to terms with a complex loss generally not appreciated or acknowledged by anyone except those who have experienced it. A small percentage of these patients might go to a support group for comfort, but even so their questions and confusion would not necessarily be resolved. In this indifferent environment, how could these people begin to piece together their lives? So, we began simply by stating, "We need to institute a level of standard care for all our patients, private or clinic, young or old, who experience ectopic pregnancy, miscarriage, stillbirth, or neonatal death."

Our plan for comprehensive extended care had to wait, important as it was. The first task was to define a patient's needs while she is hospitalized. This basic task alone seemed overwhelming. At the University of Cincinnati during 1982, we had encountered 50 stillbirths. During that same period, 250 miscarriages and 40 neonatal deaths occurred, all from among a high-risk delivery population of 3200 patients. We painstakingly formalized in-hospital care of patients experiencing a pregnancy loss, only to become more frustrated as each was discharged into a nonsystem environment. From the beginning, we realized that an inpatient system without outpatient follow-up was analogous to seeing the tip of the iceberg but missing what lies beneath the water's surface.

Commitment to Long-Term Outpatient Care

Commitment to long-term outpatient care became our primary challenge, once our inpatient care had been organized. It was not enough just to provide intensive care by physicians, nurses, social workers, and the chaplain while these patients were in labor and for 2 or 3 days after delivery. Any patient who has experienced the death of her baby remembers the shock and numbness that dominate those first few days. Only a portion of what we could say would be remembered by someone immediately following a stillbirth or neonatal death. A formal

**When, Where, and
by Whom Should
Couples Be
Counseled?**

outpatient support service was mandatory to complement care provided the patient while she was hospitalized.

Establishing an outpatient support service raised many issues. How soon after discharge should patients and their partners (or parents) return for counseling? Where should they be seen? Who should counsel them? What should we say to them?

We designated a Wednesday morning in June as our first formal Outpatient Perinatal Support Service. On that day, we arrived at 9 A.M., knowing that 2 patients on the ward the previous week had been given appointments for this new clinic. We waited until noon. Neither patient appeared. We were stunned. What was wrong with our idea? Why hadn't these and other patients flocked to us? After all, we had made the initial overture.

**Expectations Must
Be Tempered**

The next week we had 1 patient scheduled, an older woman who had experienced delivery of her late-gestational stillborn daughter. The patient arrived about 10 A.M. and we counseled her for $1\frac{1}{2}$ hours. We were filled with energy. We overplayed our roles, falling all over ourselves in our eagerness to help this patient. Because neither of us had previous counseling experience, we failed to address or even recognize her immediate needs. Consequently, we counseled her not just about what she was going to experience over the next few days, but we flooded her with information about the year to come and even about events that might arise 2 or 3 years later as well. Of course, we now realize that, in our enthusiasm, we tried to accomplish in 1 visit that which we have learned to extend over several counseling sessions. But the most important aspect of this first encounter was that, before she left our office, the patient said, "I am so grateful that you have set up this kind of system. I hope you stay with this idea and give this opportunity to everyone who goes through this experience." That single statement of encouragement has sustained us through 3 years and for well over 200 patients. Our collective experience with that many patients experiencing pregnancy loss has been invaluable in allowing us to pass on what we have learned from the earliest patients to more recent ones.

PERINATAL SUPPORT SERVICE (PSS)

**Addressing Medical
and Psychologic
Needs**

In June 1983, the Perinatal Support Service (PSS) was initiated at the University of Cincinnati as an integrated model for inpatient and outpatient care of patients experiencing pregnancy loss. The program was designed to meet medical and psychologic needs of the patient having an ectopic pregnancy, a miscarriage, a stillbirth, or a neonatal death. The PSS also provides the opportunity for patients experiencing a neonatal death after discharge from the hospital to be contacted and brought back into the center's support network. They are seen on a schedule similar to that by which patients experiencing an antepartum or intrapartum perinatal death are seen. Likewise, referral patients diagnosed with a severe fetal anomaly or an intrauterine fetal death that does not lend itself to induction of labor are seen and cared for by the PSS. When an antepartum patient is admitted to labor and delivery for subsequent management, she is incorporated into the inpatient segment of our perinatal support model. On discharge, she returns to the outpatient PSS for outpatient counseling. The PSS model incorporates the expertise of the perinatologist, nurse, social worker, and chaplain, each of whom has a distinct role in the care of these patients.

Counseling by a Perinatologist and a Chaplain

Although it encompasses many techniques previously published for care during initial hospitalization, the program is unique in that all outpatient counseling is carried out by a perinatologist and a hospital chaplain. The outpatient component of this program has provided the authors a unique opportunity to evaluate (1) types of patients who seek this kind of care, (2) types of patients who refuse outpatient care and who therefore are lost to follow-up, (3) patient responses to intensive and sometimes long-term outpatient counseling, and (4) obstacles that exist in the attempt to broaden availability of this service to all patients experiencing a pregnancy loss. (See Chapter 10, "Obstetrician As Outpatient Counselor," for data.) The remainder of this chapter is devoted to a description and evaluation of the initial 3 years' PSS experience.

STUDY POPULATION

Patients with pregnancy losses seen in the initial interval of this study were drawn with few exceptions from the obstetric clinic population at the University of Cincinnati. Delivery rates at this institution in 1983, 1984, and 1985 were 3397, 3565, and 3625, respectively.

The algorithm for patient care once a pregnancy loss has occurred illustrates the major personnel components that comprise the inpatient and outpatient Perinatal Support Service (see Figure 16.1). It should be noted that commitment to outpatient care greatly expands the opportunities and responsibilities of this type of program.

Initiation of the Communication Network

When a patient in the obstetric special care unit (OBSCU) encounters a pregnancy loss, the primary nurse attending the patient initiates the communication network by informing the

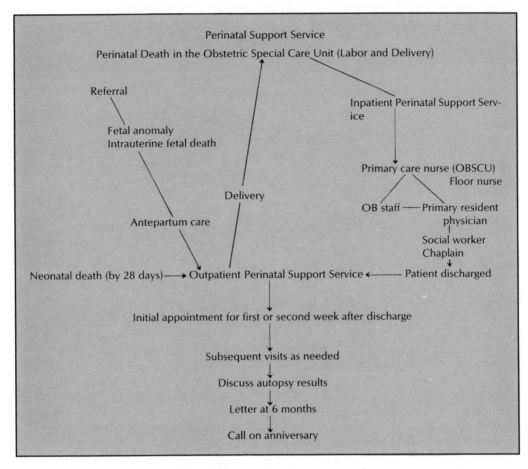

Figure 16.1. Perinatal support service.

Use of a Checklist to Identify the Pregnancy-Loss Patient

chaplain and social worker of the patient's presence in the hospital. The chaplain and/or social worker are notified as early as possible in the process, preferably before labor is induced or in the earliest stages of the patient's labor, in order to facilitate initial communication. A primary nurse, working with the resident physician, cares for the patient in the immediate, intrapartum, and postpartum periods. At this point, a checklist is inserted in the patient's chart (see Figure 16.2). The checklist details necessary items or procedures appropriate for a pregnancy loss, and it remains with the patient's chart until her discharge. After delivery, pictures are taken of the baby, the parents are encouraged to hold and spend time with their baby in a quiet room, and any other mementos of the baby are collected. The patient is given a letter, composed by the staff, that describes some events that will be occurring (see Figure 16.3). Another form explains decisions that must be made

Decisions That Must Be Made

UNIVERSITY OF CINCINNATI MEDICAL CENTER

PSS CHECKLIST

Demographic
Data:

Age:
Race:
FOB:

Primary Nurse:
Religion:
Marital Status:

Phone Number

Gestational Age:

Prenatal	G	F	P	A	L	LNMP	EDC
Care:	# visits		at				

Significant findings:

_____

_____

_____

_____

_____

Mother or sisters with prior pregnancy loss? No   Yes   If Yes, describe:

_____

Hospital
Course:

Date of admission: _____ Date of diagnosis (IUFD): _____
Date of delivery: _____ Type of delivery: _____
Date of discharge: _____ Significant findings/procedures: _____

_____

_____

Infant:	Sex	Name	Weight

Perinatal Support Service Checklist—Initiated by OBSCU 3N 3SE 3 W NBSCU PSS
Description of loss: AB_____ Stillbirth_____ Neonatal_____ Date_____
                        Weight_____   Length_____
Was Sex Determined? Yes_____   No_____   Sex_____
Previous loss?   Yes_____   No_____   If yes, type_____ at _____ weeks gestation

Parents: Named baby Yes_____   No_____   Name_____ Desires 3 W_____
Mother_____ Father_____ Other_____ saw baby at birth
Mother_____ Father_____ Other_____ saw baby after delivery
Mother_____ Father_____ Other_____ touched and/or held baby
Mother_____ Father_____ signed autopsy permit. Given appointment for PSS on_____

Keepsake Memories: P = Given to parents   E = Placed in envelope
crib card with footprints_____   booklet_____   lock of hair_____   photo (in blanket)_____
       bracelet_____   hat_____

Pastoral Care: Requests own minister-Yes_____ No_____ Name_____ called_____
Baptized? Yes_____   No_____   Certificate given_____   Memorial service_____
Burial/funeral arrangements discussed_____   Arranged_____   by_____

Social Service: CGH-309 completed   Yes_____   No_____   Sent to morgue Yes_____   No_____
Information on birth/death certificate given to parents   Yes_____   No_____

Perinatal Support Service: Private M.D. requests PSS? Yes_____   No_____   Name_____
       Seen by_____   to be phoned on_____   done_____
       Appointment on_____   Kept_____

Figure 16.2.   University of Cincinnati Hospital Perinatal Support Service (PSS) Checklist.

PERINATAL SUPPORT SERVICE UNIVERSITY HOSPITAL

Dear

We, members of the hospital staff, want to express our sincere sympathy at the death of your baby. We also want to offer you our support.

The loss of a baby is one of the most difficult and profound crises you will ever experience. In reaction to your loss you may be feeling a wide range of emotions. Shock, disbelief, numbness, anger, guilt—all of these and more are part of the pain and sadness of your grief. No one is prepared for such sorrow. Your hopes, dreams, and desires for this child will not come true. That hurts.

We want to help you as you go through this experience. Your doctor will continue to be with you, caring for you and answering your questions. The nurses will be the people with whom you will have the most direct contact. A social worker will visit to assist you in your recovery, and a chaplain will provide you with spiritual comfort and support. These staff members will follow you through your hospital stay. They are part of the Inpatient Perinatal Support Service.

You may be asked to return to the Outpatient Perinatal Support Service on the 3rd floor of the University Hospital on the first Wednesday after being discharged from the hospital, as part of your follow-up care. At that time you will be seen by an obstetrician and a least one other member of the Perinatal Support Service. We have found that couples who have lost a baby have many medical and social questions whose answers, provided by us in this early stage of grieving, help the process of recovery. This is also a time when we can share with you reactions from other couples experiencing loss of a baby who, upon returning home, have learned how to interact with family, friends, and coworkers.

Your experience is very personal, but you are not alone. We are here to support you and share your sorrow.

Sincerely,

Figure 16.3. Letter to parents experiencing a stillbirth (a slightly modified version of this letter is used for miscarriages and neonatal deaths).

during the first few days after delivery (see Figure 16.4). Sometime during the first 12 hours after delivery, the issue of performing an autopsy is carefully and compassionately introduced and the importance of the results discussed. (All of these procedures and items, so important to the care of these patients, are discussed in detail in Chapter 3.)

When the patient is transferred to the ward, she is given the choice to go to a gynecologic or an obstetric floor. Certain patients, especially those who have been hospitalized during the antepartum period, may request to return to an obstetric floor where friendships have been made and some peer support is

Some Decisions

While still in the hospital there are a few decisions that you need to make. They are your choices and whatever you decide will be accepted. There are no right decisions for everyone.

Seeing and holding your baby can be a special time that can provide you with memories, give you a chance to share your love for your baby, and help you begin to accept the reality of your baby's death. We have found this to be most helpful. (The hospital will make available a picture of your baby.)

By giving your baby a name, you acknowledge the birth, and his or her place in your family. You might find this strange but it can be meaningful, because it says to you and to the world that this was your baby.

Your doctor is going to request an autopsy. This surgical procedure is done in a professional and respectful manner. It provides you information about what went wrong and whether the baby was healthy. It may answer some of the questions you have or will have in the future. A full autopsy report is not available for a number of weeks; preliminary results, however, will be possible in 2 to 3 weeks. The preliminary and complete report will be discussed with you by an obstetrician in the Outpatient Perinatal Support Service.

The social worker will contact you regarding the disposition of your baby. If you wish, the hospital will take care of the body. You may want to consider a burial through a funeral home. The social worker and chaplain can assist you with this decision.

Some parents have chosen to have a memorial service here in the hospital. The chaplain is available for such a service. Others have had their minister conduct a service for family and friends.

These are some of the decisions you will make. It may seem impossible to decide on anything right now. Take your time. Remember, there are no "correct" decisions; whatever you decide to do is right for you.

Figure 16.4. Information sheet given to patients during their hospital stay.

already established. Most patients prefer to go to a gynecologic floor.

Early Outpatient Follow-up at the Perinatal Support Service

When the patient is ready for discharge from the hospital, the primary nurse on the ward makes an appointment for her with the outpatient Perinatal Support Service for outpatient follow-up the first Wednesday after discharge. The value of early outpatient follow-up is critical to the long-term goals of the program (see Figure 16.5).

STRUCTURING THE OUTPATIENT PROGRAM

Identifying the Role of the PSS

The initial issue that we addressed was to define the PSS team's identity as an outpatient counseling service (see Figure

Provide facts pertaining to the pregnancy loss

Provide genetic counseling

Provide psychologic support for the grieving parent

Extend counseling to include other family members, as needed

Figure 16.5.   Summary of Perinatal Support Service (PSS) Outpatient Program goals.

16.5). Identifying our role in the care of this large group of patients enabled us to focus our efforts and to minimize our level of frustration.

Provide Facts about Medical Issues

Providing Medical Facts

Our primary objective was to provide medical counseling and to reinforce information previously offered the patient during her hospitalization. We felt then, as now, that the major issue that prolongs the grieving process is a lack of information and details about the actual event. Over and over, we heard: "Why did my baby die? What are the obstetric issues surrounding my labor? Was anything found at delivery to explain 'Why'?" Regardless of the type of pregnancy loss, obstetrical and related medical questions persist (see Figure 16.6).

In offering patients a detailed account of obstetric and medical issues surrounding a pregnancy loss, we decided to provide straightforward answers to any questions. By doing so, we consciously determined not to defend substandard care; we would not attempt to cover up or defend obstetric or pediatric care that contributed to a pregnancy loss. This issue, if seemingly simple to the reader, is of primary significance for any professional dealing with patients who have suffered a pregnancy loss. The first question often raised when a baby dies is, "Who is to blame?" This question may be articulated by the patient herself. Care providers often find themselves privately wondering, "What did I do? Did I miss something? Did I contribute to the baby's death? Should I have requested a sonogram sooner? Should I have investigated earlier, when she reported vaginal spotting?" It is a natural response on the part of patient and care provider to need to learn what went wrong.

Establishing Honest Communication

Establishing honest communication early may help to dispel the anger that exists behind these questions, and it can help to establish a working relationship between care provider and patient, which is essential if the patient is to begin the process of recovery. It is the authors' belief that many malpractice suits,

The patient with a miscarriage asks:

Why did my pregnancy not continue?

Was my baby seen, and was it normal?

Was it a boy or girl?

Why did I have cramping and bleeding?

Couldn't something have been done earlier?

Was my baby genetically normal?

Did sex or my physical activity cause this?

Is it going to happen again?

What can I do differently next time?

When can I get pregnant again?"

The patient with a stillbirth asks the same questions that a miscarriage patient asks, as well as these additional questions:

Can you tell me why my baby died?

My baby didn't move much the day before I came into the hospital; were there problems then?

Why couldn't my obstetrician (or midwife) tell there were problems?

Should my obstetrician have done something more or different?

What did the autopsy show?

When can I get pregnant again?

The patient with a neonatal death has many questions regarding the pediatric care leading up to the death of her newborn. What is overlooked often in this group are the many obstetric questions that exist concurrently. Nearly every neonatal death involves important obstetric decisions.

Why did I go into labor so early?

Why did my obstetrician let me go so long past my due date?

Didn't my obstetrician know my baby had a defective heart?

Couldn't ultrasound have been used to let someone know my baby was sick before I delivered?

Will this happen again if I get pregnant?

Figure 16.6. Questions asked by parents after a pregnancy loss.

which develop out of these types of cases (and outcomes), originate because the patient and her care provider do not establish this level of communication early in the patient's grieving process. Anger and suspicion, which develop subsequently, eventuate in malpractice suits as the patient lashes out at what she and/or her family interpret as an uncaring and neglectful medical community (see Chapter 5).

Provide Facts about Genetic Issues

**Providing Genetic
Counseling**

Genetic counseling is an integral part of medical counseling following a pregnancy loss. The nonmedical public will readily accept the explanation that a certain percentage of miscarriages are genetically abnormal. Unfortunately, because miscarriage is understood to be common, this issue creates confusion among care providers as well as for patients. Should all miscarriage material be sent for karyotyping? Which couple should undergo chromosomal evaluation, and at what point should this be considered? And how will genetic counseling contribute to answering the most common questions: "Why did it happen?" and "Will it happen again?" Late pregnancy loss also may be due to genetic abnormality, as in a case of a baby with Turner's syndrome presenting with nonimmune hydrops. And what is a family's risk of recurrence when a baby has been born with a cystic hygroma or neural tube defect? (Toward these ends, the reader is referred to Chapter 12, "Genetics and Pregnancy Loss: Value of Counseling Between Pregnancies," for a discussion of the genetic implications of pregnancy loss.)

Provide Psychologic Counseling

**Providing
Counseling**

Psychologic counseling is essential in management of patients after a pregnancy loss. This type of care must be considered an obstetric responsibility. If this task engenders anxiety among many obstetric care providers, perhaps it can be more easily accepted if it is redefined as reinforcing normal behavior. Most situations of pregnancy loss involve normal people experiencing a difficult personal tragedy. Someone must reassure these patients that they are going to be all right, that they and their relationship with their partner will survive this experience, and that they are not going to have a nervous breakdown. Fears that one's life and family relationships will be permanently altered by pregnancy loss are almost universal for patients and their partners.

Because bereavement following a pregnancy loss is an appropriate response by normal patients, we chose to involve psychiatrists or psychologists only as referral resources and not as primary care providers in the PSS outpatient program. Our rationale for this decision was simply that, because caring for these patients is truly an obstetric responsibility, the first line of care should be provided by obstetric care providers.

CLINICAL EXPERIENCES OF THE PSS

**Typical Situations
Offer a Challenge**

Our principal task as obstetric counselors was to reinforce appropriate behavior. To do so, we blended counseling and friendship in order to reduce the authoritative image that care providers often assume unconsciously in a hospital setting. The hospital's clinical population includes many young, single mothers from single-parent homes. To counsel this type of patient adequately, we had to modify our objectives for counseling sessions to accommodate her needs. Following is a typical example of the patients encountered by the PSS: The mother, a 14-year old, single female seen 2 weeks after a stillbirth at 34 weeks gestation, says, "I was nothing until I got pregnant. Then the baby died and now I am nothing again. I sit inside all day. When I go out, I sit on the porch." In this case, our primary objective had to be to befriend this very young woman. Medical details could be dealt with during later sessions. We had to reach out to meet this individual at some level.

During another counseling session, a solid hour was consumed addressing the following problem. Another 14-year-old was found at 26 weeks gestation to be pregnant with an anomalous fetus unlikely to survive after birth. Her schoolmates were excited about the girl's pregnancy. Uninformed of the baby's condition, they planned to give the girl a baby shower at school the next week. When she brought this up during a counseling session, the young girl clearly was struggling with this situation and she needed to address it immediately. She could not sort out the issues involved in order to decide what to do. Many adults would have responded similarly under the same circumstances.

By undertaking full responsibility as obstetric counselors, we knew that sometimes we would confront failure. One former patient was admitted in a catatonic state to another hospital's psychiatric ward 6 months after delivery of her stillbirth. This outcome was difficult to accept because we had seen the woman on several occasions following her stillbirth and had hoped that we had been able to help her.

Setting Limits on the Services Offered by the PSS

In defining our roles as outpatient counselors, we chose to omit certain responsibilities and to utilize resources in the community. We would not give generalized psychologic counseling to obstetric patients concerning problems unrelated to their pregnancy loss. At the same time, we acknowledged that all patients, even those whose pregnancies conclude normally, could benefit from the type of attention and caring attitude provided by our system.

We also elected not to be a peer support group. Community peer support-group networks are well established in Cincinnati, as they are in most areas. They offer parents with a pregnancy loss the important long-term support that is quite unlike any that could or should be offered by the medical community.

(The reader is referred to Chapter 14 for a detailed description of the dynamics of peer support groups.)

Ironically, we have subsequently initiated a separate peer support-group network within our own institution oriented toward the population of young, single, often minority patients from low socioeconomic backgrounds. We focused on this group of patients because of our observations that, for multiple reasons, they are unlikely to utilize community support groups. Many support groups are composed of middle-class, white, married women or couples who are 25–35 years old. We decided to concentrate our efforts to attract this other group of patients who are less capable of expressing their feelings. Unfortunately, they happen also to be the group at the highest risk for pregnancy loss. Clearly, because they typically fail to utilize the services of community support groups, a large percentage of the population with pregnancy loss was being neglected without a support group aimed explicitly at their needs.

One-to-One Counseling

We determined not to allow the Perinatal Support Service be identified as offering group counseling. Even today, many patients misunderstand our role as individual counselors and imagine that they will be asked to talk about their experiences in a group setting. This fear of being pressed to speak up among a number of strangers may explain why patients often seek peer group support months (or years) after their pregnancy losses, at a time when they can more comfortably discuss their feelings openly in front of others. We continuously reinforce our program as one-to-one counseling with a perinatologist, a social worker, and/or a chaplain. Our goal, therefore, in contrast to that of a peer support group, is to provide enough information regarding obstetric and/or pediatric care to allow the patient to say, "You can't take away my hurt, but you have given me all the information I need. I know where you are and I will call if I need you."

Finally, we chose not to provide primary obstetric care to these patients but to place them back in their medical systems for their postpartum examinations and ongoing medical care.

CONFRONTING DIFFICULT ISSUES

By entering the field of obstetrically oriented counseling, we soon realized that there were very controversial issues that are central to pregnancy but seldom discussed. Obstetricians are proud of technical advances that make it possible to offer amniocentesis for genetic counseling to women over 35 years of age. Fortunately, few patients must grapple with the terrible dilemma of discovering as a result of amniocentesis that they are carrying a baby affected by Down's syndrome. The patient who decides that she cannot knowingly bring a defective baby into the world has to choose to terminate the life of her baby. For everyone, this is a terrible conflict. Lloyd and Laurence interviewed 48 women who elected to terminate their pregnancies on the basis of a neural tube defect or chromosomal abnormality. Seventy seven per cent expressed acute grief after the pregnancy was terminated. More significantly, 46% remained symptomatic 6 months after pregnancy termination. (This topic is also discussed in Chapter 2, "Early Pregnancy Loss: Miscarriage and Ectopic Pregnancy.")

Recognizing the Complex Dynamics of Pregnancy Loss

The need for support and acceptance from healthcare professionals is paramount in cases of therapeutic abortion. Someone has to say, "I understand that this choice is a sacrifice made out of love for your baby because you cannot knowingly bear a child who will suffer from his abnormalities and who will never live a normal life." In our counseling sessions, we do not take sides on these issues; we only offer understanding. Nearly all of these patients experience intense grief and loss, once they have made such a choice. Although diagnosis of a genetically defective fetus may be an infrequent occurrence in a normal obstetric practice, it is one vivid example of the complex dynamics of pregnancy loss.

OUTPATIENT PERINATAL SUPPORT SERVICE

Medical and Obstetric Issues Discussed in Follow-up Outpatient Counseling

On discharge from the hospital, the patient and her partner are seen for outpatient counseling. If the patient is unmarried and lacking the emotional support of her baby's father, then we work case-by-case to identify a significant source of support, such as the patient's mother or other close relative. All couples are counseled by either the perinatologist or hospital chaplain or both. During the counseling sessions, the following medical and obstetric issues are discussed:

1. Medical care provided in the hospital is described in understandable terms.
2. A complete (if possible) explanation of events leading to fetal or neonatal death is offered.
3. The hospital chart is reviewed with the patient.
4. Preliminary autopsy results are discussed and a copy of the report is given to the patient.

Psychologic assessment at this time focuses on the following:

1. Events that transpired after the patient returned home.

2. Support persons with whom the patient can talk at home.
3. Changes in sleep patterns, appetite, and levels of energy.
4. Fears following a pregnancy loss.

Sessions are scheduled to last 1 hour. In most cases, this is adequate time to cover the topics listed above. Understandably, patients often may experience difficulty returning to the hospital because of memories that surface there. Frequently, patients fail to appear on time or at all. We therefore keep the appointment schedule flexible. (The reader is referred to Chapter 10 for a detailed description of the techniques applied and the issues that surface during outpatient counseling for a pregnancy loss.)

OBSTACLES TO DEVELOPING A PERINATAL SUPPORT SERVICE IN A UNIVERSITY SETTING

Lack of Acceptance: Why Is Woods, a Perinatologist, Involved in This Anyhow?

In the beginning, we drew strength from those persons actively participating in the program in order to compensate for what we perceived as a lack of professional support from colleagues in the institution. We sometimes were jeeringly referred to as the "death squad," while others referred to our efforts as the "POC [products of conception] Clinic." In a busy training institution, care providers are committed to many aspects of patient care. We interpreted any negative reactions to our physician-directed program as predictable resistance to a new idea. Because it involved direct physician involvement and was multidisciplined, the program was unique. Moreover, the nature of the subject material stirs up insecurities for care providers that, if unresolved, surface as anger, confusion, or ridicule. To mock something that is threatening establishes distance between the issue and oneself.

Peer Acceptance Over Time

With many new ideas, time brings acceptance. This was our experience. It helped that we made the concepts and our clinical experiences highly visible within the hospital setting. We received good press coverage in the Cincinnati media. We provided talks at medical conferences at our hospital and at nearby institutions. We described our experiences at patient care conferences. I interjected the topic on rounds whenever it was appropriate. At times, my enthusiasm bordered on the obnoxious, as when a clinical case would be presented to a group of staff physicians and residents, followed by my addendum, "I think you need to understand what this patient went through after her discharge from the hospital." At first, eyes would roll upward during my commentaries, as if colleagues were saying, "Oh no, here he goes again." But soon the concepts began to make sense to others. It took about a year for the program to gain general acceptance. This is not to imply that every physician-in-training, much less every attending physician, became involved with and fervently committed to this area of patient care themselves. Most began recognizing the need, however, to place these types of patients in our care. Even though they themselves were unwilling to extend such care to their pregnancy loss patients, they did begin to refer their patients to us. We perceived this change in attitude as a solid achievement.

Identifying the Patient

Checklist Used to Facilitate Outpatient Counseling

In a busy university hospital setting, patients are easily overlooked and, on discharge, are lost to follow-up or proper referral. It is a tragedy when a patient with a pregnancy loss slips unassisted through the healthcare system. To appropriately identify patients and record their experiences, we fill out the checklist, while the patient is in labor and delivery (see Figure 16.2). The checklist stays with the patient throughout her hospital stay and is removed from the chart when the patient is discharged; it then is sent to the Outpatient Perinatal Support Service. In this way, when the patient comes for her first outpatient visit, details of her hospitalization are available in easily readable form. It is difficult enough for a patient to return to the hospital for her first outpatient visit to discuss her baby's death. It can be demoralizing if the care provider must fumble around with a thick chart in front of the patient and then has to ask, "And why are you here?" Instead, provided with the concise, in-hospital checklist, the counseling physician can open the discussion with, "I see that you have gone through . . . and that you were able to view and hold your daughter. An autopsy was performed. We have a lot to talk about." This approach gives the patient the impression that she is cared for and that her case is known, even if this particular care provider has not seen this patient before.

The group of patients most often passed over in our system are those who have miscarriages. These patients typically are hospitalized only long enough to undergo dilation and curettage (D & C) to remove any residual tissue. Frequently discharged home directly from the recovery area, they seldom are transferred to a hospital ward. Unfortunately, their interaction with staff often is too brief to enable anyone to establish a good basis for communicating with them.

Patients Are Given an Appointment for PSS Counseling

How then are these patients encouraged to return for outpatient counseling? In the beginning, we gave them the telephone number for the Outpatient Perinatal Support Service and instructed them to call for an appointment when they returned home. No one with a miscarriage called. It became apparent that, as with all couples experiencing a pregnancy loss, miscarriage patients must be given an appointment to the Outpatient Perinatal Support Service while they are at the hospital. Only then will they seek out the type of ongoing postpartum care they need. Patients experiencing a miscarriage are given an appointment for the first Wednesday after hospital discharge. Of course, it is their choice whether to keep the appointment or not. By this method, though, we are not placing on them the additional burden (or guilt) of having to decide once they return home, "Should I call this number to go in for outpatient counseling?" The typical experience is that, once patients return home, they will not make an appointment for this type of early postdischarge counseling. Patients who might not hesitate to take advantage of this type of service under other circumstances find themselves, because of their pregnancy loss, less assertive, more passive, and therefore less likely to take steps actively in order to get help. Sadly enough, many of these couples may flounder for weeks or months and only later contact a community support group for help. Many of these people could be saved considerable confusion had they availed themselves of the initial follow-up counseling offered by obstetric care providers at the PSS.

For patients who remain in the hospital for at least 1 day after delivery, the system is more effective. These patients usually are seen by at least 1 member of the Perinatal Support Service during their hospitalization. This personal contact is extremely important in bridging the gap from inpatient to outpatient care. Patients will return as outpatients to discuss even as painful a subject as the death of their baby, if they know the professional to whom they are returning. When personal contact is not made in the hospital between care provider and patient, fewer patients seek follow-up outpatient care.

LONG-TERM CONTACT

Letter Sent 6 Months Postpartum to Maintain Contact

For most patients, long-term follow-up is important to assure normal recovery and to detect serious emotional problems that may surface months after a pregnancy loss. Toward this goal, we composed a letter to be mailed to all patients 6 months following their experience (see Figure 16.7). The sole purpose of the letter is to maintain comunication between

Dear

    We are writing to see how you are doing. It has been many months now since you experienced the death of your baby. Time passes and for some it brings healing. We hope this has happened for you.

    Time also brings the reality of your loss and with it a variety of thoughts and feelings. Sometimes family and friends are uncomfortable or unable to talk and listen to your reactions and recollections. You may even be somewhat surprised at your feelings of grief, that they continue to be so strong with all their sadness, anger, depression, guilt, and tears.

    There may be some questions that you now have about the death of your baby. Whether it is medical or emotional concerns that you have, we want to let you know that we are here to be of assistance to you.

    We have office hours for the Perinatal Support Service every Wednesday, from 10 A.M. to noon. If we can be of help please call the Perinatal Center to set up a time to come in. We want to be informative and supportive to you in whatever way we can.

Sincerely,

Figure 16.7. Six-month follow-up letter.

patient and care provider. The letter imparts the simple message that support is still available, if the patient feels that she needs it. "It has been some time since your baby died and we have been thinking about you. For some, time heals. For others, it does not. Please call us if you would like to talk with us." The letter is not intimidating, yet it conveys a sense of caring. We have mailed over 150 of these letters. Although patients have called back only occasionally to acknowledge receipt of this letter, these few responses to this type of contact have been very positive. We encountered 1 problem, that of mailing a letter to a young patient still living with her family. In this instance, the father opened his daughter's mail and read this letter; until that incident, he had been unaware of his daughter's pregnancy or miscarriage. We have subsequently sent letters out only to those patients over the age of 18.

THE ANNIVERSARY EVENT

    We are now in the process of drafting a letter to be mailed 1 year after the pregnancy loss. The first anniversary is commonly a very emotional time for most couples. Many patients look to that day a year later and remember the exact time, the events, and their extreme pain. One patient said, "I sat staring at the clock and could hardly move. I watched the hands of the clock pass that moment and I cried." It is this response, at a time seemingly so distant from the actual event, that serves as a poignant reminder that bereavement is a protracted process that the medical community must respect as a part of serving the true needs of the patient.

CONCLUSIONS

Need for Structured Multidisciplined Program

In the end, a physician-directed perinatal support service emerges as a new concept in obstetrics addressing a longstanding problem. This is a multidisciplined program in which physicians, nurses, social workers, chaplains, and funeral directors unite to provide dignity, education, and comprehensive care to a large group of patients whose care previously has been fragmented. The overall purpose of this program is to allow a couple to grieve with dignity for their dead baby. The methods that are utilized and the items that accumulate in the process all meld as a memorial to the baby and a statement that the love, hopes, and plans for the baby were real.

REFERENCE

1. Lloyd J and Laurence KM: Sequelae and support after termination of pregnancy for fetal malformation. *Br Med J* 290:907–909, 1985.

CHAPTER

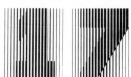

Management of Grief in a Two-Roof Perinatal Center

D. GARY BENFIELD, M.D.
JUSTIN P. LAVIN, M.D.

The Akron Perinatal Center is a two-roof tertiary care program comprising a large adult general hospital, housing the obstetric service and Levels I and II nurseries, and a children's hospital, housing the Level III Regional Neonatal Intensive Care Unit. Genetic and counseling services are available at both institutions. Although closely linked in philosophy and medical administration, the 2 institutions are separated physically by several city blocks. Therefore, the management of families experiencing grief in the neonatal period requires careful communication and coordination by the professional staff at each institution. The protocols and practicalities of this system are discussed in this chapter in the hope that they may be helpful in other situations requiring coordination among multiple institutions.

The approach to helping families suffering a perinatal death is based on a number of assumptions, many of which were adapted by the International Work Group on Death, Dying, and Bereavement in 1981 (see Figure 17.1).

GRIEF IN THE ANTEPARTUM PERIOD

Social resources and the sophistication of medical care have reached a level where the occurence of antepartum fetal death is a relatively unusual event in the United States. Recent statistics report a stillbirth rate of 8/1000 (2). In comparison to previous eras, the stillbirth rate is astonishingly low even among high-risk populations (3). In contrast, at least 15% of pregnan-

1. *When a fetus or newborn dies, parents grieve.*

2. *Grief is normal.* It is the emotional response to loss that manifests itself physically, mentally, spiritually, and behaviorally.

3. *Grief is highly personal.* What parents feel, how deeply and intensely they feel it, how they respond, and which coping mechanisms produce relief vary greatly.

4. *If people grieve, then they must also engage in a process called "grief work," "mourning," or "grieving."* The goals of the process are for grievers to resolve their feelings, to accommodate themselves to their new reality, and to get on with their lives.

5. *Failure to mourn may produce lifelong stress.*

6. *Bereaved persons, even parent-couples, have differing personal philosophies, moral and religious values, past experiences, and cultural expectations.* Those who care for parents should respect these individual differences and incorporate variations in care accordingly.

7. *Care givers who are present at the time of dying and death are in a unique position to facilitate healthy grieving.* Because parents are especially vulnerable, care givers have a responsibility to respond appropriately.

8. *Rituals and ceremonies of leave taking (for example, funerals) allow the death to be acknowledged in a symbolic and formal way and may meet many psychosocial needs.*

9. *Healthcare providers do not work alone to offer bereavement care following death.* Funeral directors become part of the care-giving team. A smooth transition may facilitate the resolution of grief.

10. *Most parents can cope positively following a stillbirth or neonatal death if they are offered and choose to receive 2 things: information and human support.*

Figure 17.1. Assumptions adapted by the International Work Group on Death, Dying, and Bereavement, Children's Hospital Medical Center, Akron, Ohio (1).

cies end in clinically recognized abortion (4), and 3 to 5% of pregnancies are complicated by severe congenital abnormalities (5). The fact that grief in response to a pregnancy loss may be associated with later psychologic problems has only recently been recognized (6, 7, 8, 9). It is our practice to consider all of these losses as potentially engendering a grief reaction.

Initial Contact with Pregnancy-Loss Patients

Patients with pregnancies possibly complicated by problems such as severe congenital abnormalities are referred (for diagnosis and/or treatment) to the antepartum fetal diagnostic center at Akron City Hospital. Diagnostic evaluation involves ultrasound, biophysical, biochemical, or cytogenetic testing. We find that most patients are much more accepting of the ultimate diagnosis, and better prepared to deal with abnormal findings, when the possibilities have been explained to them by the primary physician at the time of referral for ultrasound or other testing. We avoid comments such as, "We'll just check on the baby," or "Things are all right, but I just want to make sure." A patient is encouraged to bring her partner or someone else when she is referred to our fetal diagnostic center. This companionship can ease the patient's anxiety while she is undergoing the tests. If the feared outcome is confirmed, her partner provides an essential source of comfort. We find that many women experience a sense of guilt at having failed under such circumstances. Often, this is indicated in such comments as, "How can I tell my husband? I've let him down." This response can be addressed directly and diminished by explaining the diagnosis and etiology in the presence of both parents. Providing first-hand information to both parents can prevent subsequent misunderstanding as a result of one parent's relaying information second-hand to the other.

Minimizing Delay between Referral and Diagnosis

Most patients experience significant anxiety until a diagnosis is reached. Therefore, we make every attempt to schedule them for an appointment at the antepartum fetal diagnostic center within 24 hours of referral. Additionally, personnel at the diagnostic testing center are made aware of the suspected diagnosis so that well-meaning but inappropriate comments may be avoided.

Explaining Ultrasound Findings

In most instances, ultrasound has been our primary diagnostic tool for the detection of intrauterine fetal deaths or lethal fetal anomalies. Normal findings on ultrasound are relayed as soon as possible to the couple. Similarly, when abnormal findings are suspected, this information is provided to the couple. We have found that statements such as, "I am concerned about the possibility that there may be a problem, so the exam may take a while longer than usual," help the couple understand the process when a detailed ultrasound evaluation of the fetus is performed. Moreover, when abnormal findings are detected, this information becomes an extension of the previous statements. When a diagnosis of blighted ovum, incomplete or missed abortion, congenital abnormality, or stillbirth is made, the information is given the parents in an unemotional and gentle manner. We may begin with the statement, "I'm very sorry that this has happened," or "I'm sure that it must come as quite a shock and we're very sorry to have to tell you, but. . . ."

Typical Responses from Parents

Most of our patients react to the news of an abnormal diagnosis with disbelief. Some may say, "How could this be true? I can feel the baby moving," "My doctor heard the heartbeat just last week," or "No one in our family has ever had an abnormal baby." At this point, we will usually restate the finding and, whenever possible, show them the abnormal scan, explain the karyotype, or define the biochemical parameters in order to help the couple understand better this unwanted information. For many parents, their initial disbelief gives way rapidly to anger. The patient or her partner will accuse the physician of being wrong in the diagnosis, or they will call the physician and staff incompetent. Once they realize the significance of the diagnosis, they may weep or even scream. It is unfortunate that this acute display of profound emotion often embarrasses the patient and/or her partner, adding shame or guilt to grief. We have attempted to defuse these resultant feelings by saying, "You've suffered a terrible loss; it's normal for you to be upset, and it's okay to cry." Members of our staff try to remain with the couple for a short period of time and then suggest that they spend some time together in a quiet room. This room is equipped with a telephone for their use. A care provider is always nearby to answer questions or to amplify explanations. We find it very confusing and distressing to patients to receive abnormal findings but not know what therapeutics will be undertaken to terminate the pregnancy or deal with the anomaly. Therefore, we notify the referring physician as soon as possible after the problems have been confirmed at the fetal diagnostic center. In this way, the couple feels that their primary physician is still very involved in their care. Prior to their leaving the testing center, they are given a full explanation of the alternatives for management, even if this process requires that the patient and her partner remain at the center for a longer period of time. During this period, the physician explains the rationales for various therapeutic plans and seeks the parents' input. If fetal congenital abnormalities have been detected, further evaluation and additional therapeutic maneuvers are often required. If subsequent visits to the fetal diagnostic center are needed, specific periods of time are allotted to assess the couple's psychologic wellbeing, to allow ample discussion of prognosis and potential avenues of therapy, and to provide emotional support.

Antepartum Counseling

INTRAPARTUM CARE

Epidural Anesthesia

It is now exceptionally rare (approximately 1/1000 deliveries) for an unanticipated fetal death to occur during labor. Within our obstetric service, we have found that there is usually an opportunity to prepare the woman with an intrauterine fetal death and her partner for labor and delivery. Other situations likely to end in an unfavorable perinatal outcome are patients with an incompetent cervix and advanced cervical dilation, premature rupture of membranes, premature labor resistant to tocolytic therapy early in gestation, and those with a severely anomalous fetus. Many of these patients hope emotionally that modern medicine will save their infant. It is our policy whenever these situations arise to initiate a calm, objective discussion of the problem and its consequences, followed by a description of the various treatment options and anticipated outcomes. Frequently it is useful, for reasons of emotional support, to involve the baby's grandparents in this discussion. Additionally, a member of the neonatal team often will participate in the discussion and encourage parents to ask questions regarding neonatal management. If labor is to be allowed to continue or if induction of labor is indicated, a careful discussion of the medical procedures involved is reassuring to a patient. Many women are willing to experience significant discomfort to assure the delivery of a healthy baby. The prospect of undergoing discomfort to accomplish the birth of a baby with little chance of survival is extremely distressing for the patient and her family. In the past, the pain in such cases was alleviated with heavy sedation. But sedation depresses the woman's senses, lending a sense of unreality to the experience (7), and predisposes her to pathologic grief. We prefer epidural anesthesia as the anesthetic of choice during labor because it does not induce mental depression and it provides excellent pain relief.

Autopsy   At the time of delivery, we encourage the couple to see and hold their baby. We do not, however, coerce them to view their baby if this action is too distressing to them. If the baby is too premature to allow effective resuscitation, patients are often encouraged to hold and interact with him or her during the time their baby is alive. (Chapter 4 contains a full discussion of these concepts.) All couples are strongly encouraged to consent to an autopsy to determine the cause of death. We have found that the optimum times to discuss the matter of the autopsy of a stillbirth are prior to the induction of labor and shortly after delivery. During these discussions, we emphasize the importance of determining the etiology of the death and the implications this loss has for the parents and their other present or future children (8). At our institution autopsies are conducted by a pediatric genetic pathologist who is familiar with the many factors that may explain the perinatal loss and who is aware of the implications of the findings with regard to future childbearing (8). Medical photographs and total body x-rays are also taken. (See Chapter 13, "Value of the Perinatal Autopsy," for information on this topic.)

POSTPARTUM CARE

Recovery in a Private Labor Room   Most of our patients experiencing a pregnancy loss recover from delivery in a private labor room instead of in the general recovery room. This location provides them with privacy so that they may express their grief and emotions openly. A nurse remains available to assure the woman's wellbeing and to provide support and information. Our patients then choose whether they wish to remain on the postpartum floor near other newly delivered mothers and the regular newborn nurseries or to be moved to a gynecologic floor. Approximately 80% of women do not choose the postpartum floor. We have found, however, that some women take comfort from the presence of other women and their newborns. During the postpartum period, 1 designated nurse works closely with the patient and offers to act as a 24-hour contact person if problems or questions arise (see also Chapter 6). This nurse is to be available if the patient wishes to talk. This same nurse visits the woman daily for the remainder of her hospitalization. The medical staff attempts to schedule additional time during postpartum visits to discuss the parents' grief and any medical issues generated by their baby's death.

Continuity of Care

Format of Postpartum Responsibilities to Patient

We have found it very helpful to patients to divide the postpartum period into stages in order to address specific needs as they arise. On the first day postpartum, we review with the couple the facts related to the birth process, funeral arrangements, and burial options. We encourage parents to name their baby and inform them that the woman in particular may experience difficulty sleeping and eating or have incessant thoughts or frequent dreams concerning her baby. The woman is reassured that these events are normal and should not be mistaken as an indication that she is "going crazy." Additionally, we attempt to spend some time preparing the patient and her partner for potentially destructive comments that they may hear from family or visitors. The loss of a fetus or a newborn commonly is not viewed as an event that can cause extreme grief, so relatives and friends may seem callous or uncaring, although their comments usually are well intended.

These points are reinforced at subsequent visits as long as the patient is in the hospital. Additionally, if there are other children in the family, we advise parents as to how they may wish to discuss the loss with the siblings of the dead baby. The possibility that older children may feel a form of sibling rivalry with the dead baby is discussed. Children may imagine that their normal jealousy of an expected rival has caused the abnormal outcome. (The reader is referred to Chapter 1, "Pregnancy Loss and the Grief Process," and Chapter 8, "Social Worker: Hospital Advocate for the Immediate and Extended Family.")

Prior to discharge, the couple is offered a picture of their baby and copies of the baby's footprints. If they do not wish to accept these objects at this time, they are informed that these items will be saved for them. The couple is also provided information regarding pregnancy loss support groups in the community. After the patient's discharge, a follow-up visit is scheduled. Patients are given telephone numbers of members of the perinatal team in the interim to use if they have additional questions or emotional needs.

The follow-up visit is usually conducted in conjunction with the postpartum physical examination. It is important for the attending physician to allow ample time for this office visit. At this visit, facts regarding the pregnancy loss are reviewed. If an autopsy has been performed, the findings are explained. The implications of this information with regard to future pregnancies are discussed. The psychologic response of the family is assessed. Finally, suggestions are made for further care, as deemed necessary.

PROFESSIONAL COMMUNICATION BETWEEN FACILITIES

The second roof of our two-roof perinatal center consists of the Level III Regional Neonatal Intensive Care Unit (NICU) located at the Children's Hospital Medical Center in Akron, Ohio. In addition to receiving neonatal transports from Akron City Hospital, the NICU serves approximately 30 community hospitals within the 80-mile area east, south, and west of Akron.

The standard of neonatal care in the Regional NICU requires the continuous presence of a neonatologist as well as the resident and fellow staff. This feature is especially critical for providing continuity of care for parents when a baby is dying or has died. Furthermore, a neonatologist is available to the Perinatal Unit at Akron City Hospital to meet high-risk obstetric patients prior to delivery and to participate in the delivery room care of babies who are expected to require emergency care.

Maintaining Contact when Mother and Newborn Are in Separate Facilities

When a critically ill baby is transferred to the Regional NICU, his or her parents have access to their baby and to information via a toll-free line. There also is a 24-hour open visiting policy for parents and grandparents. Sibling visitation is permitted when requested by parents. A woman who is still hospitalized at Akron City Hospital following the transfer of a baby can see her baby and talk to the attending neonatologist via a telecommunication system, which transmits both audio and video signals through a telephone-line hook-up. This feature is especially important when a baby has been transferred directly from the delivery room at Akron City Hospital to the NICU at Children's Hospital Medical Center and the woman has had little or no chance to see her newborn baby.

RESPONSIVE CARE

Our NICU Mission Statement says, in part, "We recognize that sick newborn infants are an integral part of a family in crisis and that our caring requires that we respond by nurturing families physically, emotionally, spiritually, and mentally ... whether the baby lives (well or handicapped), or dies." What follows has been developed in response to this statement of purpose (9).

Our approach to neonatal death is based on a variety of assumptions. Many of these assumptions were adapted by the International Work Group on Death, Dying, and Bereavement in 1981 (referred to earlier; see Figure 17.1).

Responding to parents when their baby has died involves more than communicating a few facts. The responsive process can be divided into 3 phases: (1) thoughtful preparation, (2) issues for discussion, and (3) expressions to avoid. Although the process of being responsive is described from the perspective of a two-roof perinatal center, these concepts may be useful to physicians wherever they care for newborn babies. (The reader is referred to Chapter 4, "Death of a Newborn: Merging Parental Expectations and Medical Reality.")

THOUGHTFUL PREPARATION

Who Is to Inform Parents?

Thoughtful preparation involves anticipating the needs and concerns of the parents and extended family. Faced with telling parents that their baby has died, we have found it important to consider the task before us and to organize our thoughts. One of the first decisions is to determine who will inform the parents. In our setting, a neonatologist is usually the one who tells parents what has happened. At times, though, circumstances may dictate that another trusted person be chosen to fill that role. The individual who assumes this responsibility must be knowledgeable about the baby's medical history and the events leading to the baby's death, and must be able to gauge what parents have understood up to the point of death. We have found it necessary to vary our approach depending on whether the parents believed that their baby was going to die or expected that all was going well.

A question that frequently arises in our setting is when and where should parents be told. We believe that the attending physician or his or her designee should inform parents promptly when their baby has died. Although it is preferable to provide this information in person, this is not always possible when the baby dies in a regional center soon after birth, while the mother remains confined in a distant community hospital. We discourage the practice of calling parents to tell them that their baby's condition has worsened (when in fact the baby has already died), and we do not tell them that they should come immediately to the hospital while the baby remains "alive" artificially on a respirator. There is no substitute for telling the truth. Lying undermines trust. Moreover, lying may create the needless risk of an accident if parents rush to the hospital to be with their presumably alive, but actually dead, baby.

In all of our conversations with parents about their baby, we attempt to use the baby's name. In our follow-up discussions with parents, we have observed that they remember and appreciate that their baby's name was used in discussions with medical staff.

ISSUES FOR DISCUSSIONS WITH PARENTS

As a result of our experiences with families of many critically ill or dying newborns, we have found it unnecessary to dictate the precise words used by the doctor to tell parents that their baby has died. We have, however, established a clearer sense of the type of information that parents want. Both parents want first-hand information. We do not assume that 1 parent can communicate accurately to the other what he or she has been told. Even when both parents have been informed of their baby's death together, 1 may interpret what is said differently than the other does. If the woman remains hospitalized in her community hospital, we make every attempt to inform her physician and the nurses caring for her about her baby's clinical course.

Describing the Baby's Appearance

We always offer parents the option to be with their baby at or shortly after death. To assist parents in making this decision, we gently describe the baby's appearance and reassure the parents that the decision whether or not to see the baby is not necessary immediately. Also, we point out that sometimes parents have differing individual needs. One might want to see the baby, the other not. Subsequently, the discussion is expanded to explore whether or not parents want us to perform an autopsy and to discuss burial issues.

Accepting Unusual Parental Requests As Normal

Some may regard a woman's request to handle, caress, and dress her dead newborn as bizarre. Others view it as normal behavior and support her request. We feel that we should accept the possibility that not all parents will want or choose the options that we offer. We recognize that some parents may request options that we have not mentioned or even thought of. If a request is within the bounds of a reality that acknowledges that the baby was alive for a short while and then died, our response should be, "Why not?" We wrap the baby in a blanket before handing him or her to the parents. If 1 or both parents are absent when the baby dies, their desire to hold their baby may necessitate transporting the baby's body to the parents at the hospital of delivery or waiting for the parents to come to the NICU. Whichever site is chosen, parents must be permitted the opportunity to be alone together with their baby.

Before or after the baby dies, we take a photograph and offer it to parents. If parents refuse to accept it, the photo is marked for identification and filed away, in case they desire later to take it. When parents are ready, the discussion shifts to the question, "Where do we go from here?"

"Where Do We Go from Here?"

"Where do we go from here?" first includes a discussion of how and what to tell the other partner if he or she is absent. It may involve a description of the dynamics of grief or suggestions for how and what to tell siblings about what has happened. "Where do we go from here?" requires decisions to be made about disposition of the baby's body and the funeral service. Our healthcare providers are familiar with information about the following topics:

Ground burial, cremation, or entombment;

Calling hours, visitation, and the wake;

Whether or not to hold a service; whether to have a service at the church, the synagogue, the funeral home, the hospital, or at the graveside.

We discuss parents' choice of a funeral home and ask that they call us back after they have selected their funeral director, to keep us informed regarding the plans they have made. The attending physician calls the funeral home to alert them that the family will be calling. In order to facilitate a smooth transition for the family and funeral director, we obtain parents' permission to relay the following information to the funeral director:

A list of the baby's problems;

Whether or not an autopsy is planned;

How the family seems to be doing with their grief;

To what extent the family has been able to see, touch, or hold their baby.

Helping the Family with Funeral Plans

Whether or not a funeral service is part of the parents' culture, we are often asked for advice about this issue. When a newborn dies, there is a tendency for the father and funeral director to get together and make all of the plans to "get it over with." This collaboration is often part of a conscious, well-meant effort to protect the mother from the discomfort of coordinating events surrounding her baby's death. Unfortunately, mothers have reported later that being left out made them angry. Moreover, their lack of involvement further complicated their adjustment to the baby's death. We warn parents that this type of communication breakdown can occur and recommend that they discuss the funeral arrangements together before calling the funeral director. Likewise, we recommend to funeral directors that they meet with both parents to agree on the final arrangements. At times, this meeting must occur while the mother remains hospitalized. Cooperation among health-care providers permits both parents to remain involved in the decisions about their child's care. As a consequence, the couple stands a better chance of having their individual and joint needs met. (See Chapter 9, "Funeral Director.")

Facilitating Autopsy Consent

"Where do we go from here?" also includes a discussion about performing an autopsy. We request permission to perform an autopsy on almost all of the babies who die in the NICU. We explain to parents that the primary reason for performing an autopsy is to answer their questions such as, "Why did it happen?" and "Will it happen again?" We inform parents that an autopsy need not delay funeral arrangements, nor should it prevent the family's viewing their baby afterward at the time of the funeral. We accept witnessed telephone permission for autopsies rather than requiring written permission every time. This decision results from our experience on several occasions in which we were unable to obtain written permission for an autopsy. For example, a father may need to stay with his partner in a distant hospital. Requiring him to travel a great distance just to provide written consent for the autopsy is unreasonable. Whether or not an autopsy is performed, it is imperative that a follow-up meeting with parents be scheduled. We believe that a physician's obligation does not end with the baby's death, but instead continues throughout the recovery period as parents respond and adjust to the death of their baby.

When parents return for their follow-up appointment, each is asked first to fill out a brief questionnaire, which we use to assess how the individual is reacting to the loss and to identify problem areas for discussion.

In addition to the attending neonatologist, a variety of other professionals may join in for the follow-up meeting with parents. Depending on circumstances, parents may bring a trusted relative or friend. Usually, the neonatologist is joined by our coordinator of regional bereavement services. In addition, the pathologist who conducted the autopsy, a geneticist, the involved social worker, our family-care coordinator, or the baby's primary nurse may also take part. At a minimum, the follow-up discussion includes the following issues:

A review of the baby's hospital course and postdeath care;

Autopsy results, if an autopsy was performed;

How the death has affected the entire family;

Implications of this death for future pregnancies.

At the end of the meeting, we inform parents that we will continue to be available should the need arise for them to discuss any lingering issues or new ones that surface as time passes.

CONCLUSIONS

Most parents strive to comprehend the fact that their baby was born, lived for a short time, was a person, and then died.

---

1. Speak openly, candidly, and gently about the baby.

2. Use the baby's first name, if one has been selected; otherwise be careful to refer to the baby by the correct sex.

3. Support the need to recall memories; after all, when a loved one dies, memories are a significant part of what remains.

4. Offer opportunities for parents to see, touch, hold, talk to, give something to, or in other ways "parent" their sick newborn or their dying, newly dead, or embalmed baby (deformed or not).

5. Provide parents with tangible mementos; a lock of hair, footprints, photographs, birth and death certificates, a burial site, a name, or a death notice in the newspaper.

6. Be sensitive to funeral rituals and methods of disposing of the body that are in keeping with the family's cultural values.

7. Recognize the value of the support offered by significant others, especially in the case of single mothers, and be sensitive to their presence.

8. Avoid, if possible, medications that distort the mother's perception of events or postpone attaining results.

Figure 17.2. Ways to help parents accept the reality of their baby's death.

Our task, as care providers, is to assist parents as they work toward accepting this reality. We can provide such opportunities in a variety of ways (see Figure 17.2), all of which recognize parents' right to grieve for their baby. Most important is for primary care providers to remain involved with and available to families who have suffered the loss of a baby. We must bear in mind that our responsibilities toward patients with a pregnancy loss extend through their process of grief.

REFERENCES

1. Jane Nichols, Convener of the International Work Group on Death, Dying and Bereavement, Children's Hospital Medical Center, Akron, Ohio, Personal communication.
2. U.S. Government Statistician, 1983.
3. Lavin JP, Lovelace DR, Miodovnik M, Knowles HC, Barden TP: Clinical experience with 107 diabetic pregnancies. *Am J Obstet Gynecol* 147:742–752, 1983.
4. Glass R and Globus M: Pregnancy wastage. In Creasy R and Resnik R (eds), *Maternal-Fetal Medicine—Principles and Practice*. Philadelphia, WB Saunders, Co., 1984, pp 385–394.
5. Bennett P, Weber C, Miller M: Congenital anomalies and the diabetic and prediabetic pregnancy. In *Diabetes and the Fetus*, CIBA Foundation Symposium 63. Amsterdam, Excerpts Media, 1979.
6. Cornery RT and Horton FT: Pathological grief following spontaneous abortion. *Am J Psychiatry* 131(2):825–827, 1974.
7. Leppert P and Pahlka B: Grieving characteristics after spontaneous abortion: a management approach. *Obstet Gynecol* 64:119–122, 1984.
8. Furlong RM and Hobbins JC: Grief in the perintal period. *Obstet Gynecol* 61:497–500, 1983.
9. Benfield DG, Leib SA, Vollman JH: Grief response of parents to neonatal death and parent participation in deciding care. *Pediatrics* 62:171–177, 1978.

The Patient Speaks Out

PART

A Couple's Perspective

A Mother's Stillbirth Experience

JENIFER L. ESPOSITO

I had tried all night to make my baby move. In the morning, I told my husband Paul that the baby was not moving. I explained to him that this might mean that the baby was dead. He thought that was a horrible thing to say and he was very angry with me. I burst into tears.

It was the first time that I had voiced my fear that something was very wrong with this baby. All the anxiety I had kept bottled up inside suddenly spilled out. It seemed impossible, but at the same time I was convinced that the baby was dead. Off and on for almost a week I had sat still for long periods of time, waiting for a flicker of movement. Every time I had felt a faint stirring, I had been enormously relieved. But by now 24 hours had passed, and I was poking and pushing at my baby to no avail. It was time to tell Paul, time to call the doctor. I cried terribly hard.

CONFIRMING THE BABY'S DEATH

We calmed down and quietly arranged for me to be seen by a resident at the Family Practice Center, where I had elected to go for my prenatal care. In spite of a miscarriage right before this baby had been conceived, I had been confident that this pregnancy would be perfect. I did not bother to find an obstetrician, as I was satisfied with the level of care available at the Family Practice Center.

A resident physician saw me at 10 A.M. No one had warned this young man about what we were there for. He turned absolutely grey as we listened in vain with the doppler. He avoided looking me in the eye. Paul had never heard the fetal heartbeat before, so he was unsure about what was happening. The doctor left the examining room to talk with his advisor. When he came back, he said that he had arranged for me to have an ultrasound at the Perinatal Center, in the main part of the hospital. He told us, "Don't leap to conclusions. Wait until you've had the sonogram." But he was openly crying.

We waited at the Perinatal Center for the ultrasound. It took more than an hour to work me in. No one spoke to us. Pregnant women came and went. Finally, at lunchtime, I was taken in for the sonogram.

Ultrasound Confirmation

The technician did not speak to us. She took one look at the screen and left the room. Paul looked at the screen and saw that the baby's heart was not beating. That was the moment when he became convinced of the truth. I was hoping desperately that a doctor would come in and tell us that the baby was all right. Paul looked at me, horrified at his realization. I looked at him only for a moment. This was the instant of the purest shock I have ever experienced. I turned my head away toward the wall.

I lay on the table passively, not looking at Paul, at the doctor when he came in, nor at the screen when the doctor took a look for himself. I never did see my baby's dead image on the screen. If I had it to do over, I would not only look but would also ask for a photograph.

The doctor held the scanner on my stomach only briefly. He sighed loudly. He flipped off the switch on the ultrasound. I did look at him then. He said, "There is no cardiac activity. This means that your baby has died." That was all he said. He gave us instructions to come across the hall to an examining room. I got dressed. Paul guided me down the hall. I was blind and deaf with shock. I am sure he was, too.

DECISIONS AND PREPARATION FOR LABOR AND DELIVERY

The nurse outside in the hall greeted us very gravely and warmly. She led us into one of the examining rooms and stayed with us. She also asked us if we would like the hospital chaplain to come talk with us, and she sent for him when we agreed.

Urge to Get Delivery over with

The doctor came in and sat at a little desk in the corner. Two of the doctors from Family Practice were present and they hovered in the background. We were given some choices about what to do. We could wait for labor to begin; we could wait until my regular Family Practice doctor got back from his vacation and see what he had to say; or we could elect to begin inducing labor right away. Without discussion, Paul and I jumped at the last option. We both felt that we had to get this miserable business out of the way quickly. We had no idea how we were going to feel about the fact that our baby had died. The doctor told me to get undressed so that he could insert laminaria, to start dilating my cervix. I had had that done once before, and I remembered the needle-like discomfort of having something in my cervix overnight. I began to regret agreeing to be induced, because I was afraid of the pain. But I did not say anything. I had been expecting to experience the physical pain of my baby's delivery. It had to be accomplished somehow. I shut out my fears about the physical pain.

Paul was allowed to remain with me. It was perhaps more than he was quite ready for. He certainly got an eyeful, seeing his wife spread open with a speculum and probed by a complete stranger. This was one aspect that disturbed him throughout my hospitalization. He had never thought about the mechanical treatment that a woman must accept as routine. Having total strangers enter the room and poke gloved fingers into my vagina was hard for him to get used to. I was oblivious to it.

I got dressed, and then I had to give my history to be admitted. The doctor told the nurse to have a private room held for me. After a phone call, the nurse came back and reported that there were no private rooms available. He was adamant. "This patient *must* have a private room," he insisted. "Go tell them that." I got my private room. I was glad.

Choice of a Room on Obstetric or Gynecologic Floor

I chose to be on the obstetric floor. I was asked several times while I was in the hospital if I would prefer the gynecologic floor. But, already, I dimly had the feeling that I had failed as a mother. I wanted to be on the obstetric floor because I was having a baby. Maybe it was dead, but I was an obstetric patient. I was still a mother, wasn't I?

At some point, the chaplain came into the examining room to meet us. I liked him instantly and felt that he was someone whom I could really ask questions. The doctor spoke with a heavy accent, which compounded for me the feeling that I could not talk with him. The chaplain was like an interpreter and a buffer, too.

The doctor came back and suggested that we go home and pack a suitcase before I was admitted as a patient. As we got ready to leave, he said, "You may want to bring a camera with you. Some people want photographs later on."

Desire to Have Taken Pictures

I was repelled by the notion. Previously, of course, we had planned to photograph the birth of our baby. But who on earth would want to photograph the grim proceedings we were about to undergo? Who would want a picture of a dead baby? Now I wish that we had taken millions of pictures. It just had not occurred to me that this was all I ever was going to get in the way of time spent with this baby. I did not understand what all of this would come to mean to me. I wish so much that I had pictures.

We had to wait in the admitting office. I wondered what other people thought about us. Did they look on us as a happy couple here to have a baby? I thought I caught fond glances and knowing smiles from other women. I wanted to scream out, "This baby is dead!" to everyone. But, of course, I did not do that. The employee who processed my admitting forms was so businesslike and impersonal. After I had been admitted and had samples taken for lab work, someone with a wheelchair came for me. I felt absurd being wheeled around the hospital. I did not feel sick. It felt so wrong to be in a wheelchair in a hospital with a bracelet on my wrist.

There was an unfortunate misunderstanding about where I was supposed to be taken. Someone had told the man pushing me in my wheelchair to take me to the Labor and Delivery Unit. Actually, the plan was to begin inducing me at 6 the next morning, a Friday. But we were taken to Labor and Delivery, and at the reception desk there was a discussion about who I was—I was the patient whose baby had died; they knew about me—and about where I was supposed to be taken. I sat in my wheelchair and began to cry loudly while they talked about me. Someone called upstairs and learned that they were waiting for me up there to go in my private room.

When we got upstairs, a nurse at the desk came around to greet us. She said that my father and brother were waiting in my room. I could not be engaged in conversation. I crawled from the wheelchair onto the bed and sobbed and sobbed. No one knew where to look. Everyone wanted me to stop crying.

The word was getting out. The news had spread like a brushfire amongst our family, friends, and co-workers. Continuous telephone calls started the minute we got to the room. One call I made was to a teacher from our childbirth class. It had dawned on me that we would no longer be showing up for class, and I wanted them to know what had happened. Furthermore, I wanted the teacher to give Paul a crash course in prepared childbirth over the telephone. We had just started on the breathing business in class. I wanted my poor "coach" to do his job. I had no idea what was involved with inducing labor. I must have thought that they would push a button and there we would be, dilating and effacing and doing the proper breathing. This teacher was not able to handle the situation. She was flustered and upset and told me that she would call back after dinner.

My dinner arrived. I looked at it without interest, but someone had warned me that I would not be allowed to eat or drink in Labor and Delivery; so I ate a little. I skipped the milk. Obviously, the baby did not need it anymore, and I had choked down gallons of it for 7 months. It was a tiny rebellion.

After visiting hours, a nurse came in and talked with us until the end of her shift. It was a relief never to have to be alone. She told us that she had had a miscarriage, and she spoke about her reaction to that experience.

Common Reaction of Outsiders

Late in the evening, the head nurse came in and told us that a phone call had been routed through the switchboard for us at the nurses' station. It was my father-in-law, who was on a business trip. He had just received the news at his hotel. I remember he said to me, "It's one of those things, Jen. You can't be angry at anyone for this. You'll just have to put it behind you." I agreed with him fully. That was how I expected to feel about it, too. I still was in shock and not yet able to comprehend that what had happened was connected with the fact that we would not have this child now. There is no way to put into words the irrational way I was thinking. It was due to the shock and need for denial.

The doctor had prescribed some horsepill-sized tranquilizer to ensure that I would get some rest. The nurse who brought it to me assured me that this pill would knock me out so fast that I would never know what hit me. It did not. I was awake all night, crying. I cried loudly, in stormy bursts. Paul was so exhausted. He was trying to get some sleep, and he was not too comfortable on a lounge chair next to my bed. At one point during the long night, he said to me, "Could you please just stop? I'm too tired. I can't do anything more tonight."

I tried to stop sobbing. But lying there in the dark in that alien place, carrying the knowledge that my baby was dead, was just overwhelming. It was a lump of raw pain. I was literally in agony that night and I helplessly continued to cry. I did wonder what the maternity patients in their rooms nearby must be thinking. I worried that I might be keeping them awake. But, I also thought, "So what? They have their babies. What do I care if I wake them up?" No nurse came in to comfort me or to ask me to be quiet. They must have figured my husband was trying to quiet me, to no avail. If he could not, how could they? But Paul was simply too spent. So I just cried. I was awake all night, for the second night in a row.

FIRST DAY OF INDUCTION OF LABOR

At 6 A.M., an orderly burst into my room to wheel me down to labor and delivery. Paul scrambled to shave, and we both brushed our teeth. I did not have time to take a shower. I did not have any time for personal hygiene for several days.

Necessity for Privacy and Consideration

I was taken downstairs and put directly into a labor room where another patient lay. She was moaning. The fetal heart monitor attached to her living baby was beeping away loudly. Paul was still at the nurses' desk. I threw an absolute fit. I screamed for a nurse, completely unconcerned about the effect my behavior had on the poor woman across the room from me. I beat my hands on the bed. I was nearly incoherent by the time that a nurse came in and asked, "What on earth is the matter, honey?"

"Get me out of here. Get me out of here." That was all I could say. The nurse pushed me out into the hall, where a number of people, including Paul, converged on me. They demanded to know what was the matter. I had just gotten there. They had not even touched me yet. And here I was, hysterical already.

I informed them that there was no way I was going to lie there with that woman having her baby, accompanied by the gay little beeps from the monitor. There was no argument. I could almost see comprehension dawning on these people's faces. But, I found it hard to believe that these circumstances were so unusual that this had not come up before. Did other women in my situation meekly lie there listening to that? I was not going to. I could stand having a room on the maternity floor, hearing far-off baby cries from my bed behind a closed door in a private room. But I did not have to have my nose rubbed in it like this. I was wheeled to an empty labor room around the corner.

The doctor who had admitted me the day before arrived after a nurse had started my I.V. He removed the laminaria, which I had completely forgotten about. He was disappointed with the lack of results. Secretly, I was satisfied to know that my cervix was unripe and tightly shut. In the normal course of things, we would not have wanted it to be so malleable, anyway. It made me feel that I was healthy, normal. The doctor had the nurse begin with the pitocin. My contractions began at a promising rate. Things seemed to start well.

Allowing Family Members into the Labor Room

The atmosphere was surprisingly pleasant. I shut out the knowledge that my baby was dead. There were plenty of people around to talk with—a blessing. We liked the nurse taking care of me. She was supposed to stay with me exclusively. But, there was nothing much to do with me and the unit was too busy to spare her. She told us all about herself and gave us interesting bulletins about the progress of other patients. My father and sister came to the hospital and were permitted to sit in the labor room with us. The chaplain was in to meet family members and to talk with us. The young doctors from Family Practice kept showing up in pairs. One of them told me that my contractions looked really good. He added, "We ought to be out of here by 2 or 3."

"*P.M.*?" I asked incredulously. "You mean, today?"

He said, "Yep!" very cheerfully, and I wondered how this could be. It was all happening so quickly. Was it really possible for them to juice me up with pitocin and then I would deliver the baby today, this afternoon? The miracles of modern medicine! Paul and I were very impressed.

To myself, I speculated with some alarm about the necessary sequence of events. I knew about the stages of labor and so on, and it seemed like an awful lot would have to take place within the next 4 or 5 hours, especially since nothing had happened so far. Things would have to get terribly busy. I was frightened.

I need not have concerned myself. During the course of the day, nothing happened. My cervix was not responding as they had hoped. I had strong, regular contractions. To my surprise, I was not uncomfortable with them. My doctor checked me frequently and, shaking his head, would give orders to step up the drip. I was getting the maximum dosage.

There Should Be Reasonably Flexible Rules

My sister Jan had thoughtfully brought apples for Paul and lollipops for me. Paul gratefully devoured his apples, but my lollipops were vetoed by my doctor. I was being kept on the ice-chips-only regimen. Personally, I thought he was being a little tough, in light of the sluggish progress of my labor, and it seemed entirely unlikely that I would be rushing off for a cesarean section needing general anesthesia (the reason I was told not to eat or drink). Jan was miffed about this, too.

By 4 P.M., the doctors began to plan what to do next, since my cervix had not dilated at all. Gradually, I gathered that they would try something else to start my labor the next morning. An anesthesiologist and a nurse anesthetist visited us late in the afternoon to discuss epidurals. They told me that I was going to need one when they got my labor going the next day. I was going to get a different drug, which they expected would be more effective.

Sense That No One Would Want to Handle This Case

Around 5 P.M., a new doctor walked in and said that he was taking over my case. He would be on call all weekend and so had inherited me. I expected that the first doctor was glad to be rid of me. He could go home and forget the whole business. And now this poor new guy was stuck with me for the whole weekend. I felt distinctly like a hot potato.

At 6:30, they shut off the pitocin. Any dilation that may have been achieved during the last 12 hours was negligible. I requested that the nurse pull out the I.V. She was reluctant, warning me that they would have to start a new one in the morning. I hated having that "needle" in my hand—where the morning nurse had unaccountably stuck it—and I wanted it out of there. The nurse took the catheter out of my hand and I was moved back upstairs to my room.

My dinner had been sitting on my table for an hour or more. We did not care. We picked at the food and fielded more phone calls. Everyone called. The nurse at the desk told us that people had been calling all day for news. I did not pay much attention. In an abstract way, I appreciated my friends' concern. But I was far too self-absorbed to think of all the people who would be upset about what had happened. I did not want to call anyone. I had nothing to say. I was utterly exhausted and focused only on giving birth to my baby.

I should have showered, but I did not think of it. I walked up and down the hall of the maternity floor, leaning on Paul's arm and looking as pathetic as possible. I felt tragic amid the smiles of visitors, but I insisted on walking. My books at home all stated that it is helpful to ambulate when you are in labor. I erroneously believed that I was "in labor" because I had been on pitocin all day. It was pointless, but it made me feel like I was doing something productive.

That night, the medication I received helped me to sleep. My doctor had been surprised to hear that the horsepill he had left for me the night before had failed. So, he ordered something else, 2 small, white pills that knocked me out cold. Of course, I had not slept for 3 nights, either.

Irrational Concerns for Baby's Health

I had qualms about taking sleeping pills. I was irrationally afraid that the drug would hurt the baby. It was odd that this thought lingered in my mind the whole time that I was in the hospital. Even though intellectually I accepted what had happened, on other levels it obviously still had not sunk in.

SECOND DAY OF INDUCTION OF LABOR

The next morning was a repeat of the previous one: the predawn scramble to brush our teeth and the ride to a labor room, insertion of the I.V., and the enema. My new doctor did not arrive until nearly 8 A.M. I dozed on the bed in the labor room. When the doctor arrived, he placed Prostaglandin E2 suppositories up next to my cervix, which was an uncomfortable procedure. The doctor was wearing a suit and tie, and he explained that because a seminar was being held in the hospital he would be in and out all day. But, he said, there were residents on duty to take care of me.

When the first suppository began to take hold, I started

Side Effects of Prostaglandins

experiencing a multitude of side effects, all of which I had been told to anticipate. I became very ill. I felt miserable. I was having strong contractions. The epidural that I had been given provided some relief. The only problem I perceived as a result of the epidural was that it put my feet and legs to sleep. I thought I should move them around to get blood circulating, and I made Paul massage them endlessly. Everyone—the staff and then my family, repeating this for them—reassured me that my legs were supposed to be numb, but it did not register with me. The medications I was given intravenously to counteract the pros-taglandins' side effects made me vague and woozy.

I was sick and incoherent, and I began to suffer terribly from back labor. I vomited often. With nothing in my stomach, however, all there was to vomit was bile. It left a terrible taste in my mouth, and the dark greenish-brown liquid in a silver pan scared me. I could not see well. The room's lighting was dim, and I thought I was throwing up blood. I had a fever, too. And I also had what the nurse called "flash diarrhea." Fortunately, the enemas I had received previously somewhat alleviated the problem, but I felt as if I had sunk to the depths of humiliation, getting myself and my bed so soiled and filthy in front of my husband and my mother and sister, as well as the staff and the residents from the Family Practice service.

My new doctor returned every few hours to insert prosta-glandin suppositories. Once, he arrived as I was realizing the need to vomit again. He and Paul lifted me up and held me upright. I was too anesthetized to sit up on my own. Someone held my hair away from my face as I vomited. I thought that was very kind—I felt repugnant and was surprised that anyone could stand to touch me.

Physical and Mental Anguish

I slipped in and out of the conversation carried on by Paul and my mother and sister. I remember saying aloud crazy, disconnected things that startled my family but that made perfect sense in the context of my hallucinations and dreams. I was in a semiconscious stupor. It was a nightmare. I cried periodically that day, in physical and mental anguish. It was the worst time I had ever endured, overwhelmed with the physical discomfort and knowing that my baby was dead.

The biggest disappointment at that moment was that this process had not accomplished anything. I was not dilating at all, in spite of the contractions which—unlike the ones the day before—hurt although I still had the epidural anesthesia. The doctor came in late in the afternoon wearing scrubs. The seminar had ended and he was ready to turn his attention to me. He inserted the prostaglandin suppositories at regular intervals; I got them 4 or 5 times, at least.

During most of the day I was hardly aware of what was

Husband's Experience

going on around me. I do remember asking someone to take Paul for something to eat. He had spent the whole day on his feet by my bed, massaging my legs, applying pressure to my sacroiliac because of the back labor, and holding bedpans for me to throw up in, urinate in, or have explosive diarrhea in. I almost think his experience as a hands-on observer and distraught husband might have been worse than my experience was.

My mother and sister left without my being aware of their going. The doctor, the anesthesiologist, and Paul spent the evening talking, from about 8 P.M. onward, seated on chairs with their legs up, near the foot of my bed. The room was darkened, and they spoke softly. An employee brought them pieces of someone's birthday cake, and the 3 of them ate it there. Paul told me in an aside that the anesthesiologist was the "Pain Fellow"—a title which sounded funny—and a member of the History Book Club, to which Paul also belongs. The doctors and Paul found that they had common interests and they got along well. I sensed that their evening was not unpleasant, the surroundings and my circumstances notwithstanding.

FAILURE TO PROGRESS

At about 1:30 A.M. I was due to receive more prostaglandins. I was awake and reasonably alert. I understood that my cervix had not dilated. The doctor said that I was "maybe a finger dilated." He could not even insert laminaria into my cervix, which he attempted to do in an effort to soften my cervix.

It seemed there was a crowd in my room, nurses and the doctor and the chief resident and the "Pain Fellow." Everyone was venturing an opinion about what should be done with me, and I was piping in, too, with my own observations about my case.

Rethinking the Methods Being Used

"We have not burned any bridges yet," the doctor said thoughtfully. "Your water hasn't broken. We don't have to rush our thinking here. You are not especially vulnerable to infection. I think we should stop for tonight, let everyone get some rest, and in the morning we will figure out where to go from here." Later, I learned that the doctor considered sending me home to wait for labor to begin on its own. I would have been horrified if I had learned that night that he was contemplating this course of action.

As it was, I hastily came to the conclusion that he was thinking of doing a cesarean section. No one had said anything to that effect, and there was no valid reason to conclude that.

But I was frazzled and very tired. I had been through a harrowing day. I thought a cesarean section was the only option left. It was simply ignorance on my part, but that was what I was sure he had in mind. This was a breaking point for me.

I imagined that I waited until he was out of the room, but he must have been in the doorway when I burst into a rage, albeit a whispered one. "I am furious!" I hissed at Paul. I went on at length, using the worst vocabulary, to explain to Paul how enraged I was that "they" would put me through all this and then turn around anyway and do a cesarean section, which they should have done in the first place. Actually, I had asked at the outset why we could not do a cesarean section and get this over with as fast as possible. I had been told that it was not appropriate to do this. Now, I thought that they were going to perform a cesarean. I was livid.

Paul let me talk. I know that the doctor heard at least part of what I said because, shortly afterward, he approached Paul in the hallway and told him, "Don't worry. I've had women say far worse things to me." Later on, Paul heard him tell the resident, "This is the last time we attempt an induction of labor this long." He did not like what "they" had put me through any more than I did. After one more attempt with another patient to induce labor in a case of intrauterine fetal death, the hospital changed its policy and began to send selected patients home to wait for more favorable conditions to develop, so that labor would be more spontaneous and as brief as possible.

Allowing the Patient a Drink of Water

Meanwhile, I had been waging a campaign to get some lemonade. I was dying of thirst and had a craving for the lemonade that the hospital dispensed in the evenings on the maternity floor. We had been given a container of it in my room upstairs the previous evening. The nurses hesitated to grant my request because I was not supposed to have anything by mouth. But I could not get it out of my mind; I begged for a drink. My second doctor was less exacting about the rule that I could not have fluids, because in my case it was clear that labor was going to last many hours longer. He gave his permission for me to have a drink, and one of the nurses got the lemonade for me. I must have drunk most of the small carton myself. It was the most satisfying drink I had ever had.

The pain fellow came along to put some more drugs in my I.V. that would put me to sleep. He selected Demerol from his pharmacopoeia and told me what he was going to give me. I watched him do it, saying, "Now I'll find out what it's like to mainline . . ." That was it. I was out before I could complete the sentence. The scene was highly amusing to Paul, and it became one of the stories he told people later on.

Paul was finally allowed to lie down on the other bed in

my room. He had not sat on the bed all day because some of the staff members seemed to be reserving the right to claim that half of my room for another patient. The unit was very busy. But I encouraged Paul to lie down, as a means of stalling in case they wanted to bring someone in. I was prepared to protest strongly if the staff tried to bring another laboring patient into "my" labor room.

THIRD DAY: ONSET OF TRUE LABOR

Fortunately, Paul got a little sleep. About 2 hours after everything had quieted down, 4 or 4:30 in the morning, I suddenly awoke, in spite of the Demerol. My bed was soaking wet and I had come to consciousness aware of that, as well as of strong, painful contractions that the epidural was not masking.

My doped, initial reaction was to think that I had wet my bed. It would not have surprised me, really, since I had drunk a carton of lemonade. Besides, the I.V. had kept me hydrated and I could not remember the last time anyone had let me use a bedpan. It had probably been 10–12 hours.

I woke Paul. "Something's happening," I called to him. He came to me, looked at my sheets, and went for the nurse. She came back with him and looked, too. She told me that the membranes had ruptured. That was good news.

Tracing of Contractions Could Be Given to Woman As a Memento

My contractions, real ones this time and to the best of my knowledge not being augmented by drugs, were increasing. For the past 2 days, the staff had monitored my contractions. Ironically, at this point, the paper ran out, and it was time to insert a new roll. The night nurse was not adept at reloading the roll of paper on the monitor. She struggled to do so, but could not, and she turned the monitor off. I was extremely annoyed. I wanted to watch the pattern of my contractions, now that it really mattered and I finally seemed to be getting somewhere. But there was no fetal heart to monitor as a legal precaution, so they were not worried about it. I would have liked to see the tracing later when I was putting all the pieces of my experience together, and I am sorry that none was made.

Around 6 A.M., someone woke my doctor. He came in and checked to see how things were going. They were going well. I was dilating beautifully. My contractions were very strong and regular. It looked like things were coming to a head, so to speak. The doctor was cheerful about this. He rubbed his hands together and turned to Paul. "Let's go take a shower and get some breakfast." Paul went up to my room on the third floor and took his shower, and then the two of them met and went off to eat in the cafeteria.

Meanwhile, my contractions were coming one on top of the other. There was no pause between the end of one and the beginning of the next.

Make Sure the Patient's Anesthesia Is Effective

I was keenly aware of sensations on my left side. I could wiggle my toes in my left foot, move that leg at will, and feel every single contraction, beginning all the way in my back and swinging around in the front to a squeezing point down in the lowest part. It was almost like the wringing of a wet rag. It was an endless series of steady, drawn-out contractions, and I found it very interesting to experience it. It never for an instant occurred to me that I should mention the sensations I was feeling to a nurse or my anesthesiologist. I thought that this was the way an epidural worked.

I have the impression that I was alone for a good hour and a half, except for the visits of the nurse, the same one who had taken care of me on Friday. It was now Sunday morning, and she expressed surprise to see me still there.

My contractions kept me very busy. I had my eyes shut and I fell into a natural rhythm of breathing my way through each one. I did it instinctively. My well-fed, showered husband reappeared sometime around 8:30 A.M. The doctor went in and out, being kept apprised of my progress. I just kept my eyes squeezed shut and breathed through the contractions. Paul timed them and told me that they were coming every minute and lasting the whole minute. I was totally absorbed by them and not able to listen to him as he offered encouragement.

DELIVERY

At 9 A.M., I felt something solid in my vagina. It was unmistakably some part of my baby. I had Paul get the nurse. She lifted the top sheet off me, and Paul and I both watched her as she squinted with concentration. Paul looked at me, looked between my legs, and, pointing, looked at the nurse. "Is . . . is that a hand?" he asked with disbelief in his voice. She nodded, still staring. Then she got my doctor. He ran in and took a look.

There was a bustle and flurry of activity. People came and went. Sterile drapes were arranged all around me. I kept my eyes shut and breathed through each contraction. I felt like I was completely alone, even in that crowd of people.

The bed was a new one, a prototype for the ones they were purchasing for the new labor and delivery unit scheduled to open in 6 months. It converted into a delivery table, with sections being removed and adjusted. The unfamiliar table kept them all busy for several minutes more. My legs were inserted in very high stirrups. My right leg was a dead weight, and my left I could move however I wanted to.

The doctor asked someone to get a bowl. He sat on the foot of the bed and started pressing my uterus. "I can't . . . There's something blocking . . .," he said. He sounded puzzled.

I suddenly spoke up. "I think my bladder may be full."

He looked like he was ready to laugh. We all saw the humor in it, momentarily. Then someone quickly supplied a catheter and bedpan, and my bladder was emptied. The catheter hurt. We were amazed at how much urine there was. The doctor was provoked that my bladder had been neglected for what was obviously a long time. They positioned some fresh sterile drapes. Everyone got very quiet again, and I felt the doctor pulling my baby from me.

After Delivery, Only Silence

It was a wrenching, painless kind of sensation, as of pulling against a strong suction. I could feel the baby in my vagina, and I could feel the resistance; I could feel him pulling, and after a few moments the resistance faltered and then I felt the whole baby sliding out and then gone. I kept my eyes tightly shut the entire time. As he pulled the baby out, I thought, "It will be a whole year until I can do this again and have a live baby."

He put my baby directly into the big stainless steel bowl that was waiting right there between my legs. He squeezed my left knee very gently and said, "Jenifer, it's over. Your baby has been born."

Suddenly, everyone was leaving the room, and the doctor picked up the bowl and walked away, too. I opened my eyes in time to see him going out the door, bearing the bowl with my baby in it high up in front of his chest.

"What is it?" I called out to him. "Is it a boy or a girl?"

He turned and said, "We don't know." Then, he vanished into the hallway.

I have no idea where Paul was when all this was happening. After the doctor's answer, "We don't know," I was on a new level of shock. I sank back into my pillow and shut up inside myself completely, trying to take in the implications of that answer.

Patient's Need for Information at Delivery

They could not tell what sex the baby was. I must have had a monster. I could not imagine what horrors we now were going to hear about our baby. It must be awful. I was so shocked. Nothing in any of the 3 ultrasounds I had been given had indicated any abnormalities. I was so unprepared for this.

I was still quiet when they wheeled me up the hall several minutes later, to have the placenta delivered. I was lifted onto the delivery table. People fixed me up for the procedure. The anesthesiologist fiddled with the epidural catheter, and then suddenly I was anesthetized with a vengeance. I was dead from the waist down to my toes. It was like the lower half of my body had been removed. While he was at it, the anesthesiologist also put some Valium into my I.V. I became suddenly loquacious and amusing. I cracked jokes. The nurses and anesthesia people were laughing and cracking jokes with me.

My doctor came in and delivered the placenta without difficulty. He decided to give me a D & C. I spoke up as they started to move me out. I asked the doctor, "Well, what did I have? Was it a boy or a girl?"

He was talking to the nurse, but when I asked this he turned around to me with a very surprised look on his face, like "Oh, didn't you hear?" He said, "You had a girl."

"See," I called euphorically to Paul. "I told you it was a girl all along." I had insisted for a couple of months that it was a girl. Paul did not respond, and I sank back into myself to think and doze. I still was terrified that she was grossly abnormal. They must have done some test in that bowl to determine the sex. I was wheeled to the recovery room.

RECOVERY ROOM: SEEING THE BABY

When I first got to the recovery room, I was the only patient present. I was put in the far corner. It was a dingy, bleak room, and the nurses stayed away from me. I lay there, looking at the ceiling.

Sense of Exhilaration Still Possible

Unbelievable as it may seem, I had a wonderful sense of exhilaration at that moment. Nothing about my baby's death had really hit me, and so I was able to appreciate the miracle of what I had just done. I had had a baby. A little girl had grown inside me and I had given birth. It was a miracle in and of itself, the outcome aside.

Patient's Need for Accurate Information

Soon, Paul came in, with the doctor right behind him carrying our little girl wrapped in a blue cloth. I was totally unprepared for their abrupt appearance. I had been assured that I would see my baby, but I did not expect it so soon. I had imagined that it would be later, in my room or something. But, I supposed then that maybe there was a rush to do the autopsy. Maybe they could get more, or better, information if they did the autopsy right away, and so that was why they were in a hurry for me to see her and give her back to them. The doctor set her down on my bed and fetched a chair for Paul. Then, he pulled the curtain around to the foot of my bed and disappeared.

Too Anesthetized to Hold the Baby

She was on my bed, to my right, by my shoulder. I was still so anesthetized. In fact, the catheter was still in. I had been told that the pain fellow was on his way to come take it out. I could not turn over. I could not sit up. I could not pick my baby up, and I wanted to so badly. I wanted to feel her weight and hold her as I had waited all those months to do. I almost literally had never held a baby before. During my pregnancy, I became superstitious about not holding any baby until I got to hold my own. And I never got to hold her.

We were still just positioning me to look at her when the doctor returned. He handed a snapshot of her to me. It was a blurry Polaroid. He said, "It's not a very clear picture; I'm sorry. But we took 2 more, and if they come out better, we'll let you have those."

Photograph Should Be Clear

I later tried to track down those other 2 pictures. I was so glad to have the one, and I desperately wanted the other 2. But, they were lost. This picture showed her face. An arm was in the picture, holding her head. It was a very blurry photo, as if the person taking the picture had been jarred just as he snapped the shutter. Paul took the picture after we looked at it and put it in his pocket for safekeeping.

We were alone with our baby. Paul pulled the blue sheet away from her body, and there she was.

Appearance of a Stillborn Baby

She was not a monster at all. She was perfect, except for her color, which I ignored, and except for her peeling abdomen. I figured that her skin was peeled there because they had already taken samples of skin for tests, to grow cells. It seemed that they had needed a big patch, because the whole left side of her abdomen was peeled. I did not know that the peeling was in fact due to her being dead in utero. In the autopsy, it was characterized as "superficial erosion."

Her hair was still a little wet. It was dark and matted. She was limp and her hands were unnaturally straightened, not curled up like you always see an infant's hands. I picked up her left hand and it dropped back on the bed, still straightened out.

It was so hard for me even to lie on my side to look at her. The anesthesia was still numbing me and incapacitating me. But I made a huge effort to lie sideways, half-propped up on an elbow, because I knew this was the only chance I would ever have to be with my baby.

Paul and I cried hard while we looked at her. He pointed out things to me that the doctor had pointed out to him. Anatomically, she was perfectly normal. I was overwhelmed with awe and misery. She was a beautiful baby; it was a miracle that we had produced this beautiful little girl. But, she was dead, and I was stunned and could not possibly imagine what could have caused this perfect little girl to die.

It would have been simpler if someone could have come in and said, "This was what was wrong with her. She died because of this and that." But, no one could give us any information. This complete enigma began to haunt me there in the recovery room. What killed her?

I was grief-stricken that my baby never opened her eyes and saw the world. Those half-opened eyes disturbed me. I was afraid to touch her much, but I had a desire to pull up an eyelid and see what color her eyes were. I did not, though. Her skin was very tacky. When I did touch her once, the top layer of skin peeled away on my finger. It was ghastly.

Mother's Sense of Responsibility

It was profoundly sad. I felt as if I were to blame. She looked fine. I felt like some failure on my part had killed her. My body had shut down on this beautiful, healthy baby. My body must have quit on her. She would have had a whole lifetime ahead of her, and my body had somehow annihilated her.

We were with her for about 10 minutes. Someone came for her, appearing around the edge of the curtain. I was incredibly weary and numb, both emotionally and physically. I was ready to have them take her away, at the time, and I said, "Yes, fine. Take her away now." But I wish I had asked to see her again. I wish I had asked to have her brought back in later, when the anesthesia had worn off. I wish I had asked if I could let my mother hold her. She wanted to, but did not dare speak up, either. I thought as soon as they took her away from me in the recovery room she was taken downstairs for the autopsy. I wish someone had told me I could see her again.

Signing Autopsy Consent Form

Paul left when they took our baby away. Even though it was early on a Sunday morning, the chaplain came to visit. It was not until months later that I realized that the hospital had paged him at home and he had driven into the city to come see me after my baby had been delivered. I took his presence for granted. He had me sign the autopsy consent form and the stillbirth certificate, and I told him our baby's name, Edith Rose. The chaplain went off to baptize Edie. I wished later that I had asked him to do that in my presence.

My mother arrived and was permitted to come back to the recovery room to see me. It would have been so easy for me to get Edie back and let my mother see her. It never crossed my mind. My mother wishes she had seen Edie. We both regret that lost opportunity.

One of the Family Practice residents came in to see me. I showed him my picture of Edie, but told him jocularly that it did not do her justice. I told him she was a beautiful baby. He said he knew, he had just seen her. I wondered what was going on outside the recovery room. It seemed that a lot of people were seeing her out of my presence. The labor nurse told me that she had my mouth. The doctor showed Paul that she had a normal, perforated anus. It confused me when people came in and told me these things, because I thought that the doctors were in a hurry to take her to the morgue for her autopsy.

The Family Practice resident was the one who told me that her skin was peeled just as a natural development following death. I complained to him that they had taken such a large skin sample to grow a culture. He explained that, in fact, they would only need a little scraping and that the patch on her abdomen was like that because she had been dead for 4 or 5 days.

Need for Privacy—Insulation From More Fortunate Patients

The room suddenly filled up with patients. There were too many all at once for it to be just by chance. The staff must have kept them outside while we saw our baby. I was so glad that no one else had been around while we were with Edie. Now, my curtain had been drawn back, and there were 2 patients on my side and 3 on the other, across from me. I was sure that all 5 of the others had just had live babies. The wiped-out new fathers sat next to them. It was so unfair. I began to cry loudly.

A nurse approached the foot of my bed and said, "What's wrong, dear?"

I said, very emphatically and loudly, "My baby died."

She said, "I know." She turned and left the recovery room. In my state, I suspected that she could not deal with me. Actually, though, she must have judged that it was time to get me out of there, both for my sake and for the sake of the other patients, one of whom was coughing like she was on her deathbed. The nurse must have left to arrange to have me moved to my room. I lay there, crying harder than ever.

Very soon, Paul came back in and sat with me. He made disparaging remarks about the coughing woman, saying that we were being exposed to something dreadful. Really, I think we were both jealous of all these folks whose babies were fine, and we directed our anger at this one person in this way. The anesthesiologist came to take out my epidural, and then I was wheeled back upstairs to my room.

Total Loss of Memory after Delivery

I staggered across the room, poked in my suitcase to find my toilet articles, and brushed my teeth. It felt so good to brush my teeth; it had been more than 24 hours since I had last brushed them, and I had been vomiting bile the day before. Brushing my teeth sapped me of any energy I had remaining. This was noon, at the latest. All of that day and night are a complete blank. Even close to 4 years later, I cannot recall anything about that time.

FIRST DAY POSTPARTUM

The next thing I remember is that, bright and early at 7:45

A.M. on Monday, my doctor strode into the room. Paul and I were sound asleep. Paul was in his underwear, covered with a sheet on that unwieldy lounge chair. He was very embarrassed, unshaved and lying there like a slob, while the doctor, all chipper and fresh and on the job, palpated my uterus and gave me a quick check.

Desire to Prolong the Experience

The doctor said, "Do you want to go home?" I said, stridently, "No!" I could not face being home yet. It was too soon to have to leave and be home, with the whole experience in the past. If I remained in the hospital, the event would still be happening. I had to buy all the time I could.

As soon as the doctor left Paul did, too. He wanted to teach his classes as usual. My sister came to spend the day with me so that I would not be alone. I stayed in bed all day, and I still did not think to take a shower. I must have been awfully ripe by that time, but no one hinted at it. It was talk, talk, talk, all day. I was not left alone much, and that was absolutely the best thing for me that day.

Being Educated about the Process of Grief

A social worker came in to have me sign the form to let them cremate Edie. I put her off, telling her I had to talk about that with my husband. She stayed and talked with me for some time. She, like my doctor and the chaplain, talked with me about grief. I knew nothing about the process. Their concerted effort at educating me about it, reassuring me that all the feelings I would have would be normal, was the most important service I received at the hospital. I think it saved my sanity. It saved me from losing myself in depression, thinking that I was going out of my mind. The whole time I was hospitalized, I was busy talking; so it may have seemed that what the doctor and the others told me could get lost in the shuffle. But, later on, when I was home and all alone, everything they said came back to me and helped me a lot.

The chaplain came to make arrangements for the private service that Paul and I wanted to have in the hospital chapel, just before I was supposed to go home the next morning. The nurse I had had in Labor and Delivery on Saturday came to visit, even though it was her day off. The nurse who had met us at the Perinatal Center after the ultrasound on Thursday came in to give me the names and phone numbers of people who ran support groups. I took the information, but I could not imagine that I would *ever* call on them. Three weeks later, when I became acutely depressed, they were the people who sustained me.

Difficult to Accept the Term "Stillbirth"

A woman from the Bureau of Vital Statistics came to obtain information. She gave me a printed sheet entitled, "Filing for a Birth Certificate." On my copy, she ran her pen through the words "Birth Certificate" and wrote above the line "Or Stillbirth." It took me almost a year to call the delivery of my baby a "stillbirth," and I cringed when she wrote that. I asked her how many babies had been delivered over the weekend (she was complaining because she was so busy that day). She said 36 babies had been born. I asked how many babies had died. She said one. Mine, and 35 live babies. Why did mine have to be the one who died?

An employee came in to clean my room and change the bed while my sister went to get herself a sandwich. The woman was over by the window, cleaning the sill. Her back was to me, and she said, just being pleasant, "And how's that beautiful new baby of yours?" I said flatly, "My baby died." She walked straight out of the room. It must have been awful for her.

Fortunately, I did not have time to think because there were always people around or phone calls to answer. I had visitors during both visiting hours. We kept the door to my room shut, and I was unaware of all the joy up and down the rest of the floor. If I had been aware of what a normal stay there is like, being on the obstetric floor would have been intolerable. But I did not know, not having had a baby before this experience. It must have been hard on my family and friends to weave their way through all that scenery to come to my closed door and be there with me.

SECOND DAY POSTPARTUM: DISCHARGE HOME

The next morning, Paul left before the doctor arrived. He went home to change and to get my clothes to wear for the service in the chapel. I could not wear the clothes I had worn the previous Thursday when I was admitted. After Paul had gone, the doctor came in to check me. I did not feel like I was ready to go home. But, when the doctor repeated his question from the day before, "Do you want to go home," I said, "Yes." So, I was discharged.

Physician's Suggestions for Understanding the Feelings

He sat and talked with me for quite a while, until Paul got back. He recommended some helpful actions, such as writing a letter to the baby and keeping a journal. He said, "I know it's a cliché, but today is the first day of the rest of your life." It sounded corny, but it turned out to be true. In the hospital, along with all the other things I heard from him and the others, I sort of filed it and forgot it. I remembered it later, though. I found that this stillbirth had gouged an irrevocable chasm in my life. Everything from that day onward was permanently classified as either "Before Edie Died" or "After Edie Died." I even thought of trivial and irrelevant things in this way.

The social worker returned with the consent form to do the cremation. I made Paul sign it. I did not want to shoulder the responsibility myself. I had signed the autopsy consent form, and that was bad enough.

Paul made several preliminary trips to the car, carrying down my stuff. While he was in and out, one of the floor nurses came in with a supply of breastpads. She had realized that my breasts were going to start getting engorged, and she delivered a thoughtfully worded lecture on how I could suppress the milk supply.

I asked Paul to take the flowers and plants we had received down to the chapel. I did not want them home with me. It bothered me to think that the plants would live, although our baby had not. We agreed that it would be nice to see the flowers there in the chapel anyway, while we had our memorial service.

I walked off the obstetric floor. They did not have to wheel me out in a wheelchair, because there was no baby to hold.

Memorial Service in the Hospital

Paul and I met the chaplain at the appointed time in the chapel. That was the way we had decided to do it. We had not even told our families. It was a rash decision. I wish I had not had Edie cremated. I wish that we had buried her and had a funeral service which included everyone who would have wanted to attend. Our private memorial service was brief, tailored insightfully by the chaplain for Paul's and my religious beliefs. We sat in the front with him and we sobbed the entire time. I used up the small box of tissues that I had brought from my room.

Paul and I thanked the chaplain and left. I waited in the lobby while Paul got the car and drove it to the door. I was physically weak, and I was emotionally drained after the symbolic service we had just walked away from. I sat looking out the window at the street, waiting for Paul. All I could think about was that it was the worst thing in the world to have to go home from the hospital without your baby. It was hopeless.

General Lack of Understanding in the Real World

The first time I went into the grocery store, 4 days later, Paul and I met one of the couples from our childbirth class. She was enormous. Her baby was due a week before Edie was to have been due. We saw each other from across the store. Paul and I quickly decided to get out of sight, but they came up to us. They said they were very sorry. I started to cry. The husband said to me, "I guess it still bothers you, huh?" I got out of the store as fast as possible, and Paul stood and hugged me while I wailed in the parking lot. It was part of life. I was back in the real world.

WHAT HELPED ME

Having my own labor room—hearing a healthy baby's heart on the monitor was awful;

Seeing my baby;

Being given a choice of private rooms on the maternity or the gynecology floor;

Receiving tangible memories (bracelet, photo);

Having my husband with me for my entire hospital stay;

Having my doctor express his sympathy and remain involved, instead of avoiding us;

Having the hospital chaplain baptize my baby and give a memorial service in the hospital for her;

Being educated about the normal process of grief;

Being advised about possible marital stress:

> "It is not possible to synchronize your grieving, although the 2 of you are grieving for your dead child."

> "Feelings about the sexual relationship and contraception may cause great tension."

Getting a referral to a support group—that is the best way to deal with all the feelings over the long term, when the medical professionals are no longer available;

Being advised to write, to capture intense feelings while they are fresh (letter to the baby, record of dreams, journal);

Receiving a follow-up phone call from my doctor and having a series of office calls in the next few weeks.

The hospital experience is something that I will remember in great detail all my life. It is so important that the experience be as positive as possible. A bad experience can cause much pain and anger and can complicate the grieving process. My experience was handled quite well, at the time. Healthcare professionals are even more knowledgeable now about what will help someone later on. I want to list some observations that I have made, things I noticed and things I wish had been told to me at the time, in the hope that other women will benefit.

WHAT WOULD HAVE HELPED ME

Being told immediately the baby's apparent condition and the baby's sex. I did not see Edie being delivered. It took place in a dimly lit labor room, and she was delivered directly into a large stainless steel bowl that was on the bed to catch her as she came out. I wish that someone would have told me right away what sex she was and that she was normal in appearance. Not hearing anything about her made me imagine all kinds of horrors.

Being told explicitly that there was no rush to see my baby. I had the mistaken impression that they hurried to get that part over with, to get Edie to the morgue so they could perform the autopsy immediately. No one said anything to that effect; but, in the absence of information, I had to rationalize. I wish that someone would have told me to keep her as long as I liked and that someone would have offered to bring her to me a second time, some hours later, after I was rested and after the anesthesia had worn off.

Recovery Room Stressful

Being taken to my room, instead of making me lie in the recovery room. My delivery was technically normal without complications. I did not require any care from the nurses in the recovery room. I wish that I could have had privacy in my own room, with a nurse nearby to do the monitoring. It was stressful to be in the presence of other women, all of whom I was sure had just had healthy, live babies. Also, I think my visit with my baby was brought to a close prematurely so that the other patients could be brought into the room. If it is unacceptable to release a patient directly to her room, then taking her to a private labor and delivery room should be standard procedure. Every woman I know who has had a miscarriage or stillbirth has hated being in the recovery room. It is always mentioned as a stressful, painful experience.

Being provided with more keepsakes. I did get a bracelet and a photo, which I treasure and always will. I wish I had gotten more. I did not get footprints or a lock of hair or a record of birth or a baptismal certificate, all of which are simple to obtain. Probably, a nurse would have given me a lock of hair if I had thought to ask. In this situation, I did not think clearly enough and I was shy about speaking up. Someone should ask the patient if she wants things like this. Footprints should be taken, so that they will be available later on, when the woman thinks of such things and wants them.

Being given a good clear photograph of the baby. I am inexpressibly grateful that someone at the hospital took the photograph which I possess. But ... I have heard that these photographs are deliberately made fuzzy and unclear, to blur the dead baby's appearance and thus cushion the blow. I wish I had a very clear image, with fine detail visible. I knew that Edie was dead and I knew that she would not look like a model, healthy baby. I wish now that I could clearly see what my baby looked like.

Having a symbol or codeword unobtrusively posted so that hospital staff could avoid painful blunders. Some poor woman from the housekeeping staff asked me how my "beautiful new baby" was. I did not beat around the bush about it. I told her my baby had died. She must have felt awful about the whole thing. She walked out of my room without saying another word. A mark or coded notation should be visible outside the room and perhaps on the chart so that this type of encounter will occur less often.

Being shown the autopsy report and discussing it with the doctor. I was uncertain about whether or not I would be given a copy of the autopsy report. No information about it was given to me and I was afraid that it was official— something that I did not have a right to request. I very much wanted to see the report. I brought it up with my doctor, who then read me a sentence from the preliminary report, 2 weeks later, which said that the cause of death was at that point undetermined. I never heard another word about it. I finally called a secretary many weeks later and timidly asked her if she would mail me a copy of the full report. I wish someone had told me it was perfectly reasonable to request a copy. I also felt awkward much later on, requesting a copy of the hospital records.

LACK OF PREPARATION

I wish that I could have known somehow that I would suffer a stillbirth. Then, I could have signed up for a seminar and learned beforehand all the things I was going to need to know when my baby died. I could have examined the options ahead of time and known that I wanted to have a funeral and that I wanted to videotape or photograph the delivery and that I wanted to wait until the epidural had worn off to hold my baby and maybe stand by the window holding her just once.

Care Providers Can Offer Memorable Services

It does not work that way, though. I did not become an expert until it was all over. Parents of stillborns come to the hospital as greenhorns. What happened to me while I was in the hospital will remain with me for the rest of my life. What you [hospital staff] did for me in particular, you will forget in a day or two, while I will remember it always. I will remember your name and what you looked like, what you did, what you said, and how much you helped me. You may not have to deal with patients like me every day, but you brought a lot of experience and insight with you when you walked into my room. You can be a patient's eyes and ears. Please ask your patients like me if they want things to be done, because later on they, like me, will wish that they had had the presence of mind or the nerve to speak up and ask for them.

THE FEELINGS

I was 7 months pregnant when Edie died in utero. It was the most unexpected shock to me that she died. I had never heard that such a thing was possible—the baby just plain dying in utero. I was on top of the world at the time that Edie died. I had slammed shut my pregnancy books when I got through the 28th week. That is the age of viability. I told Paul, "Even if our baby were born now, it would be okay. They could save it." And then, suddenly, during the 30th week, she was dead.

Shock

The shock lasted quite a while and only diminished over time. I left the hospital and was confronted by reality. I had the usual postpartum physical processes to deal with—bleeding, breastmilk, even hemorrhoids—but no baby. All pain, no gain. I received mounds of hospital bills and the junk mail that pregnant women get themselves in for when they buy maternity clothes. The shops take your name from your charge or get your address from your check, and then you are on every mailing list in the country.

The Baby's Nursery

There was the baby's room at home, too. We had not begun fixing it up; we had just accumulated things we were going to need. We had bought the crib the weekend before the baby died. It was in its carton, leaning against the wall in the baby's room. There were clothes, a bathtub, a playpen, all kinds of things piled up on the floor. I had to pack it all away.

I still identified with pregnant women. I still wanted to talk about pregnancy. I still wanted to browse in the infants department in stores. I still wanted to be a mother. I did not want to go back to just being a couple with my husband. I did not want to be free to go out to dinner.

Coming to Terms with the Loss

I became obsessed with pregnancy. I wanted to finish being pregnant, and I had to come to terms with the fact that the pregnancy with Edie was concluded. That was simple to say, but on other levels I did not grasp it for a while. All I could think about was getting pregnant, and it was all jumbled up— somehow finishing Edie's pregnancy the "right" way, but at the same time having a separate, different person who was not Edie.

Intercourse was no fun at all. I did not want to have to be there, contemplating conception all over again. I cried while Paul made love. I did not participate; I could not respond to him.

Importance of the Support Group

After 3 weeks, I contacted a support group that my doctor had told me about. I found very sympathetic and dedicated people there who sustained me in the long, slow months while I grieved for Edie. They were the only people who knew how I felt, and I leaned on them heavily.

As time passed, I gradually moved through my grief and

then even came to the point where I could begin to help others with more recent experiences. I felt an obligation to be there for others, as the people before me had been there for me. And then, many months later, I became satisfied that I had paid in kind sufficiently, and I moved away from the support group and on in life with our new baby.

Trying Again

The doctor had advised us to wait 6 months to a year before again trying to conceive, in order to give us time to grieve and say good-bye to Edie. I could not find any medical reason to wait that long. Paul and I felt that the waiting would make us more depressed. At the beginning, when we decided not to wait (I got pregnant during the next cycle), I felt like we had nothing to lose. I subconsciously believed that if I got pregnant and lost the pregnancy, it would not make a difference. The baby was already dead. It is complex and difficult to word, but in any case I was soon shaken to my senses on that subject. I was pregnant again, I had bleeding 4 times during the first 8 weeks, and I rapidly realized that what I had to lose was another baby. I feel very lucky that I had a healthy baby the next time, because I was not emotionally strong enough to cope with another failed pregnancy.

Depression

Three months after Edie died, I realized that I was quite depressed. Life had gone on. I was back at work, although my plan had been to quit before Edie would have been born. My friends who were pregnant before Edie died were having their babies without mishap. Everything was the same, except that my baby was dead. I missed her. I was lonely for her, and the rest of the world had forgotten all about her and certainly did not want to hear me talk about it anymore. And I had a sense of failure.

Sense of Failure

I struggled with the feelings about failure. I heard myself saying things such as, "I flunked out of childbirth class," and "I'm going to get pregnant again and do it right this time." I was surprised at how much my ego was bruised. I never mentioned it to anyone because it was not something I thought was very admirable to admit. It was hard to look closely at myself, to acknowledge the jealousy and bitterness I felt toward other parents and the anger I eventually came to feel toward my baby.

Blaming the Baby

That really felt bad, being angry at my poor baby for dying. But everyone said it was not my fault, so it must have been her fault.

I was used to "controlling" my life. It was difficult to accept my lack of control over my own body. Even when I came to terms with that, I had a residual sense of guilt for letting my baby die. I sensed that I had "let" Edie die inside my own body, where I thought she should have been safest. I could have alerted the doctor 2 days earlier than I did, and probably they

Sense of Responsibility for the Baby's Death

could have safely delivered Edie by cesarean section and treated her in the NICU. Feeling that I was "in charge" made me feel that her death was my fault.

Being pregnant again added to my burdens, because I knew that I had to make the distinction between the 2 children. It was a continual effort. I was so pessimistic because of Edie's death that I never enjoyed my pregnancy with Teddy. I was always afraid that the baby would die while I was sleeping. I had to be vigilant all the time, to catch this baby before he could die. I monitored his movements for hours every day, and the days between doctor visits were filled with despair, grief for Edie, fear for Teddy, and the conviction that he would not live to the next check-up, which my doctor began to schedule weekly at the 20th week. He knew how rough it was.

Responses on Subsequent Anniversaries

A year after Edie had died, I had a 2-month-old son. I was wrapped up in Teddy. I could see what we had missed with Edie. I wanted both of my babies. I was sad for Edie. The intensity had lessened. I no longer noticed when it was 9:18 on Sunday mornings, which was the time of Edie's delivery. I still longed to know how Edie had died. When I did not have anything else to think about, my mind always turned to that topic.

Two years after Edie had died, I was hard on myself. I was frustrated with the feelings that surfaced in the weeks before the anniversary date. I told myself I could not fall apart every May. But, I caught myself recalling exactly what had been going on at the same hour 2 years previously.

Three years later, I did not attach great significance to the anniversary date. I had many other concerns and activities in my life, including my healthy 2-year-old son. But still, occasionally, something I heard or read could grip me, and momentarily I would recall my grief and sadness about Edie. But, I did not cry.

As Teddy grows, I learn more and more how precious and unique each baby is. That is what continues to sadden me most about Edie—that she is not here to be Teddy's big sister, our daughter, my mother's granddaughter, my friends' kids' playmate. . . .

Often, though, I am hardnosed about the whole experience and tell myself that, unless I die at a young age, I am going to have other, worse losses in my life. Is that true? Who would believe that a stillborn baby could generate so much grief and sadness and leave such a trail of sorrow? She was like a shooting star—gone before I was sure she was there, but indelibly imprinted in my memory and leaving a sense of wonder and deep emotion.

CHAPTER

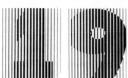

A Father's Experience

F. PAUL ESPOSITO, Ph.D.

It has been 4 years since our daughter died. She was stillborn at her 30th week. The autopsy did not reveal the cause of her death, and we will never know why she died. It is difficult for me to describe everything that I felt when our baby died and during the months that followed, but I will try to describe those things that have had the most lasting effects on my wife and me.

The initial shock of finding out that our baby had died in utero was like a lightning bolt. I did not have even a hint that there was a serious problem at any time during Jen's pregnancy. The sudden suggestion and rapidly confirmed fact that our baby was dead had a devastating effect on me. However, my concern that morning was for Jen. Right after the ultrasound had shown conclusively that our baby was dead, we elected to remain in the hospital to induce delivery of our baby. I was very relieved that we could do this. At the time, I only wanted to get the entire experience behind us as quickly as possible. I thought that we would be done with the whole issue as soon as the baby was born and we could leave the hospital.

I will elaborate on several points concerning what happened to us in the hospital, what happened to us since we went home, and what ramifications from our daughter's death I still feel are of significance in the years since she died. We now are parents of a happy, healthy little boy who was born by cesarean section 10 months after his sister's death.

334

HOSPITAL EXPERIENCE

**Shattered
Expectations**

That morning in May 1983 when Jen told me something was very wrong with our baby was, in many ways, the end of a whole way of life for us. We would go on from that day and develop a different life from the one that had been unfolding. It is fortunate that shock can produce such complete numbness, because we probably benefited from the insulation it provided in the terrible time that followed the baby's death. We expected to have a smooth pregnancy, an easy delivery, and a healthy baby. That is the standard way that babies are born and that families come into existence. It was our turn for it. The problem was that it did not happen in the standard way for us. At the time, it made us angry and jealous toward others who were luckier. Now, we are both sorry that it had to be that way.

**The "Baby" Was Still
an Abstraction**

When I saw during the ultrasound that the baby's heart was not beating, I accepted that fact and knew that there was no question that the baby was dead. I had not had many glimpses at the baby before, via Jen's ultrasounds; "the baby" was just Jen's stomach growing bigger and the initial 5 months of morning sickness and my happily assuming a larger burden for doing chores and fixing meals. If it happened now, after I have been a father, I am sure that I would be fully devastated right away. But, back then, I was not yet a father and the whole issue of having a baby was an abstraction to me. While I knew that "the baby" had died, it did not really hit me.

**Urge to Get the
Experience over with**

That day, all I wanted to do after we conferred with the hospital staff was to get the baby delivered. I wanted to get out of the hospital. It was very important to me to get Jen through the hospital experience and then home as soon as possible. This seemed to me to be the best way to get what happened behind us, to forget about it, to move on to the future, and to go back to the way we were before the death. These urges, some of which were contradictory in the extreme, were what I felt at the time. As I look back now, they appear to be all wrong.

The effects of the loss were worsened for Jen, and probably for me also, by my trying to rush through those days at the hospital. In a significant way, that experience was Jen's. It was she who felt the baby die inside her and she who had to deliver. I had no right to impose my wishes on her. No matter what a husband or doctor does, there are aspects about pregnancy and birth that are known only to the mother. The husband may be very involved, and the doctor may be quite sensitive; but in the end, it is the mother who lives with the baby growing inside her. It is she who experiences the movements and the changes the baby's growth produces on her own body. Until after the baby's birth, it is only the mother who really knows the baby.

The mother-fetus development is a symbiotic relationship which, at its most profound level, excludes the father and all others.

In retrospect, I think that it was very important that, however bad the circumstances, the experience in the hospital was as normal as possible. I now know from our son's birth that even with an emergency cesarean section a woman can feel cheated out of one of the most important events in her life, giving birth. Jen has lamented many times that she was under general anesthesia during our son's delivery. And that delivery resulted in the miracle of our son. How much more "cheated" a woman must be when she has to go through a pregnancy and all the physical pain of labor only to deliver a stillborn baby.

Desire for as Much Normalcy as Possible

It is difficult for me to articulate everything that I mean by a "normal" experience in the context of a delivery such as our daughter's. In our case, we had knowledge of the death to confront before we started anything. So what was normal and why was it important? To me, "normal" meant that, except for the baby's being dead, everything went the same as in a healthy delivery. The delivery itself was uncomplicated and uneventful. In a way, it was a confirmation that our daughter was a real person, that she mattered, and that something about her brief existence was all right. The hospital staff treated Jen well, and somehow Jen came away from the experience with many positive feelings about having given birth. She found the delivery itself wonderful, an incredible experience, which I find hard to believe. I think she was able to be open to that natural exhilaration only because the doctor and rest of the staff were thoughtful about the way they acted toward her, us, and our dead baby.

I did not think of our baby while we were in the hospital. During that time, I tried to ease Jen through the difficulties she had in being induced in to labor. I felt so sorry for her. She had to go through labor and delivery with a terrible outcome known beforehand. I did not think about our baby or our loss. I was very glad to have our daughter delivered. I was glad to get safely back home with Jen.

AFTERMATH

Taking In What Had Happened

Although many people—the doctor, nurses, social worker, and hospital chaplain—had advised us about what it would be like when we got home, I still was not prepared for that time. It was only at home that I fully realized what had happened. We both cried a lot, especially when we went into the nursery or found something we had bought for the baby. We talked about bad luck, what might have happened, what we did on the days just before our daughter Edith had died, our guilt feelings, and many other things. We talked over what happened in the hospital during labor and delivery, and we talked about the people who helped us. We went over these memories many times. We wanted to remember what had happened and who had been involved. It was an integral part of our grieving. When an older person dies, there are other kinds of memories. This was all we had in the way of "memories" about Edith.

Returning Home

The house now seemed emptier even though both of us were there. It was emptier because Edith was missing. We had planned to have her there with us. We had bought things we thought we would need, and we had planned for our family's future. These and all of the things we had enjoyed doing together before Edith's death seemed pointless after she died.

I thought that I could get rid of the terrible feeling of emptiness by immersing myself in my work. That did not happen. In fact, I could not put anything behind me. It was always there, right beneath the surface. It was unsettling to realize that the life Jen and I had lived before Edith's death could not be resumed. It was even more unsettling to think that Jen was no longer enough. I wanted more now, and we had less. And this feeling applied to everything—our marriage, friendships, family, and work.

Lack of Support from Colleagues and Friends

After a day or so, no one at work talked about Edith or her death with me. The graduate students sent a card that they all signed. A few other expressions of sympathy trickled in from the wives of my colleagues. Jen was deluged by cards and flowers and baskets of fruit and whole meals from her friends and co-workers. I could not talk much about the baby with people in my department. I remembered guiltily that a colleague's wife had miscarried at 5 months several years before. I had never told them I was sorry. I had never noticed if my colleague was at all affected by that loss. Now, I knew that he must have felt the way I did, and I knew that no one had much interest in what I was going through.

Reluctance to Talk About or Reexamine the Event

There were only 2 things that provided any solace to me then. These were the very long conversations that Jen and I had and the fact that she got pregnant as soon as possible. The conversations were, as I recall, of vital importance. Initially, they were to me a duty or an obligation I thought I had for Jen's sake. I also felt that they were repetitious. The question, "Why did she die?" came up over and over. I was not interested in speculation that was fruitless. The autopsy shed no light on why she died, and that was the end of any investigation into the cause of her death. There was no answer except that we had rotten luck. For me, the fact that someone might have been able to determine that there was a specific cause for Edith's death did not seem very important anyway. For Jen, it was very important because, in searching for a cause and not finding an external one, she often blamed herself. It was hard for her not to believe, "If only I had done this and this, she would not have died."

Jealousy toward Other Families

These discussions were very long and very trying for both of us, but in different ways. My attitude at first was very frustrating for Jen. She wanted to talk and talk, and I felt that there was not much point in talking. The talks became important to me only as I realized our loss. The feelings I began to have made me want to talk, too. We talked about our feelings of guilt and the need to blame something. We talked about us, our anticipations, our marriage; about our friends and about how some of them reacted to our loss. Jen was back at work and a few times she came home upset about something someone had rather thoughtlessly said. We were in full accord about our feelings of jealousy toward other couples who had babies. It was always painful to run into people who had been in childbirth class with us. We were jealous of complete strangers, as well. It was so hard to accept the statistics and be shut out of the kind of life we wanted, which all these other people, friends and strangers alike, were enjoying.

As I said, at first I did not think that all of this talk was necessary. Talks were a source of friction and irritation at times between Jen and me. Aside from the fact that we did not always agree, she was always eager to talk and I was not. After all, how could you put things behind you if you continually talked and thought about them? I was slow to change this attitude, and now I sorely regret that I was not sensitive enough with Jen and with myself.

TRYING AGAIN

Strain during Subsequent Pregnancy

Jen's immediate pregnancy was very important to us. Her doctor had advised us to wait for some time before attempting another pregnancy. But, as soon as we found out that there were no medical impediments to getting pregnant again right away, we thought that it would be best for us to start immediately. Pregnancy should be a time of joy and happy expectation, as was our previous experience until our baby died. This new pregnancy was not a happy time. In fact, it was a very hard time for us. Although it provided a hope and a focus for our frustrated energies, it was also a constant source of tension. Could it happen again that the baby would die like that? Could something else terrible happen? We were too experienced not to believe that something could indeed happen.

I was learning about grief and it was not pleasant. It was hard to be sensitive to Jen's needs. Sometimes, they seemed to change from one extreme to the other, for no reason. How do you deal with that, and with your own grief, and with the feeling that your job and your life are not holding up under the scrutiny that a devastating life experience causes you to undertake?

A Range of Emotions

I became irascible and found that I had to force myself at times to be tolerant of Jen. This was not an easy time for either of us. It led to many irreversible changes in our relationship. I was on a sea of emotions and feelings, overwhelmed with grief and responsibilities, anticipation, frustration, emptiness, loyalty, loneliness, loss, hope, and love. Things variously emerged from that muddle in one combination or another, sometimes diffusing into one another and sometimes abruptly changing. Jen was going through the same thing, and our emotions necessarily impinged on one another and were influenced or changed by what the other was feeling. Our emotions seemed to have their own logic, which was confusing and difficult to deal with. I am still struggling with these feelings.

The one thing about which I felt no confusion was jealousy. I was jealous of everybody—people at work, friends, even my family. I put severe strains on these relationships because of those feelings, and I am sorry to say that some of the relationships have not survived that time.

Support Group Meetings Not a Source of Comfort

For some time, I have questioned if all that talk and support really helped. Support group meetings were not a solution for me as they were for Jen. Going to a large group of people whose babies had all died did not appeal to me in the least. I never went to a meeting. It would not have comforted me to hear someone else's miserable story. That would have made me feel worse, especially after Jen got pregnant again. It was clear enough to me that any number of terrible things could go wrong. I did not want to know any more details.

Advice from Doctor and Chaplain

The kind of advice that we received at the hospital was, for me, more to the point. The doctor and chaplain described common reactions to stillbirth. They gave us a rough description of the grief period that we could reasonably anticipate. Much of what we were told at the hospital was directed more toward Jen. That turned out to be appropriate, because there is no doubt for me that she had a much more intense, prolonged, shocked response to the loss than I did at the time.

We have healed differently. In the end, I have come to feel very sad about my daughter. I miss her and think about her more often than Jen realizes. Sometimes, I say I wish that Edith were alive. Jen points out that we most certainly would not have had our son if our daughter had not died, because of the timing involved. But, the fact is that we had a daughter and a son, and our daughter is dead. She will always be missing from our family. I would love now to have both of our children around, with their whole lives ahead of them. I worry about my son more than I think I would have otherwise. Sometimes at the happiest of moments with him I have begun to cry because I know that he is as vulnerable as Edith was.

Index